GOVERNING THE FEMALE BODY

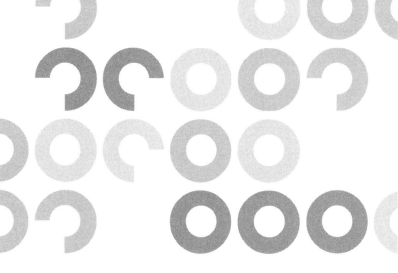

GOVERNING
the Female Body

GENDER, HEALTH, AND NETWORKS OF POWER

EDITED BY

LORI REED & PAULA SAUKKO

SUNY
PRESS

Chapter 11 has been reprinted with permission from Palgrave, London, and has been published in B. Mennel (2007), *The Representation of Masochism and Queer Desire in Film and Literature*. London: Palgrave.

Published by State University of New York Press, Albany

Printed in the United States of America

For information, contact State University of New York Press, Albany, NY
www.sunypress.edu

Production by Robert Puchalik
Marketing by Anne M. Valentine

Library of Congress Cataloging-in-Publication Data

Governing the female body : gender, health, and networks of power /
edited by Lori Reed and Paula Saukko.
     p.   cm.
Includes bibliographical references and index.
ISBN 978-1-4384-2953-3 (hardcover : alk. paper) — ISBN 978-1-4384-2952-6
(pbk. : alk. paper)
1. Women—Health and hygiene. 2. Women—Psychology. 3. Women's studies.
4. Feminism—United States. I. Reed, Lori Stephens. II. Saukko, Paula.
RA778.G735 2010
613'.04244–dc22
                                        2009015475

10   9   8   7   6   5   4   3   2   1

CONTENTS

Introduction

Governing the Female Body

Three Dimensions of Power

PAULA SAUKKO & LORI REED

Loughborough University and Independent Scholar

IN 1973 BOSTON WOMEN'S HEALTH COLLECTIVE published the book *Our Bodies, Ourselves: A Book by and for Women*, which was to become second-wave feminism's health manifesto. The book articulated a women-centered health agenda, drawing on expert, scientific, and medical knowledge as well as personal experience. It had its origins in the collective's workshops that applied the consciousness-raising method, which started from the premise that by exploring together personal experiences of oppression women could begin to see that their troubles were not personal issues but were shared by other women speaking about social subordination of women and requiring political responses. As discussed by Echols (1989) consciousness-raising was a method shared by many 1960s' radical movements, such as the civil rights movement and the Guatemalan guerrillas, but the feminist version was unique in its aim to politicize intimate, embodied feelings and issues, such as sexuality, health, and family.

The opening paragraphs of *Our Bodies, Ourselves* relate moments of recognition the women of the collective experienced when they had gone through the same embodied experiences, such as feeling that their first menstruation was scary, mysterious, and embarrassing (Boston Women's Health Collective, 1973, p. 2). Overall, the second-wave feminist movement's goal was to bring to the surface and challenge long-sedimented patriarchal myths, such as the association between menstruation and shame, which layered women's sense of themselves. The aim was to pave the way for alternative or more emancipatory modes of relating to the female self, body, and health.

Around the same time, Michel Foucault (1978) published the first volume of his *History of Sexuality*, offering a highly original theory on the production of various "perverse" bodies, such as the masturbating child, hysterical woman, and the homosexual. The book offered a detailed account of how what had previously been considered aberrant behaviors were constituted as "specimens" by the early modern sciences of psychiatry and sexology. The conditions, such as masturbation, homosexuality, and female hysteria, were positioned in scientific classificatory tableaux and associated with detailed lists of symptoms, photographs, and methods of intervention. These diagnostic categories isolated and intensified certain behaviors not only as objects of diagnosis and often cruel treatments, but also as sources of pleasures, identification, and emotional and political investments.

What united the feminist politics and Foucault's oeuvre was a strong liberatory agenda that was in keeping with the radicalism of the late 1960s and early 1970s. Both the feminist health collective and Foucault explored and attacked the way in which the bodies of women, gay men, and children were inscribed as always potentially eruptive and pathological by expert gazes of medicine and science, accounting for the sense of shame and mystery that they associated with their bodies. The feminists and Foucault parted company, however, in their understanding of emancipation. The Boston Women's Health Collective (1973) set out to discover and construct a "more whole" or "more self-confident" and "stronger" femininity (p. 3). On the contrary, Foucault was circumspect about any attempt to recuperate a "more whole" identity, arguing such a project was always bound to recreate a dogma of "true self," which deciphers and classifies certain behaviors and dispositions as the true and the norm, and others as false and wrong (Foucault, 1984; also Sawicki, 1992).

The title of this book, *Governing the Female Body*, refers to both the feminist and Foucauldian critical traditions of analyzing discourses that have constituted female bodies and selves. The term *governance*, derived from Foucault's (1991) middle works, both bridges and clarifies these two traditions. Governance has three dimensions that usefully highlight and trouble classical ways of understanding the relation between power, gender, and the body. The first and most obvious dimension is the reference to political power or the art of governing nations and populations. One of the red threads running through Foucault's work is an examination of the link between political governance of populations and the intimate governance of bodies and selves, which is crystallized in the feminist slogan "personal is political." Thus, as King discusses in this volume, the self-identification of women with breast cancer as "survivors," who empower themselves by taking charge of their health and self, not only articulates an attempt to deconstruct the stigma of pollution, passivity, and victimization associated with cancer, but also embodies the contemporary individualist, self-enterprising political sensitivity and identity.

The second aspect of Foucault's theory on governmentality is that it highlights the Janus-faced nature of power, which is never simply a force of dominance. Rather, governance always refers to both the process of becoming an object of governance of a social institution and a discourse and of becoming a subject of governing oneself. The way in which discourses both subjugate individuals to their agenda and constitute them as individuals capable of enacting their own agenda often cannot be separated from one another as exemplified by the contradictions of the breast cancer survivor movement.

The third aspect of governance is that it points toward a less hierarchical and more horizontal or network-like notion of power. Foucault's dearest objects of attack, as well as sources of inspiration, were Marxism and Freudian psychoanalysis, both of which are grounded in a hierarchical metaphor of "foundations." These foundations, such as the economic base or the unconscious, are seen as explaining social or personal life and being the true object of investigation for political-economic and psychoanalytic science. Rather than look for a final explanation an analysis of governance pays attention to networks and circuits of power that traverse different spheres of life or, to use Appadurai's (1997) term, "scapes." To continue using King's chapter as an example, the breast cancer survivor movement has a strong emotional dimension to it, both for the women who take part in it and for the various audiences that purchase pink ribbons or follow events, such as the Race for the Cure, through the media or from the sidewalks. Breast cancer activism is also big business, and major corporations, from BMW and Avon to National Football League, have adopted breast cancer awareness as a particularly "safe" form of corporate philanthropy and image-building. However, the movement's upbeat message of empowerment, in tune with contemporary liberal, individualist self-empowerment zeitgeist, does not address the glaring and widening disparities in survival rates from breast cancer between women of different races and social classes. This case illustrates the way in which emotional, economic, and political agendas and gendered and racial inequalities mix in breast cancer activism producing a disconcerting political cocktail. None of these dimensions is more fundamental or explanatory than others, but it is rather the intertwining of these politics that accounts for the appeal of breast cancer activism and its contradictions.

The goal of *Governing the Female Body* is to disentangle and critically analyze the multidimensional networks of power or governance that traverse the female body and through which the female body traverses. The poststructuralist framework has inspired many excellent works and collections on gender, health, and the body. Some of this work has focused on theory (McWhorter, 1999; Ramazanoglu, 1993; Sawicki, 1992;) methodology (Clarke & Olesen, 1998), reproduction (Davis-Floyd & Dumit, 1999; Ginsburg & Rapp, 1995; Inhorn & Van Balen 2002), science and new technologies (Goodman, Lindee, & Heath, 2003; Terry & Urla, 1995; Treichler, Cartwright, & Penley, 1998), family and kinship (Franklin & McKinnon, 2002) and psychology, (Henriques, Holloway, Urwin, Venn, & Walkerdine, 1998). This collection builds on this exciting work. However, we do not focus on theory or a particular area of health and science. Rather, we explore a variety of new and emerging gendered discourses and practices around health, such as genomics; in-vitro fertilization (IVF); development and marketing of various psychotropic and hormonal drugs; formation of advocacy groups and identities; and new popular, interactive, and online modes of communication and (self)-diagnosis. The framework or backbone that ties together the chapters of the book and accounts for its specificity is the application of Foucault's three-dimensional notion of power or governance. This framework guides our objective of providing timely, empirically grounded, and theoretically sophisticated analyses on the personal and political, subjugating and enabling, and many dimensional (mediated, economic, political, and diagnostic) aspects of power, and how they play out in the contemporary ways of governing the female body with a view of advancing its health. By showcasing the diverse case analyses together we hope to draw attention to the similarities between the contemporary coworkings of power, gender, and health on the Internet, in the IVF-clinic, and in debates on lesbian sadomasochism, while also exploring their specificities and disjunctures between them.

Before moving on to the case studies themselves, however, we will discuss the three dimensions of governance.

Between the Micro and the Macro

To start with the first dimension of governance, the linking between the personal and the political, it is useful to define the concept that has become synonymous with Foucault's work: discipline. In colloquial language *discipline* refers to techniques adopted to modify the behavior of a person, usually that of a child. Foucault distinguishes three elements of discipline: (1) the embodied element, which refers to harnessing the body's capacities to operate in a certain way, such as sit still or walk with a particular gait; (2) the symbolic element, which refers to meanings attached to certain behaviors and modes of communicating those meanings, for example, diagnosing children who cannot sit still as having ADHD (Singh, 2005); and (3) the power-relations it establishes between individuals, such as the one between a parent and a child or a doctor and a patient (see Foucault, 1991). The concept of discipline was central to Foucault's early works on medicine, psychiatry and the prison system.

In his later essay on governmentality Foucault (1991) defines *discipline* as referring to the management of states as well as the closely associated management of populations, such as children, the sick, families, and communities (221). Governmentality bridges the micropolitics of disciplining the body and mind and the macropolitics of governing the nation-state via management of populations by various programs and institutions, such as education and health care. Doing so draws attention to parallels between historical modes of political governance and the way in which we govern our bodies and selves in our everyday intimate lives. The aim of Foucault's works on clinics, asylums, prisons, and sexuality was to delineate a particular mode of governing people's bodies and minds or souls typical of the modern period. The modern way of governing states, populations, bodies, and selves, however, is currently giving way to something new. Trying to make sense of this emergent development, commentators have begun to talk about, for example, postdisciplinary (Deleuze, 1992) and neo-liberal (Rose, 1999) societies.

Emily Martin (1994) has termed the new mode of governance the era of the "flexible" body. In the postwar period the ideal individual was imagined in terms of an impermeable fortress with solid boundaries that kept its body and mind intact from outside invaders bc they bacteria, viruses, or dangerous social ideologies or propaganda. Lately, however, a new ideal has begun to emerge, that of a body and mind that are open to the outside world, dynamically transforming themselves in interaction with it. A "robust" immune system is no longer imagined as a fortress but a system that has been exposed to a variety of external stimuli and learned to react and adapt to them. Similarly in the workplace the ideal manager and worker no longer follow orders and pursue stability but rather seek to perpetually innovate, reorganize, and retrain themselves and their companies in response to turbulent business environment. As Martin notes, while the new ideals of connectivity and fluidity may appear fresh in comparison to the stale old ideals of isolation and stability, their newness masquerades the fact that they are also strictly normative and often perpetuate same old inequalities. Thus, the ideal of continuous self-innovation is not only liberating. Rather, it often connotes an obligation to readapt oneself.

In this scenario those with less flexible work portfolios, immune systems, and less economic and symbolic capital to opt for reeducation and complex drugs wilt away in the brave new world of continuous economic and psychological restructuring.

Martin's (1994) work highlights the way in which our relation with our bodies is shaped by wider social regimes. One of the specific focuses of *Governing the Female Body* is to examine the links between the micropolitics of enhancing the health of individual bodies and the macropolitics of maintaining and re-creating social, political, and often global regimes of power. We are particularly interested in investigating new forms of governance that challenge the old bulwarks of institutionalized medicine and linear health communication from experts to the public and give rise to a contradictory mosaic of "flexible," self-help and self-health movements, groups, interactive forums, tests, and internationally funded but locally participatory telenovelas.

Indicative of this new regime of self-adaptation is that while the second-wave feminism questioned the patriarchal myths and shame attached to menstruation, the postfeminist drug Seasonale promises to help women by eliminating menstruation and the associated "toxic estrogen surge" altogether, as discussed by Gunn and Vavrus in this volume. In a similar vein, in the twentieth-century, genetics and gender frequently came together in prenatal testing, a technology designed to detect and eliminate fetuses deemed "defective." As analyzed by Saukko in this collection, in the twenty-first century women may have a genetic testing for a susceptibility to deep vein thrombosis and miscarriage to carry to term a fetus, which will always also potentially have genetic susceptibility. This new application of genetics blunts its eugenistic edge, yet, it also commits women to lifelong monitoring and modifying of their own, their child's, and family's lifestyle and medical treatment based on genetic information.

In these cases an old interpretation and practice around gender and health seems to be giving way to a new way of relating to the body, self, health, and the polity. Rather than simply impose a diagnostic norm, such as a genetic diagnosis, or invite a straightforward opposition or resistance to it, the new mode of governance invites individuals to use new medical technologies to re-create their postfeminist presents and genetic futures. *Governing the Female Body* investigates the problems and possibilities embedded in these new micropolitics around health and bodily conduct and the personal meanings, uses, abuses, and fantasies as well as historical, political agendas, and regimes attached to them.

Power as Productive

Even if *Governing the Female Body* is driven by critical interrogation, our aim is not simply to denounce contemporary discourses on health and gender. Foucault frequently underlines that governmentality should not be conflated with domination, just as power should not be conflated with force. As Foucault (1982) famously put it, violence "bends, breaks on the wheel and destroys, closing the door to all possibilities" (p. 220). Rather differently, power refers to "actions upon actions"; instead of treating an individual as an object or a thing, the way violence does, power engages with a subject or a person who acts. Thus, unlike the concept of discipline, governance not only refers to modifying individuals to fit institutional agendas, but also to an active practice of self-governance. Self-governance encompasses the way in which discipline is internalized or owned by individuals so that children internalize parental discipline and become "good." Still, self-governance also encompasses the way in which individuals detach themselves from or problematize their being and actions, thereby opening a space that allows some freedom to govern themselves differently, the way the Boston Women's Health Collective did (see Foucault, 1985). Thus, the relation of power with action opens a "whole field of responses, reactions, results, and possible inventions" (Foucault, 1982, p. 220).

In his late works Foucault (1988) conceptualized a mode or ethos of governing self and others, which would enable the productive exercise of power with minimum domination. Foucault envisioned this ethos as consisting of reflexive, conceptual, as well as practical, techniques that aimed to distance the self from the discourses and practices that had constituted it. This critically reflexive technology of the self (and the body) forms the methodology of this collection in that all chapters interrogate an existing discourse and practice, aiming to open up a space to think and act about it differently. This critical reflexive methodology moves away from a dichotomous notion of power, emphasizing the Janus-faced nature of power, as always both constraining and enabling. Interpreting power in simple terms as domination produces a dilemma that has been extensively debated in feminism: emancipatory politics, which is oblivious of its own dominating elements. From early on, White middle-class feminists were reminded of their race and class based omissions, silences, and silencing (e.g., Moraga & Anzaldua, 1984). In the late 1980s and 1990s the dilemma resurfaced in debates on whether feminist condemnation of beauty practices and pornography were patronizing and quick to pass judgments on "correct" forms of beauty and sex (e.g., Chancer, 1998; Davis, 1995; Rubin, 1993). These criticisms have led to their own excesses, such as the postfeminist "Grrrl Power" advertisements that suggest that young women dress in highly sexualized fashion gear "for themselves" (e.g., Gill, 2003). All and all, these debates and counterdebates have highlighted the danger embedded in emancipatory, antirepressive politics, which does not consider its own potentially subjugating elements.

The complicated play of power, gender, the body, and politics is illuminated by many of the chapters in the book that tackle the beguiling nature of phenomena, such as pink-ribbon breast cancer activism or the way in which women's and men's lifestyle magazines understand "control." The multifaceted nature of power becomes particularly clear in Mennel's analysis of the feminist debates in the late 1980s and early 1990s on lesbian sadomasochism (S/M). She points out how the anti-S/M feminists missed the theatrical and parodical nature of lesbian S/M, condemning it as "real" while the pro-S/M feminists interpreted the fantasy-like aspect of S/M as "authentic." Reading this debate against the original historical works of Sacher-Masoch (1870), Mennel points out how the anti-S/M stance reinforces the idea that women are naturally masochists (and cannot parodically mimic it), whereas the pro-S/M stance denies the fluidity of the border between the private theater of S/M and the public arena of institutionalized sadism. As a whole, both the proponents and critics of lesbian S/M missed the main point of S/M, which is the play with the precarious difference between power and violence.

Bearing this complicated nature of power closely in mind this volume hopes to analyze the way in which power is used and mobilized in contemporary discourses and practices on health and gender in an often bewilderingly contradictory way.

Network of Sites and Scapes

The third specific feature of this volume is that it examines how power, gender, the body, and health come together in different sites or locales articulating diverse areas or spheres of life (see Appadurai, 1997; Marcus, 1998). The causal model of reasoning informing natural and social sciences tends to direct inquiry into seeking "origins" of social structure, psyche, or life in some predestined or prioritized sphere, such as economy, the unconscious, or DNA. Different times and different disciplines have held significantly different beliefs about what is the fundamental sphere or loci that explains the object of study. For example, in the early twentieth century personality was understood to be reflected in body shape (e.g., Sheldon, 1940). After World War II the psychoanalytic boom viewed the unconscious as the hidden abode of individuality. In the early twenty-first century brain-imaging technologies, such as magnetic resonance imaging, are increasingly seen as the method par excellence to reveal the essence of personhood and its aberrations (see Dumit, 2003).

Governing the Female Body is not informed by a vertical notion of scientific endeavor in terms of seeking origins. On the contrary, the chapters of the volume question assumptions about origins of personality or pathology in mothering, gender, hormones, or genes. Rather the collection follows a network-like model of analysis, or to use Deleuze and Guattari's (1987) metaphor, imagines analysis not in terms of "roots" or tracing causalities but in terms of "crabgrass" or mapping connections between sometimes seemingly disparate entities or issues. One of the themes running through the chapters in the anthology is how different issues, such as meanings, emotions, economics, politics, and science, intertwine to produce the messy politics characterizing many of the phenomena we are analyzing.

Many of the chapters in *Governing the Female Body* analyze meanings, such as diagnostic categories, including computer addiction (CA). However, as Reed demonstrates in her chapter, the discourse on CA does not have a merely symbolic or stigmatizing function. Illustrated by an analysis of two talk shows the discourse on CA is associated with regulating the activities and movement of female bodies. The scandal of the Internet is that it literally provides a "space" of escape from domestic duty and conjugal fidelity, while allowing the woman to remain within the safe confines of the home. As such, regardless of its "virtual" referent, CA participates in the time-worn regulation of the location of female bodies, which has traditionally been the task of the decidedly material profession of town planning that separated the spheres of public production, political deliberation, private unpaid production, and familial devotion.

One of the goals of this volume is to explore how the practices of health link from the outset separate agendas or processes together. Mapping these connections allows the chapters to use medical terminology to provide a "multifactorial" analysis of various contemporary discourses and practices around health and the female body.

Outline of the Book

In the spirit of exploring the spheres and dimensions of governance and their interaction, this volume is divided into four parts, which address the mediated, economic, political, and scientific dimensions of governing the female body.

Part one on mediated self-health begins with "'It's Down to You': Psychology, Magazine Culture, and Governing Female Bodies" by Lisa Blackman. She examines how we are currently invited to become self-enterprising or neo-liberal individuals who are willing and able to judge and amend our own psychology to achieve success, satisfaction, mental health, and happiness (see Beck & Beck-Gernsheim, 2001; Rose, 1999). Blackman investigates women's and men's lifestyle magazines and how they address the "problem of relationships." Her analysis reveals that women's magazines employ the postfeminist narrative of empowerment, where a woman overcomes one's self and her dependency on others in order to achieve autonomous selfhood. On the contrary, men's magazines do not discuss relationships in terms of learning to master and manipulate oneself but in terms of learning to master and manipulate the bodies and selves of women. Reflecting on these differences, Blackman concludes that theories on the entrepreneurial self presume its universality, which obliterates the fact that the new subjecthood may have very different implications for women and men. The following chapter by Paula Saukko, "Beyond Pill Scares? Internet Discussions on Genetic Thrombophilia and Gendered Contradictions of Bioindividuality," analyzes an Internet support group for people, mainly women, who have usually a low-risk genetic susceptibility to deep vein thrombosis or blood clots. Doctors may recommend this genetic test for women before going on the Pill or when they are pregnant, and so some may choose not to take the Pill, which increases the risk of clotting, or may take anticoagulants, which help to prevent clotting-related miscarriage. The new test no longer frames genes as "fate" but as something we can "do" something about. However, what passes unnoticed is that this "doing" refers to women's unending private labor of love, framed as "choosing" their own and their families' contraception (when there are no equal alternatives to the Pill), prophylactic medications (with potentially fatal side effects), health care, diet, exercise, vacationing, making love, having children, and obtaining insurance.

Chapter 3, the last chapter in part one, "Gender, Pathology, Spectacle: Internet Addiction and the Cultural Organization of 'Healthy' Computer Use" by Lori Reed, discusses the politics around the new diagnostic category of CA, or computer addiction. Analyzing two talk shows on the topic Reed concludes that even if computers are associated with masculinity CA as a diagnostic technology regulates female bodies. The most notorious cases of CA involve women who have neglected their children and spouses by escaping their domestic confinement and responsibilities to the virtual reality. While male computer nerds or hackers are romanticized as eccentric geniuses or Robin Hoods of the contemporary Microsoft world, women's and children's virtual journeys are associated with social problems, abuse, neglect, and pathology.

Part two concerns the privatization and the body proper-ty focuses on the ways in which economic incentives and programs intertwine in the production of healthy female bodies. It opens with chapter 4, "Pink Ribbons Inc.: The Emergence of Cause-Related Marketing and the Corporatization of the Breast Cancer Movement" by Samantha King, which examines how breast cancer has been reconfigured from a stigmatized disease and individual tragedy best dealt with privately and in isolation, to a neglected epidemic worthy of public debate and political organizing, to an enriching and affirming experience that is best responded to by charitable giving. King reflects how the discourses and practices of volunteerism and privatization have shifted the attention away from more mundane issues of cancer screening, mortality, and inequality, rendering the pink ribbon donned by many women an eerie ring. Chapter 5, "Regulation Through the Postfeminist Pharmacy: Promotional Discourse and Menstruation" by Joshua Gunn and Mary Vavrus, focuses on another marketing campaign, namely the launch, more or less at the same time in early 2000, of three pharmaceutical products regulating menstruation: Remifem for menopause, Sarafem for premenstruation, and Seasonale for cessation of menstruation. Gunn and Vavrus analyze how the advertisements for these drugs unabashedly used feminism, such as being a "Remifemin-ist," in their campaigns to reaffirm a familiar postfeminist discourse on self-empowerment. What Gunn and Vavrus argue is that these drugs belong to the commercial end of a wider "gyniatric apparatus," which includes practices as varied as self-breast exams and affirmative action that focus on defining and acting on a pathology or disadvantage specific to the female body. The last chapter in part two by Kristin Swenson, "Productive Bodies: Women, Work, and Depression," also examines drugs marketed predominantly to women: antidepressants. Starting from Metzl's (2003) analysis of advertisements for antidepressants Swenson argues that while the early psychotropic drugs for women, such as Valium, addressed the depressed women as agitated and full of tension and frustration, the contemporary advertisements for products such as Zoloft depict depression in terms of listlessness and sadness. Swenson argues that the change in the marketing of the drugs is symptomatic of wider changes in economy, where women have not only moved from the domestic sphere into the labor force but have also become the ideal worker, who is flexible, able to multitask, and orientated to fulfilling the expectations of others. In this situation antidepressants become the trendy remedy that helps women and men to embody this active, agile, and endlessly helpful worker.

Part three addresses the political aspect of governing female bodies and health, particularly from the point of view of transnational inequalities. Chapter 7, "'The Pill' in Puerto Rico and the Mainland United States: Negotiating Discourses of Risk and Decolonization by Laura Briggs, rereads the narrative on the testing of the Pill on Puerto Rican women, which has been argued to epitomize the way in which science subjected vulnerable women of Third World countries to dangerous side effects in order to develop a drug for middle-class White women. Reading the original documents, Briggs contends that the Pill was never primarily intended for middle-class use, but that it was deliberately designed as a drug to solve a cold war political and economic problem: Third World poverty and Communism. Revisiting the mythology about the early development of the Pill underlines the continuous need of feminism to be wary of making claims about "women's" oppression and analyze how different women are differently imbricated in webs of power, gender, race, and nation. Chapter 8, "Biopolitical Media: Population Communications International and the Governing of Reproductive Health" by Ron Greene and David Breshears, continues the story that Briggs starts and analyzes a new genre of communication designed by Population Communications International (PCI): participatory soap operas that educate about sexual health, contraception, and women's rights. Greene and Breshears argue that this form of media is usually lauded for being locally sensitive, feminist, and, most of all, effective. Rather than focusing on the contents of these soap operas, Greene and Breshears analyze the methods they are using, predicated on turning women into audiences. They argue that this method forces communication-scholarship, hoping to be funded, to focus on measurable outcomes, such as uptake of contraception, and gears development communication into a machinery that trains and incorporates women into the management of themselves and others. At the same time, structures of inequality underpinning both health communication and women's health in the Third World pass unnoticed. Discussing similar issues in a different context, Angharad Valdivia and Isabel Molina explore the representations of Latinidad in Hollywood films featuring prominent Latina actresses such as Salma Hayek and Jennifer Lopez in chapter 9, "Disciplining the Ethnic Body: Latinidad, Hybridized Bodies, and Transnational Identity." They argue that the films read Latina (not Latino) bodies through the tropes exoticization, racialization, and sexualization, depicting them as both seductive and hypersexual as well as foreign, out of control, and threatening to social order, the body politic, and the health of the country. As Latinas are becoming increasingly prominent in contemporary American popular culture, they are often commodified and branded using classical tropical symbols, such as hoop earrings, big hair, ruffles, and bright colors, which are nevertheless underpinned by grimmer associations between Latinidad and the menace of overpopulation, contagion, and non-White hegemony.

Part four discusses the way in which scientific discourses govern female bodies with reference to nature. Chapter 10, "'Doing What Comes Naturally . . .': Negotiating Normality in Accounts of IVF Failure" by Karen Throsby, discusses how women who have unsuccessfully tried IVF articulate their experience in terms of normality and naturalness. In her interviews these women distinguished themselves from figures, such as the "selfish" woman, who decides not to have children; the "IVF-junkie," who goes for more and more cycles in a desperate bid to have a baby; or couples, who try for the "designer baby," the mongrel sibling of the IVF "miracle baby." These narratives of normalcy highlight how women using this new technology had to walk on a narrow tightrope demonstrating they were still behaving as good mothers or did "everything possible" to become mothers without trying "too hard" or going too far. The most disheartening finding of the interviews was, however, that, regardless of whether IVF was used for reasons of female or male infertility, women tended to blame their bodies, not the technology, for the lack of success in a situation where 80% of IVF cycles are unsuccessful. Throsby concludes that while debates on IVF have often focused on the new ethical implications, much less attention has been paid to how discourses and practices surrounding the technology frequently confirm old discourses on normality, nature, and motherhood. Chapter 11, "Sado/Masochism and the Re/Production of Femininity" by Barbara Mennel, discusses feminist debates on lesbian S/M. Going back to Sacher-Masoch's original text (1870), she notes that the scenario he constructs ends in the female, a Russian woman called Wanda who was trained to theatrically abuse the hero, becoming violent and calling a Greek man to whip the hero. The feminist debates, Mennel argues, miss this fluidity between the theater of sadomasochism and real violence by arguing that the violence of sadomasochism is "real" or that it is always "authentic." The simplicity of both feminist and psychological discourses on S/M acts as a general reminder of the lack of nuance in much analysis of power that apply the diagnostic logic. The last chapter of the book, "Beyond XX and XY: Living Genomic Sex" by Ingrid Holme, discusses the ultimate frontier in the governance of female bodies: the biology of sex. Holme discusses how genomics, as opposed to genetics, has begun to discover processes that highlight that DNA is not the stable "blueprint" it was once thought to be but that the genome modifies itself in interaction with different parts of the genome, the cell, the organism, and the outside environment. Research on one of these processes, methylation, has shed new light on what used to be called "sex determination," but which has proved out to be much more processual and precarious development. These interesting findings have, however, been interpreted through old gendered narratives that frame the methylation processes involved in sex development using old gendered metaphors, such as "gagging" the X chromosome or the "battle between sexes." These stale metaphors have distracted from the radicalness of this cutting-edge research, which is that it provides new evidence of the way in which embryos do not "have a sex" but are "sexed," so that we are governed into becoming, rather than being, men and women not only culturally and socially but also biologically.

The four parts of this book highlight different mediated, economic, political, and scientific dimensions of the process of governing female bodies through health. However, similar themes and issues repeat throughout. The most recurrent theme is the discourse on self-empowerment, which pervades health-related discourses from women's magazines and breast cancer charities to marketing of antidepressants and menstruation suppressants. The issue of contraception also recurs in the global but mostly U.S. Internet chat rooms on genetic susceptibility to the side effects of the Pill, in the development of the Pill using Puerto Rican women, and in Third World family-planning campaigns that operate through soap operas. The most interesting and enjoyable aspect of editing this volume has been discovering how similar issues recur in diverse practices that govern women and their health in various settings as well as becoming aware of how similar issues are articulated differently in different contexts. Our hope is that—in the spirit of feminist consciousness-raising—the resonances and occasional discords between the chapters also evoke moments of recognition and rethinking in the reader.

References

Appadurai, A. (1997). *Modernity at large: Cultural dimensions of globalization.* Minneapolis: University of Minnesota Press.
Beck, U., & Beck-Gernsheim, E. (2001). *Individualization.* London: Sage.
Boston Women's Health Collective (1973). *Our bodies, ourselves: A book for and by women.* New York: Simon & Schuster.
Chancer, L. (1998). *Reconcilable differences: Confronting beauty, pornography, and the future of feminism.* Berkeley: University of California Press.
Clarke, A., & Olesen, V. (Eds.). (1998). *Revising women, health, and history: Feminist, cultural, and technoscientific perspectives.* New York: Routledge.
Davis, K. (1995). Reshaping the female body. New York: Routledge.

Davis-Floyd, R., & Dumit, J. (Eds.). (1998). *Cyborg babies: From techno-sex to techno-tots*. New York: Routledge.

Deleuze, G. (1992). Postscript on the societies of control. *October, 59*, 3–7.

Deleuze, G., & Guattari, F. (1987). *A thousand plateaus: On capitalism and schizophrenia*. Minneapolis: University of Minnesota Press.

Dumit, J. (2003). *Picturing personhood: Brain scans and biomedical identity*. Princeton, NJ: Princeton University Press.

Echols, A. (1989). *Daring to be bad: Radical feminism in America 1967–1975*. Minneapolis, MN: University of Minnesota Press.

Foucault, M. (1978). *History of sexuality: Vol. 1. An introduction*. New York: Vintage.

Foucault, M. (1982). Afterword: The subject and power. In H. Dreyfus & P. Rabinow (Eds.), *Michel Foucault: Beyond structuralism and hermeneutics* (pp. 208–226). Chicago: University of Chicago Press.

Foucault, M. (1984). On the genealogy of ethics: An overview of a work in progress. In D. Dreyfus & P. Rabinow (Eds.), *Michel Foucault: Beyond structuralism and hermeneutics* (pp. 229–252). Chicago: University of Chicago Press.

Foucault, M. (1985). *History of sexuality: Vol. 2. The use of pleasure*. New York: Vintage.

Foucault, M. (1988). The ethic of care for the self as practice of freedom. In J. Bernauer & D. Rasmussen (Eds.), *The final Foucault* (pp. 1–17). Cambridge, MA: MIT Press.

Foucault, M. (1991). Governmentality. In G. Burchell, C. Gordon, & P. Miller (Eds.), The Foucault effect: Studies in governmentality (pp. 87–104). Chicago: University of Chicago Press.

Franklin, S., & McKinnon, S. (Eds.) (2002). *Relative values: Reconfiguring kinship*. Durham, NC: Duke University Press.

Gill, R. (2003). From sexual objectification to sexual subjectification: The resexualisation of women's bodies in the media. Retrieved June 15, 2004, from http://www.lse.ac.uk/collections/genderInstitute/pdf/sexual Objectification.pdf

Ginsburg, F., & Rapp, R. (Eds.). (1995). *Conceiving the new world order: The global politics of reproduction*. Berkeley: University of California Press.

Goodman, A., Heath, D., & Lindee, S. (Eds.). (2003). *Genetic nature/culture: Anthropology and science beyond the two-culture divide*. Berkeley: University of California Press.

Henriques, J., Holloway, W., Urwin, C., Venn, C., & Walkerdine, V. (Eds.). (1998). *Changing the subject: Psychology, social regulation and subjectivity* (reissued ed.). London: Routledge.

Inhorn, M., & Van Balen, F. (Eds.). (2002). *Infertility around the globe: New thinking on childlessness, gender, and reproductive technologies*. Berkeley: University of California Press.

Marcus, G. (1998). *Ethnography through thick and thin*. Princeton, NJ: Princeton University Press.

Martin, E. (1994). *Flexible bodies: The role of immunity in American culture from the days of polio to the age of AIDS*. Boston: Beacon.

McWhorter, L. (1999). *Foucault and the politics of sexual normalization*. Bloomington: Indiana University Press.

Metzl, J. (2003). *Prozac on the couch: Prescribing gender in the era of wonder drugs*. Durham, NC: Duke University Press.

Moraga, S., & Anzaldua, G. (Eds.). (1984). *This bridge called my back: Writings by radical women of color.* San Francisco, CA: Kitchen Table Books.

Ramazanoglu, C. (Ed.). (1993) *Up against Foucault: Explorations of some tensions between Foucault and feminism.* New York: Routledge.

Rose, N. (1999). *Powers of freedom.* Cambridge, UK: Cambridge University Press.

Rubin, G. (1993). Misguided, dangerous, and wrong: An analysis of antipornography politics. In A. Assiter & C. Avedon (Eds.), *Bad girls and dirty pictures: The challenge to reclaim feminism* (pp. 18–40). London: Pluto.

Sacher-Masoch, R. L. (1870). *Venus in Furs.* Available at Project Gutenberg, Retrieved June 23, 2007 at: http://www.gutenberg.org/etext/6852.

Sawicki, J. (1992). *Disciplining Foucault: Feminism, power and the body.* New York: Routledge.

Sheldon, W. *(1940). The varieties of human physique: An introduction to constitutional psychology.* New York: Harpers.

Singh, I. (2005). Will the "real boy" please behave: Dosing dilemmas for parents of boys with ADHD. *American Journal of Bioethics* 5(3), 24–47.

Terry, J., & Urla, J. (Eds.). (1995). *Deviant bodies: Critical perspectives on difference in science and popular culture.* Bloomington: Indiana University Press.

Treichler, P., Cartwright, J., & Penley, C. (Eds.). (1998). *The visible woman: Imaging technologies, gender, and science.* New York: New York University Press.

PART I

Mediated Self-Health

1

"It's Down To You"

Psychology, Magazine Culture, and the Governing of Female Bodies

LISA BLACKMAN
Goldsmiths College

"Applying the art of social conduct at the level on which the individual was constituted and regulated meant that power had to find a way into the minute and mundane reaches of the habits, desires, interests, and daily lives of individuals" (Cruikshank, 1999, p. 8).

Throughout the last two centuries, particularly within the United States and United Kingdom, interrogations and understandings of the complex links between practices of self-help and arts of government, are now recognized as being integral to how populations were defined, specified, addressed, and transformed into particular kinds of citizen (Brown, 1995; Cruikshank, 1999; Joyce, 1994; Rose, 1990). In the nineteenth century, key sites for these "technologies of citizenship" to circulate and proliferate included welfare, education, the church, social reform, charity, and philanthropy (Smiles, 1864). However, it is now accepted among many contemporary commentators that "self-help" as a particular kind of cultural logic—and set of practices of self-production and understanding—has extended across almost all aspects of our public and private lives (Furedi, 2004; Rimke, 2000; Rose, 1996). Nikolas Rose (1996) argues that neoliberal or democratic forms of government presuppose the very kind of "citizen-subject" (Cruikshank, 1999, p. 22) that is assumed within the psychological sciences. He refers to this subject as the "fiction of autonomous self-hood," and through a compelling genealogical investigation links its production more explicitly to the discourses of counseling and therapy. This psychotherapeutic logic, he argues, demands and requires people to take on increasing personal responsibility for their own health and psychological well-being. This logic appeals to the individual's desires to exercise choice, autonomy, and self-control across a range of sites in which they are subjects, through the alignment of their own ability and capacities to transform themselves with their possible achievement of success, happiness, health, and so forth. The desire to empower oneself, some argue, becomes a key process through which the democratic citizen is produced, maintained, and encouraged. One key question emerging from the range of studies investigating this link is one that seeks to understand why individuals comply with certain technologies without seeing them as cultural dupes. This framing has a long history and has been central to specific understandings of mass psychology, which have framed particular ways of understanding the so-called masses through a specific trope of social influence (cf. Blackman & Walkerdine, 2001).

This chapter seeks to contribute to these debates by considering magazine culture as one key contemporary site where self-help practices have multiplied, framing problems of everyday life through what Ferguson (1983) has termed the "responsibility ethic" (p. 189). This ethic is one that presupposes that the resolution to problems, for women, is to be found through their own hard work, effort, and labor. These resolutions are such that "self-help" is the axiomatic set of practices proffered as the way out of misery, suffering, bad luck, and psychological and bodily troubles. The link between self-help and women's magazine culture (and popular culture more generally) has raised questions about the relation between the psychology of women and the cultural purchase and potency of particular practices.[1] However, cultural analysts' understandings of the production of female subjectivities have often been hindered by essentialism, even when these reductive approaches have been most vehemently opposed. Implied psychologies are often brought in through the back door within accounts, which fail to engage adequately with how women cope with the competing ways in which they are addressed across the various practices, which "make up" their lives (Beetham, 1996; Walkerdine, Lucey, & Melody, 2001). The question of how to understand the production of psychology and the relation of the psychological to consumer culture is a key focus of this chapter.

Inventing the Psychological

The question of how to approach the psychological in light of the mantra of antiessentialism is one that has engaged many sociologists (Beck & Beck-Gernsheim, 2001; Rose, 1996). These arguments focus on the production of particular kinds of psychology through the ways in which institutional practices and the discourses that help to support them create particular kinds of self-practice and understanding.

Although this work is useful when exploring the relation between government objectives and practices of self-management, what is never given any serious analytic focus is the way in which cultural logics are translated across the categories of gender, class, race, and sexuality. The eliding of these processes of translation also obscures the place of psychology in understanding the relation between discourse and identity. This chapter develops this work by exploring how the injunction to understand one's life as an autonomous individual is culturally translated within the realm of popular discourse and can come to mean something entirely different when we look across the designation of gender. The chapter focuses specifically on magazine culture and what I term the *cultural production of psychopathology*. The focus of the study I recount was on the realm of intimate relationships, and how intimacy, its potential pitfalls and problems, were articulated and resolved across men's and women's lifestyle magazines. What is striking and raises important questions about the regulation of women's bodies, health, and well-being is the way in which women were addressed in markedly different ways to men.

Magazine Culture

Magazines at different historical moments have been credited with the power to dupe, particularly women's lives; to provide forms of escapism to lives shot through with patriarchal fantasies; or to provide meaningless recipes of advice, confession, and injunctions to consume, which are picked up and put down, but which do not significantly shape how people (mainly women) think about their own aspirations, fears, and desires (Ballaster, 1991; Ferguson, 1983; Hermes 1995). In line with the shift from structuralism to culturalism that is played out in the shift from text to audience within Anglo American cultural studies, there is now more of a commitment to crediting audiences with the agency to resist media influence, often underpinned by an American discourse of empowerment. This shift is evident in the work of Angela McRobbie (1999), who within her own work on women's magazine culture has moved from a structuralist position to one where alongside a change in media representations of femininity in such forms, women are now seen as both being enabled by and having increasing choice as to how they define themselves as women within neoliberal societies. She argues that magazines' increasing engagement with feminist issues and themes have transformed the genre to such an extent that the new fictional identities offered are indicative of the newfound choices women have.

One issue then is the extent to which the contradictions and fractured themes through which "new femininities" are articulated within the pages of these magazines represent an "unfixing of femininity." This suggests that new ways of being female, which the cultural industries may be helping to produce, are indicative of the choice apparently underpinning consumer culture more generally. As a critical psychologist concerned with the "psychological," no easy or straightforward inhabiting of any new cultural categories or identities exists and the unease, linguistic or otherwise, which is part of how categories function, create hesitancies rather than any simple identification on the part of readers or subjects (cf. Riley 2000). McRobbie herself, although celebratory in tone, also points to the ways in which most representations are raced, sexed, and classed, excluding different sexualities as "Other" while representations of Black female subjectivities are relegated to a "Black genre," and class is almost entirely absent. The postfeminist woman may stand alone, single, happy, working on her self-confidence, and achievements in her relationships and the workplace, while the stories of her sisters who cannot or who are unable to achieve such success stand as cautionary tales, marked out as pathological and seen to lack the psychological and emotional capacities to effect their own self-transformation.

I maintain that the gaps, contradictions, and silences in these new fictions of femininity can also tell us something significant about the dilemmas that face women in the twenty-first century (Blackman, 2004). That these dilemmas are also still very much regulated and mediated by particular racialized, sexed, classed, and gendered discourses also raises further questions about how to understand media consumption beyond an active/passive dichotomy. Rather than viewing the contradictions within and between representations as part of a fractured address opening up more choice, the issue of what dilemmas are created, for whom, and how these are resolved and made intelligible is an important part of understanding how popular discourse functions in relation to identities and subjectivities. These issues, which are concerned as much with the reproduction of inequalities and oppressions, as with increasing choice, are often glossed over in much of the work in cultural studies, which makes particular assumptions about identity, popular discourse, and the emergence of new kinds of subjectivity. We celebrate at our peril when there is little real understanding of the complex ways in which different individuals live those injunctions, which have become part of the landscape (psychological and political) of how we think about social and psychological change and the role that the project of media and cultural studies may play in understanding these issues.

'It's down to you'

Through therapy, I've learned how hard it is for me to express my displeasure to others. My family has always brushed things under the carpet and we talked about how this had made me nervous of confrontation. When Will felt bad and tried to manipulate me, I would react by trying to make things better. I responded to his mood rather than concentrating on how I was feeling. Anything to avoid a scene. I remember once being really chuffed when he told me I was a low maintenance girlfriend. Now I see that as an insult. After ten years of acting the same way, it's a relief when you realize it doesn't have to be like that any more. A year ago, the worst thing that could have happened to me was to lose Will. Now I'm glad it's finished and feel sad that I thought so little of myself I didn't leave before. I've been in therapy for six months now. Some weeks I'm ready to finish; others, I can't imagine life without it. I don't feel dependent on my therapist. I know this is something I'm doing for myself to make my life better. (*Marie Claire*, "Relationship Rescue," 2002)

In the pages of women's magazines the most significant pattern to emerge was one in which women were faced with the necessity of self-transformation and psychological reinvention to achieve success, happiness, and satisfaction in their intimate relationships. The kinds of injunctions contained within men's magazines were attempts to shore up and defend masculine independence, where women were constituted as both a threat to this independence and the person within relationships who was required to undergo emotional and psychological self-transformation (cf. Stevenson, Jackson, & Brooks, 2000). What was significant about the kinds of discourses that govern relations of self-invention for women are that in the presentation of the female self as independent, in control, standing alone, and forward looking (the self-made or postfeminist woman), for example, there was a warrant or refuting of the kinds of discourses that Hollway (1984) characterizes as traditionally aligning women with certain signifiers of relationship—the need for emotional closeness, security, commitment, and so forth. These concepts can also be differentiated through divisions that mark them as signs of a person's emotional inferiority and weakness, that is, as neediness, dependence, weakness, and desperation; when they are read through some of the other discourses that govern what it means to be in relationship, that is, the permissiveness and sexual drive discourse. These discourses are profoundly gendered and have consequences and implications depending on the person positioning and being positioned (cf. Stenner, 1993).

> We dated for a year and I never knew if I was his girlfriend proper or not, but I didn't care. On one level, I felt slightly intimidated by him, but it was incredibly interesting and engaging being with him, which excused a lot. He'd call at 8 P.M. and say, "Hey, how about dinner?" and I'd always go. My friends said, "Don't make yourself so available," but I'd drop everything. I felt desperate about it at the time, completely insecure. He held all the strings. (*Marie Claire*, "Is She," 2002)

Many of the examples analyzed found that presentations of the female self as what we might term the "self-made woman" also function as refutations of the pejorative readings of the "have-hold" discourse. This positioning and marking of what is problematic and to be avoided, rejected, and so on, are those very concepts that articulate relationships through constructing the woman as waiting for a man to complete her. Although we might want to celebrate this move as one of increasing choice to women, what rhetorical psychology (Billig, 1988, 1997) focuses on are the kinds of dilemmas that are managed through particular presentational strategies and how these dilemmas are always "in dialogue" with a particular argumentative context—one in this case where the injunction to understand self-invention as the key to success and happiness is articulated alongside competing injunctions that require women to also refute and distance themselves from discourses that have traditionally aligned women with a need for emotional closeness, intimacy, and commitment in relationships. These concepts and the discourses they regulate appeared in the argumentative context as the unspeakable and yet affirmed categories.

The dilemmas, and indeed the potential psychopathology created for women by the ambivalence and contradiction produced through these tensions, are managed within the pages of women's magazines primarily by presenting women with the necessity of self-transformation and psychological reinvention as the means to improve satisfaction and success in intimate relationships. This is in line with previous work on women's magazine culture that emphasizes the ways in which women are required to resolve the glaring contradictions in how they are addressed through their own efforts and hard work; what Ferguson (1983) has termed the "responsibility ethic" (p. 189). The notion of "labor" as a metaphor for thinking through the governing of female bodies and psychologies within magazine culture, resonates with studies of biotechnologies such as IVF, which as Franklin (1997) has argued, requires women to engage in particular kinds of self-management practices to "hold" or contain the uncertainty and contradiction that governs their encounter and experience of this technique. Franklin (1997) aligns this with the "work of femininity" more generally, which involves "consumption, bodywork, emotional and psychological work" (p. 125). This "labor of femininity" extends to women's magazine culture where women were primarily urged to work on relationships through an injunction that privileged their engagement in practices of self-monitoring, evaluation, scrutiny and bodily, emotional, and/or psychological transformation to achieve certain desired ends. This project of self-transformation was also subsumed within a consumer discourse where diet programs, fitness, cosmetics, health-oriented foods, cosmetic surgery, and other body techniques were promoted and valorized through a vocabulary of choice that addressed the (female) reader as being able to achieve success and happiness through her choice among a range of options and preferences.

Strategies of Psychological Survival

As we have seen, what governs the kinds of discourses that frame the concerns of femininity within women's magazines is their inherently dilemmatic nature. Rather than simply competing with each other, discourses are dialogic, speaking to each other most visibly at their moments of disavowal or denial. The defensive organization of the interconnections between those discourses that govern the production of modern femininities also reveals something about the embodiment of these discourses in actual women's lives. Franklin (1997) examines the strategies and practices of "psychological preparedness," which women adopt to endure the irresolution produced by the experience of IVF: the endless cycle of hope and failure that characterizes many women's experience (p. 161). As she argues, "to negotiate a successful passage through IVF requires physical, emotional, and psychological self-management" (p. 192).

I want to contrast this study of the embodied experience of IVF with a study of how educated working-class women endure and survive the contradictory ways they are positioned as subjects across a range of practices in which they are subjects; educational, familial, scientific, popular, and so forth (Walkerdine, 1996). What characterizes the emotional landscape and psychological economies of these women who have entered typically middle-class professions through educational opportunities are a range of irreconcilable dilemmas and ambivalences.

Walkerdine (1996) characterizes this experience as one of being positioned as the "object of hopelessly contradictory discourses." This

includes a general injunction of autonomy, choice, independence, and
control through practices of consumption, leisure, and advertising, as
well as being positioned as stupid, animal, reactionary, dependent, and
pathological through discourses, cultural, and scientific, which construct
the working class as Other (cf. Blackman & Walkerdine, 2001). Walkerdine develops Bhabha's (1994) concept of the "colonial stereotype" to
explore how class is feared and desired, denigrated and envied. These
ambivalences exist beside the more normative addresses of consumer
culture where selfhood is produced as a project of self-transformation
and development (Rose, 1996).

She explores how these contradictions are lived by these women
through their own private sufferings and miseries, which are revealed
through painful disclosure of the guilt, shame, humiliation, and feelings
of powerlessness and persecution they have experienced in wanting to
"get out," to leave the working classes behind. What her study reveals
are both the routinized and habituated ways that these women attempt
to cope with the contradiction and dilemmas, but also what failure
produces in terms of its own psychopathology: depression, paranoia,
self-harm, neurosis, and so forth. These forms of psychopathology are
those that are then read within scientific discourses and practices as signs
of working-class inadequacy, inferiority, or even biological/psychiatric
illness (Blackman, 1996).

I argue, as I have elsewhere (Blackman, 2004), that women's magazines work beside and in conjunction with these very culturally produced
forms of psychopathology. Particular problems of social existence such
as losing one's job, health, beauty, relationships, and friendships are
constituted as stimuli for self-improvement. The autonomous woman
who does not lean on or need others and who above all can "believe in
herself" stands as the regulatory ideal in these addresses (Blackman,
1999). The self-made woman waits for nobody and through her own hard
work, effort, and positivity makes things happen. The "modern woman"
gets, does, improves, and rationalizes her emotions on her path of self-
transformation. Jackie Stacey (1997) talking about the kinds of personal
narratives that tend to structure "cancer stories" similarly argues that
self-help or "self-health" constructs suffering in a particular kind of
way. Failure in these practices is constituted as a temporary obstacle to
overcome, and as we have seen, these practices map onto the very kinds
of embodied experience that "make up" many women's subjectivities.[2]
Rather than simply viewing these resolutions and the practices promul-
gated on the basis of these self-relations as progressive and "unfixing"
femininity, I suggest that the dilemmatic quality of feminine discourses
and the regulative practices proffered as resolutions condense a range

of bodily sensations, anxieties, tensions, and forms of psychopathology that are "already-constituted" lived realities for many of the readers of these magazines. This work brings together much work in media studies analyzing women's magazine culture, which both emphasizes its fragmentary quality, but also the more systematic and repeated ways in which women are encouraged to see and understand themselves as subjects (Ferguson, 1986). It allows us to explore the cultural purchase and potency of particular practices, as well as highlighting the need to reformulate studies of media consumption in relation to the embodied negotiation of the kinds of cultural anxieties and personal tensions that readers bring to the text.

The Blob

Blame our education. Young women, you see, were schooled in the blob as a matter of necessity. While we were being savagely beaten on the rugby pitch, they were herded into special PE lessons, where a mustached lesbian rounders coach explained that the vending machine in the changing room did not, after all, dispense Revels. The closest we got to menstrual instruction, however, was a mumbling half-hour chat with the science teacher, where the alarming similarity between IUD coils and fishhooks stuck in the mind. Consequently, surfing the crimson wave became a mystifying feminine preserve just like going to the toilet in twos, or the enduring popularity of *Ally McBeal*. But the wise man realizes this is a hormonal cycle for two. (*FHM,* "Periods," 2001)

The dilemmatic argumentative context, which shapes women's magazines, exists alongside injunctions within men's magazines, which fix women and their bodies within essentialist discourses, which emphasize their unruly and unpredictable bodies. In the pages of men's magazines when men were presented with an injunction to work on relationships, the kinds of practice they were encouraged to engage in were what I have termed "practices of self-mastery." These practices encouraged men to acquire knowledge about women's bodies, usually as the article suggests, women's menstruating bodies, understood through scientific knowledge sanctioned within biological essentialist discourses. Where relation-ship is constructed as work, it is through techniques and practices that privilege particular kinds of knowledge acquisition, which authorize and validate male authority and commentary. This is not about psychological reinvention or self-transformation, but intellectual mastery of the Other. These kinds of knowledge acquisition tended toward intellectual mastery of women's bodies that authorized and validated male authority and commentary. An important aspect of this construction of female subjectivity is the positioning of women through understandings of biology that emphasize the kinds of wild and animalistic outbursts most likely to occur at the time of her periods.

Know Tampons, Know Girls

When she trundles down the "feminine hygiene" racks at the supermarket, don't dart down the next aisle and feign an interest in noodles. Observe what she buys and enter a whole new world of lady psychology. . . . (*FHM*, "Sex Tips," 2001)

Even though at one level success and satisfaction in a relationship with an intimate other (woman) is presented as subject to the efforts, work, and willingness of the men to engage in certain activities, the kinds of self-practice and self-understanding that govern what it means to "work" at a relationship are radically different to those that address and govern women's concerns. This is in line with previous work on men's magazines that underscore the way in which leisure is the trope through which relationships are generally understood and articulated and that the kinds of injunctions proffered operate as defenses against male vulnerability thus shoring up a particular version of masculine autonomy and independence (Stevenson et al., 2000).

Within these kinds of formulations male sexuality is constituted as "simply biological" (male sexual drive discourse) in contrast to what is characterized as the more complex feminine sexuality located within the very signifiers of relationship, which the postfeminist woman is required to disavow. In the following extract from *FHM*, a popular men's lifestyle magazine, the complexity of female sexuality is invoked through metaphors of nature where femininity is aligned with delicate flowers requiring the men to learn sexual techniques, which can be attuned to feminine sensitivity.

Unexpected neck kissing—This full-frontal mouth move is sexual, but women often prefer a more oblique approach. Take her off-guard as she stands at the sink, and trail your tongue lightly down her neck just below her ear. Why it works: Your attention to this neglected sector will have her nerve endings jangling like a cutlery waterfall. Do: Use a gentle stroking motion with the tip of your tongue so delicately that she can barely feel it. You can insert your tongue in her ear, but only in the manner of a svelte bee entering a lotus flower. Any other way and she'll feel like you've shoved a mop down there. Don't: Bite her neck. Are you twelve? (*FHM*, "Girl Talk," 2001)

Many of the warrants for the kinds of sexual techniques proffered to men, to become better lovers and increase their own sexual pleasure, are warranted through the use of female, and often lesbian authors, to authenticate the advice given. The following extract is just one example of the ways in which the lesbian woman is credited with a special knowledge of women's bodily and sexual pleasure, which can be imparted to men to improve their own mastery of the complexity of female sexuality.

The Lesbian Workshop No. 23

How to . . . Drink from the fishpot without fear.

If going down disgusts you, don't panic. You can learn to crave giving oral sex. . . .

FACE THE FACTS. Fifty years ago, you could get away with denying your girl oral sex, and still keep her around to wash your socks. Not any more. In today's world, only the most weak-willed women will stay with a man who won't go south. (*Marie Claire*, "Lesbian," 2002)

The article goes on to suggest ways the man can become accustomed to the idea and practice of oral sex, including reading a chapter on oral sex in *The Whole Lesbian Sex Book* (Newman, 2004) and buying Nina Hartley's *Advanced Guide to Oral Sex Video* from www.goodvibes.com. If this fails, the reader is introduced to a variety of strategies to habituate the man to oral sex, including forms of negative reinforcement such as burning a £20 note each day oral sex is avoided and taking deep breaths to quell any fears and anxieties. In line with the argument made thus far, when men are required to work at a relationship, the techniques of self-production they are invited to engage in are based on an intellectual mastery of female bodies, through divisions and dichotomies, which reproduce some of the most essentialized discourses associated with masculinity and femininity. These include the location of men's sexuality within a basic sexuality, contrasted from women's complex sexuality; that men are active and women are passive; women want commitment, men want sex; men are always ready for sex and women are unavailable and need encouragement. These divisions are further differentiated through the madonna/whore dichotomy where good women are distinguished from those who are viewed as "too available" for sex and who threaten the above dichotomies. This short analysis[3] reveals just some of the complex dilemmas and anxieties that govern heterosexual relations within neoliberalism and that require men and women to relate to themselves and others in radically different ways. Thus the kinds of injunctions that social and cultural theorists have identified as characterizing lived subjectivities under neoliberalism, are culturally translated very differently when we look across the categories of gender. The kinds of argumentative spaces that govern what it means to be both an autonomous agent and desiring to be in a relationship with an intimate Other are governed through very different discourses and authoritative institutions and create very different dilemmas and resolutions to possible conflicts and struggles for men and women. This focus on both dilemma and the kinds of strategies of psychological survival that women need to develop to cope are those which are obscured by much of the work in cultural studies and sociology, which seeks to understand the authoritative status of self-help as an essential component of the ways in which we live the complexity of global cultures (Franklin, Lury, & Stacey, 2000).

Self Health

Franklin et al. (2000) have argued that the proliferation and rise of self-health practices is characteristic of global cultures. These are cultures whereby individuals are increasingly taking on more responsibility for the management of their lives and of the concomitant risks and uncertainties created by the global flows of people, information, knowledge, images, and risks that do not respect national borders or boundaries. Rather than focus on the well-rehearsed sociological analyses of these distinctive cultural forms, they are interested in the more subjective dimensions of transnational communications and their implications for how we shape and act on ourselves as subjects. They characterize these "contemporary cultures of self-management" (p. 113) as attempts to regulate and manage the risks and uncertainties of global flows through engaging in narrativizing practices that understand individuals as agents of their own transformation. One focus of these analyses has been on the ways in which "nature" is used as a concept and distinction, which authenticates particular ways of being, doing, and maximizing one's life. Non-Western beliefs and practices are invoked and constructed as being more authentic showing, they argue, the dependence of global cultures on new forms of spirituality. The kinds of self-to-self relations constructed through these practices are those that promote particular practices of self-decipherment (you have the power within), self-reliance, self-management, and self-discipline that they argue produce particular kinds of "biographical biologies" (p. 126) and fantasies of a "pan-humanity" (p. 125).

Self-health narratives and practices are therefore linked to the kinds of narratives of progress and redemption authorized within scientific discourse. Rather than the schizophrenic-overload Fredric Jameson viewed as salient to postmodern subjectivities, Franklin et al. (2000) explore how those metaphors and narratives that structure science as the liberator of humanity have increasingly become individualized and lived as part of individual's own practices of the self.[4] Their focus on "modes of subjective commitment" (p. 97) and the forms of embodied subjectivity, fantasy, and desire created through the cultural discourses and narratives that tend to characterize global cultures intersects with the concerns of critical psychology. As a discipline, critical psychology focuses on the cultural and scientific production of subjectivity and identity, and pays particular attention to how cultural narratives and practices shape and construct embodied experiences (Blackman, 2001). As we have seen in my discussion of magazine culture, there is a particular concern with how individuals live and embody the contradictory ways in which they are positioned as individuals (cf. Walkerdine et al., 2001). However, although there is a concern with embodiment and modes of subjective commitment within Franklin et al.'s thesis on global cultures, there is much less attention in this work to the translation of these injunctions across race, class, sexuality, and gender. The analytic attention is mainly focused on consumer markets and the kinds of systematization and significations, which underpin the strategies of global brands such as Benetton and The Body Shop.

Taking Care of Yourself

Franklin et al. (2000) suggest that these kinds of fantasies of self-control and practices of body management enable individuals to manage the increasing global risks that science can no longer guarantee safety and salvation from. The fantasy of science as protector and guardian has mutated and converged with a proliferation of narratives and practices of self-management that construct individuals as the agents of their own change, transformation, and redemption. Stacey (1997) argues that these kinds of narratives have a potency and cultural purchase because of our familiarity with their structures through filmic and cultural narratives. Narratives such as the action movie or melodrama genre are organized through codes and devices, which fictionalize the storytelling in particular kinds of linear ways. These narratives identify and contain threats produced on the basis of a fantasy of reestablishing (national) security and boundaries. This narrative structure guides Hollywood's circulation of numerous films, such as *Independence Day*, which have dealt with threats to national or even global security through unwelcome or uncontrollable threats such as asteroids or nonworldly visitors such as aliens. Although we may be more willing to accept the role of figurative language such as metaphor in the production of cultural narratives, Stacey suggests that scientific narratives similarly draw on metaphors and figurative language, but through particular rhetorical tropes and strategies are able to cover their figurative tracks. As Foucault (1972) and other analysts of the production of scientific knowledge, such as Bruno Latour (1987) have cogently shown, science uses a variety of tricks to make and produce knowledge that "functions in truth."[5] Stacey develops the analysis of figurative language by analyzing the symbiotic relation between the kinds of narratives that structure "cancer stories," biomedical discourse, and the narratives and practices valorized by the specific self-help and self-health discourses that organize "alternative" cancer care, such as the well-known Bristol Cancer Help Centre in the United Kingdom.

This attention to the interdependence between individual practices and narratives and those that organize the global and cultural imaginary goes some way in exploring the more subjective dimensions of media and cultural forms and how they work in conjunction with scientific narratives and discourses. This is a pressing concern for media and cultural theorists interested in the thorny question of how to analyze the relation between media and cultural forms, and subjectivity and identity. However, the previous discussion of global self-health, although foregrounding embodiment still relies on the body as constructed within text and does not engage with how actual subjects inhabit the kinds of positions constructed within these texts and practices. The assumption made is that they are inhabited with relative ease due to the way in which these narratives are established as true and normative through their insertion into a range of cultural and scientific practices that shape our subjectivities. There is a discourse or social determinism in this kind of work that plagues the more constructionist approaches to identity and subjectivity that tend to characterize the discipline of cultural studies. Fuss (1989) and Riley (1983) have both made calls for a move beyond the essentialist/constructionist dualism when considering the social and psychological significance of discursive formations. Many think that the move to consider embodiment to be a way forward and out of this dualism (cf. Blackman, 2001), but as we have seen with the previous discussion, often very generalist claims are made to account for the possible subjective commitment to certain practices and narratives. These claims become de-gendered, de-sexualized and de-raced as individuals become abstracted from their social and cultural locations and considered through very general injunctions and addresses.[6]

It is the question of subjective commitment, particularly to self-help cultures of consumption, which this chapter has considered in relation to femininity and magazine culture. As I have argued elsewhere (Blackman, 2004), Stuart Hall (1996) has raised the urgent need for cultural theorists to account for our investment in certain discourses, fictions, and fantasies other than passive duping, or its counterpart, the voluntarism of many culturalist perspectives (cf. Blackman & Walkerdine, 2001). This model, Hall argues, relies on a homogenization of identity at the expense of any discursive understanding of the production of individual biographies and narratives. The only knowledge we have as cultural theorists interested in these issues seems to be psychoanalysis, which Hall himself resurrects as a possible way of understanding this question. Indeed psychoanalytic concepts are the mainstay of perspectives engaging with the embodiment of cultural categories mapping out the parameters of how these categories are seen to function. Franklin et al. (2000), although not explicit about their reliance on psychoanalysis, nevertheless, invoke psychoanalytic concepts of fantasy and desire to explore the cultural purchase of self-health. Many cultural theorists developing studies of embodiment use the pioneering work of Homi Bhabha (1994) on the colonial stereotype to explore the relation between visual representation and the mediation of social encounters through fantasies and fictions of Otherness organized through both a desire for and fear of the denigrated subject/object (Ahmed, 2000). This work on raced subjects has provided an analytic vocabulary for exploring the mediation of one's relationship to one's own and another's body through the projection of certain fears and fantasies. This work is important for highlighting the interpenetration of the social and cultural with the subjective, but still for the most part engages with the body as text, rather than the ways in which actual subjects inhabit particular cultural categories. This is a more general problem with media and cultural studies that I explore with Valerie Walkerdine in *Mass Hysteria* (2001), a book that develops work in critical psychology at the intersection of media and cultural studies.

Mass Hysteria

In this book we argue that much work within cultural theory is characterized by an antipsychologism, which is often hostile to psychological and even psychoanalytic understandings, but fails to adequately engage with how subjects are both made and make themselves into particular kinds of subject. There has been a shift to sociological explanations to explore individuals as socially and historically located, rather than fixed in any way by preexisting psychological desires. This move is extremely laudable and provides one way of engaging with the regulation of individual and social bodies. However, there is a danger in much of this work that the pregiven psychological individual is brought in through the back door. As an example, in work exploring female pleasure and soap opera, which is at pains to explore the active ways in which female viewers invest in certain characters, such as the mother figure (Geraghty, 1991), the relation between televisual reality and pleasure is conceived through a social-learning perspective that is a central psychological theory of socialization derived from the behaviorist tradition (cf. Henriques et al., 1984, for a developed critique). Although this model is not explicitly drawn on, assumptions are made that women learn certain female competencies through their roles as wives and mothers, which they see positively reflected back to them on the screen. The valorizations of the kinds of skills, that is, relationship skills, which women acquire through social learning are valued within soap operas. The "realism" of these representations are what afford women pleasure in viewing, and hence their active investment in these televisual fictions and fantasies.

This body of work is important to begin to specify the particularity of viewing practices and to question the view that women are culturally duped through patriarchal fantasies of femininity. However these kinds of approaches are still reliant on psychological assumptions about how women are "made social," and what processes of socialization enable in terms of the basis of women's identifications. Geraghty (1996) herself is aware of the homogenization of women that underpin much of this work, but remains unaware of a large body of work within critical psychology, which may provide novel ways of thinking through audience investment and subjective commitment. Cultural studies seems to be at a crossroads with the danger of either inscribing the homogenization of identity to explain the social and cultural locations through which people consume media forms or invoking a voluntarist subject who can ideally resist media influence. Again psychological assumptions are made in this work although psychology is vehemently opposed (Morley, 1992). Audience research is heavily reliant on cognitive psychology and the idea of subjects as code decipherers who bring to bear their own interpretive structures on media texts (Morley, 1992). Structural understandings of identity derived largely from the work of the French sociologist Pierre Bourdieu are then used to link particular viewing competences to identity positionings such as class and gender. There is a clash between the empowering aims of audience research to find audiences who can resist media influence, alongside a commitment to exploring social location and possible fixity in different audience's consumption practices.

This work is in large part a reaction to the idea that audiences are undifferentiated masses who for the most part are vulnerable and susceptible to media influence (Blackman & Walkerdine, 2001). However, as Stuart Hall (1996) himself argues, it is equally problematic to view groups of people as homogenous, defined on the basis of their shared affiliation and access to particular cultural codes. Hall and Du Gay (1996) suggest, "identities are thus points of temporary attachment to the subject positions which discursive formations construct for us" (p. 6). The key question is how to explain and analyze audience investment and subjective commitment without imposing structural understandings of identity to read media consumption. This chapter has attempted to reformulate this problematic by working through some examples from a recent study of magazine culture.

The key focus of this work is how to understand the governing of female bodies alongside arguments that suggest that women's magazines present an "unfixing of femininity" (McRobbie, 1999). The theoretical backdrop to these arguments comes from rhetorical psychology (Billig, 1997) and the later work of Michel Foucault (1990) who was concerned with the kinds of relationships we develop with ourselves, what he termed "processes of subjectification." He focused specifically on the kinds of discourses, authoritative institutions, and explanatory structures that govern these self-to-self relations. Although some examples I have given from this study are based on what is evidently a textual form of analysis, I argue that this work has important consequences for how we might think about an individual's own engagement with popular discourse beyond discourses of choice, or their counterpart, the positing of the mass-media as a duping apparatus, particularly in the lives of those who through particular historical tropes of the mass-mind are considered more vulnerable and susceptible to media influence (cf. Blackman & Walkerdine, 2001).

Conclusion

The arguments presented in this chapter suggest first that some of the general accounts of new forms of selfhood made by sociologists such as Beck and Beck-Gernsheim (2001) and Rose (1996) do not adequately engage with how these subject positions are translated within different media and cultural forms. I have given some examples of the dilemmas that govern male and female subjectivities within neoliberalism, which show how the injunction to understand success and happiness as being subject to one's own efforts to transform oneself, is profoundly gendered, and articulated and framed very differently. This chapter has focused specifically on gender and its centrality in reconfiguring selfhood within media forms such as women's magazine culture. The injunction to understand one's life as an autonomous individual is governed through very different concepts, discourses, and broader argumentative contexts, creating very different dilemmas and conflicts for men and women. The dialogic context of these discourses is also very different showing how the kinds of generalist accounts of subject formation do not engage with how they intersect across the designations of race, class, gender, and sexuality. Michel Foucault's (1990) later work on "technologies of selfhood" was useful in exploring what kinds of concepts and categories readers were encouraged to problematize themselves in relation to, and what kinds of practices of self-transformation they were encouraged to enact on the basis of these problematizations. The assumption within this work and its development within critical psychology and related disciplines, is that what we might term body techniques and practices, condense broader cultural values and discourses bringing to light the more normative ways in which individuals' fears, desires, aspirations, and anxieties are shaped and defined (Blackman, 2001; Franklin et al., 2000). This focus can also begin to tell us about the cultural production of psychopathology and the way in which particular media and consumer cultures work in conjunction with and alongside "already-constituted" fears and desires created in other social practices that "make up" individuals' lives. This highlights the importance of developing ways of understanding the production of psychologies, as a means of analyzing the basis of the possible identifications readers may have with the contradictions and resolutions proffered within magazine culture. The governing of female bodies within neoliberalism presents women with a range of impossible dilemmas that they are invited and urged to resolve through the adoption of a variety of self-care and body techniques. The self-made woman, rather than enacting choice and freedom, is obliged to disavow any desires for emotional security and safety, and to experience these as the outcome of her own desire for personal authenticity and self-development. Within the interstices of these contradictory injunctions, self-help techniques, framed increasingly through the discourses of therapy and counseling, provide practices through which these self/self and self/other relations can be remade.

Notes

1. Beetham (1996) draws on Kristeva's account of feminine psychology to argue that the qualities of women's magazines, such as having more than one authorial voice, the mixing of medias and genres, and resisting closure, meet or reflect the psychology of its readers.
2. "In contemporary western culture, we are encouraged to think of ourselves as coherent stories of success, progress and movement. Loss and failure have their place but only as part of a broader picture of ascendance" (Stacey, 1997, p. 9).
3. This analysis is taken from a study funded by the Arts and Humanities Research Board, "Inventing the Psychological: Lifestyle Magazines and the Fiction of Autonomous Selfhood," AN6596/APN10894. My thanks extend to the research assistant, Dr. Laura Miller.
4. "Anchored in the familiar stories of progress, of liberation, and of the pursuit of knowledge, individualized accounts of global self-health condense the grand metanarratives of modernity, reconnecting individuals back into the universal narrative of modernity" (Franklin et al., 2000, p. 136)
5. See a development of these ideas in relation to the concepts, explanatory structures, and "rules of truth," which psychiatry has developed to distinguish the so-called hallucination from the pseudo-hallucination (Blackman, 2001).
6. As Morley (1992) argues, the key concern is to explore, "how members of different groups and classes, sharing different cultural codes, will interpret a given message differently, not just at the personal, idiosyncratic level, but in a way systematically linked to their socio-economic position" (p. 88).

References

Ahmed, S. (2000). *Strange encounters: Embodied others in post-coloniality.* New York: Routledge.

Ballaster, R. (1991). *Women's worlds: Ideology, femininity and the women's magazine.* London: Macmillan.

Beck, U., & Beck-Gernsheim, E. (2001). *Individualization.* London: Sage.

Beetham, M. (1996). *A magazine of her own? Domesticity and desire in the women's magazine* 1800–1914. London: Routledge.

Bhabha, H. (1994). *The location of culture.* London: Routledge.

Billig, M., et al. (1988). *Ideological dilemmas. A social psychology of everyday thinking.* London: Sage.

Billig, M. (1997). From codes to utterances: Cultural studies, discourse and psychology. In P. Golding & M. Ferguson (Eds.), *Beyond cultural studies* (pp. 205–226). London: Sage.

Blackman, L. (1996). The dangerous classes: Re-telling the psychiatric story. *Feminism and Psychology, 6*(3), 361–379.

Blackman, L. (1999). An extraordinary life: The legacy of an ambivalence. In Diana and democracy [Special issue]. *New Formations, 36,* 111–124.

Blackman, L. (2001). *Hearing voices: Embodiment and experience.* London: Free Association.

Blackman, L. (2004). Self-help, media cultures and the production of female psychopathology. *Cultural Studies, 7*(2), 241–258.

Blackman, L., & Walkerdine, V. (2001). *Mass hysteria: Critical psychology and media studies.* Basingstoke, United Kingdom: Palgrave.

Brown, W. (1995). *States of injury. Power and freedom in late modernity.* Princeton, NJ: Princeton University Press.

Cruikshank, B. (1999). *The will to empower. Democratic and other subjects.* Ithaca, NY: Cornell University Press.

Ferguson, M. (1983). *Forever feminine. Women's magazines and the cult of femininity.* London: Heinemann.

Foucault, M. (1972). *The archaeology of knowledge.* London: Routledge.

Foucault, M. (1990). *The care of the self.* London: Penguin.

Franklin, S. (1997). *Embodied progress: A cultural account of assisted conception.* London: Routledge.

Franklin, S., Lury, C., & Stacey, J. (2000). *Global nature, global culture.* London: Sage.

Furedi, F. (2004). *Cultivating vulnerability in an uncertain age.* London: Routledge.

Fuss, D. (1989). *Essentially speaking: Femininity, nature and difference.* London: Routledge.

Geraghty, C. (1991). *Women and soap opera.* Cambridge: Polity.

Geraghty, C. (1996). Feminism and media consumption. In J. Curran, D. Morley, & V. Walkerdine (Eds.) *Cultural studies and communications* (pp. 306–322). London: Arnold.

Girl talk: Fire her up—Ladies spill the beans on how to push their buttons. (2001, September). *FHM*, p.117-118

Hall, S. (1996). Introduction. In S. Hall & P. Du Gay (Eds.), *Questions of cultural identity* (pp. 1–17). London: Sage.

Hall, S. & du Gay, P. (1996). *Questions of cultural identity.* London: Sage.

Henriques, J., et al. (1984). *Changing the subject. Psychology, social regulation and subjectivity.* London: Methuen.

Hollway, W. (1984). Gender difference and the production of subjectivity. In J. Henriques, et al., *Changing the subject. Psychology, social regulation and subjectivity* (pp. 227–263). London: Methuen.

Is she really going out with him? (2002, February). *Marie Claire*, 37.

Joyce, P. (1994). *Democratic subjects. The self and the social in nineteenth century England.* Cambridge, United Kingdom: Cambridge University Press.

Latour, B. (1987). *Science in action.* Milton: Open University Press.

The lesbian workshop no. 23. (2002, February). *Marie Claire*, 242-45

McRobbie, A. (1999). *In the culture society.* London: Routledge.

Morley, D. (1992). *Television audiences and cultural studies.* London: Routledge.

Newman, F. (2004). The whole lesbian sex book. 2nd edition. San Francisco: Cleis Press.

Periods: Read our essential guide to periods and battle her monthly blob no more. (2001, September). *FHM*, p.116

Relationship rescue: Would therapy improve your love life? (2001, September). *Marie Claire*, 183.

Riley, D. (1983). *War in the nursery.* London: Virago.

Riley, D. (2000). *The words of selves: Identity, solidarity, irony.* Stanford, CA: Stanford University Press.

Rimke, H. (2000). Governing citizens through self-help literature. *Cultural Studies, 14*, 61–78.

Rose, N. (1990). *Governing the soul: The shaping of the private self.* London: Routledge.

Rose, N. (1996). *Inventing ourselves. Psychology, power and personhood.* Cambridge. United Kingdom: Cambridge University Press.

Sex tips for men. (2001, September). *FHM,* p.54.

Smiles, S. (1864). *Self-help. With illustrations of character and conduct.* London: John Murray.

Stacey, J. (1997). *Teratologies. A cultural study of cancer.* London: Routledge.

Stenner, P. (1993). Discoursing jealousy. In E. Burman & I. Parker (Eds.), *Discourse analytic Research* (pp. 114–134). London: Routledge.

Stevenson, N., Jackson, P., & Brooks, K. (2000). The politics of "new" men's lifestyle magazines. *European Journal of Cultural Studies, 3*(3), 369–388.

Walkerdine, V. (1995). Subject to change without notice. In S. Pile & N. Thrift (Eds.), *Mapping the subject,* (pp. 282–301). London: Routledge.

Walkerdine, V. (1996). Psychological and social aspects of survival. In S. Wilkinson (Ed.), *Feminist social psychologies* (pp. 145–164). Buckingham, United Kingdom: Open University Press.

Walkerdine, V., Lucey, H., & Melody, J. (2001). *Growing up girl. Psychosocial explorations of gender and class.* Basingstoke, United Kingdom: Palgrave.

2

Beyond Pill Scares?

Online Discussion on Genetic Thrombophilia and Gendered Contradictions of Personalized Medicine

PAULA SAUKKO

Loughborough University

IN OCTOBER 1995 ALL U.K. DOCTORS received a letter from the Committee on the Safety of Medicines regarding a study that had identified a correlation between the use of third-generation oral contraceptives and the occurrence of deep vein thrombosis (DVT), which was widely reported in the media. Afterward the medical community, blaming the committee and sensationalist media, reported a rise in the number of abortions and births (Drife, 1996). This 1995 "Pill scare" was not the first of its kind. The association between drugs containing estrogen and DVT had been reported in 1961 (Jordan, 1961), nearly coinciding with the mass release of the Pill in 1960 and resulting in major controversy, which provoked, among others, acidic feminist remarks, which Briggs discusses in this volume.

In 1994 the University of Leiden identified a gene alteration that increased, even if not dramatically, an individual's susceptibility to DVT (Bertina et al., 1994). Some doctors were soon suggesting that women going on oral contraceptives be tested for this "factor V Leiden" (FVL) alteration. The discovery of FVL promised to resolve the mystery of the Pill and blood clots, which had made women of reproductive age nervous by identifying the minority of women who were likely to have a DVT while on the Pill. It seemed one of the first success stories in preventive genomics, which had sought to identify "at-risk" individuals and to help them to prevent common diseases from cardiovascular disease and diabetes to cancer (e.g., Collins, Green, Guttmacher, & Guyer, 2003; Department of Health, 2003; Weinshillboum, 2003). Thrombophilia was later also discovered to be associated with miscarriage and stillbirth. It was suggested that testing could help identify women, who would benefit from prophylactic anticoagulants during pregnancy to help carry the fetus to full term.

However, the genetic test for a usually low-risk susceptibility to DVTs has proved a double-edged sword. The evidence has not been strong enough to support screening all women going on the Pill or all pregnant women (Wu, 2006). The therapeutic implications of positive test results have also been uncertain (Bauer, 2003). Because no general screening is done, most women with thrombophilia are blissfully unaware of having it while on the Pill. Some of them will develop a DVT, but most of them will not. However, those women who have been tested for thrombophilia are usually recommended to avoid the combined oral contraceptive Pill. Also unclear is in what situations women with thrombophilia should be recommended prophylactic blood thinners or anticoagulants during pregnancy (Bauer, 2003).

This chapter examines how women with thrombophilia discuss the decisions about contraception and pregnancy amid uncertainty brought about by the new scientific technology in an online support group. I make sense of the discussion drawing on Deleuze's (1992) observations on a general shift in medicine and other modes of governing populations, from normalization to individualization (also Foucault, 1991). Twentieth-century modern medicine was characterized by mass products (the Pill) and screening programs (prenatal testing) that prescribed similar drugs and tests for everyone. Modern medicine typically did not respect individual differences and views, as indicated by the downplaying of the side-effects of the Pill and the controversies around prenatal screening. In the twenty-first century medicine still believes in standardization based on evidence (Timmermans & Berg, 2003). But contemporary medicine also seeks to offer "personalized" treatments, be "patient-centered" or sensitive to patient views, and to offer health-care customers more "choices" (Department of Health, 2003).

Preventive genomics and online health groups are both part of the new personalized approach to health and medicine. Preventive genomics seeks to identify genotypes, which put individuals at risk of common illnesses to provide them "personalized" advice on preventive medications and lifestyle. Online health groups have been observed to validate and support lay views and issues (for a review see, Wright & Bell, 2003), often ignored by clinicians, and to advance a more democratic approach to health and medicine. Thus, in their different ways, preventive genomics and online health groups both advance a medicine more sensitive to individual needs.

The discussions on the online thrombophilia group highlight the contradictions of this new sensitivity to individuality. The online discussion offered participants abundant views and experiences on various forms of contraception and advice on preventive medications and pregnancy. This conversation openly debated the pros and cons of alternatives and validated lay views. However, the advice provided was also contradictory, confusing, and emotionally laden, which illustrates the downside of proliferating multiple views and "choices" in a situation of uncertainty—particularly when the advice is on sensitive topics, such as sexuality and pregnancy. Furthermore, while different views were aired in the conversation, the group tended to emphasize the risk of DVTs at the expense of all else, recommending women not adopt any hormonal contraception and take preventive anticoagulants during pregnancy. This attitude was explained by the fact that the most active participants had often experienced DVTs and miscarriages, which illustrates the invested nature of lay views. It also raises the question of whether, and to what extent, the communication on the list was an act of collective empowerment or self-medicalization.

The following reviews the basic premises of preventive genomics and individualization of health, moving on to discuss the gendered contradictions in the online exchanges.

Preventive Genomics

Research on genetic susceptibility to common, blockbuster diseases, such as cardiovascular disease, has promised to enable the identification of healthy but "at-risk" individuals to offer them preventive advice and treatments. The U.K. Department of Health's White Paper on Genetics represents the future preventive genomics in an upbeat, politically correct way:

> **A patient today:** Ali has a heart attack and is lucky to survive. . . . Ali is prescribed tablets for high blood pressure and high cholesterol. He resolves to try harder to lose weight, eat more healthily, and take more exercise. Secretly, he wishes he had taken these things seriously before.

> **In the future:** . . . Although Ali does not yet have any symptoms, and his blood pressure is normal, the test shows him to be at high risk because of his genetic makeup. Ali and his doctor are then able to make more personalized decisions on lifestyle changes or drug therapy to reduce his likelihood of developing heart disease. (Department of Health, 2003, p. 15)

In this scenario genomics is imagined to decipher the genes rendering individuals, such as people of South Asian origin, vulnerable to common diseases. This information is then communicated to doctors and patients so that they can personalize their actions, such as drug treatment and lifestyles. The process seems straightforward.

Critical academics (e.g. Melzer & Zimmern, 2002) and nongovernmental organizations (GeneWatch, 2002) have taken a different view. They have argued that preventive genetics may medicalize healthy but at-risk individuals and increase the use of unnecessary preventive medications in a situation where the validity and utility of genetic susceptibility tests often remains poor.

Amid these optimistic and concerned views, this chapter explores what happens when people are detected to have a genetic susceptibility to a common illness.

Genes and Governing

To contextualize the debates on preventive genomics, we need to understand them in terms of Deleuze's (1992) distinction, based on Foucault's (1991) work, between governance through normalization or "molding" and governance through individualization or "modularizing." With this distinction Deleuze refers to the ongoing historical shift away from governing people by making them the same, through, for example, mass education, mass production, and public health initiatives. What is emerging is a way of governing people through difference, such as continuing education, customized production, and personalized medicine.

The move toward individualized modes of governing manifests itself in a new conceptualization and practice of genetics. It marks a shift away from identification of genetic "defects" to design programs, such as prenatal screening, which aim to eliminate people falling short of "normal." New genomics identifies genetic susceptibilities to fetch a personalized treatment and prevention plan (Rabinow, 1996: Novas & Rose, 2000). Rabinow has made sense of current trends in genetics by discussing them against "sociobiology," which modeled society on the basis of the metaphor of nature—social hierarchies constructed based on presumed genetic differences, giving rise to social policies perpetuating these seemingly natural differences and inequalities. Rabinow argues that what is emerging is biosociality, which models nature on the basis of the metaphor of society or as a constructed or designed social artifice. Rather than accept their biological fate, biosociality invites people to fetch individual programs to mold their biology (Novas & Rose, 2000).

Biosociality also carries the promise of democratizing medicine in that individuals form identities based on biology, such as a genetic susceptibility, and mobilize to advance their interests in relation to clinicians and other experts. Online health groups for individuals with genetic conditions are examples of biosociality. However, biosociality may also come close to sociobiology in that in its urging of people to use genetic information to "be all that they can be," it may subtly shift the responsibility for health to individuals, naturalizing inequalities, arguing they reflect the "choices" people make about taking care, or not taking care, of themselves (Petersen & Bunton, 2002). Lay communication and activism also not only represent the "lifeworld," but are often infused with biomedical knowledge (e.g. Richardson, 2003) and may fuel self-medicalization (Petersen, 2003). As discussed by Rapp, Heath, and Taussig (2001) biosociality often has both "resistant" and "dominant" aspects.

The following analysis reflects on the pros and cons of online genetic support groups in light of the social scientific discussions on the contradictions of biosociality and personalized medicine, and it investigates the gendered nature of the discussion. Statements about the psychological and social implications of genetics are often general. Yet, these technologies typically address issues, such as reproduction, families, and lifestyle, which are traditionally managed by women. Women have also been found to seek genetic testing to help their children and extended families (Hallowell, 1999), participants in genetic interest groups are often women (see Rapp et al., 2001, p. 398) and women are more likely to seek information on health online and participate in online health groups (Seale, 2006). My other goal in this chapter is to examine the specific gendered contradictions of preventive genetics in the wider context of personalized medicine.

Thrombophilia

Before moving to the analysis of the online discussion, a few words are in order about thrombophilia. In contrast with rare monogenic conditions, such as Huntington's disease, which are more or less caused by a single gene alteration, thrombophilia is a common, complex polygenic susceptibility. This means that around one in 25 Caucasian individuals have the most common allele (FVL) that predisposes to DVT. Multiple genetic (various markers), biological (age), and environmental factors (taking estrogen, surgery, pregnancy, immobility, smoking, and obesity) also contribute to the development of DVT. The risk of DVT associated with FVL is low for healthy individuals (Middledorp et al.,

2001), but individuals with thrombophilia, who have experienced a DVT or have inherited multiple thrombophilia alleles, have a more significant risk.

Whether and when individuals should be tested for thrombophilia is uncertain and controversial. No general screening program exists, and individuals are tested on an ad hoc, individual basis. Nevertheless, because thrombophilia is such a common condition, the test for it is the most common genetic test in the United Kingdom and the United States, even if it receives much less public attention than breast cancer genetics (Hellman, Leslie, & Moll, 2003; Wu et al., 2006). The preventive and therapeutic implications of the test are uncertain. Women with thrombophilia may be recommended to avoid the combined oral contraceptive and hormone replacement therapy (HRT), to take commonsense preventive measures during long flights (drinking fluids, moving, wearing flight socks) and to keep generally healthy (maintaining a healthy weight and not smoking). Women with thrombophilia who have experienced miscarriages or a DVT during pregnancy may be recommended to take a specific form of anticoagulants (Heparin/Lovenox) throughout pregnancy, but this is not generally recommended for healthy women with thrombophilia. Individuals who have developed a DVT are prescribed a course of anticoagulants (such as Warfarin/Coumadin), which contain a significant and potentially fatal risk of internal bleeding; the harms associated with the drugs far outweigh benefits for healthy individuals with thrombophilia.

Online Group

The group studied was the main online support group for people with thrombophilia and the first one to be picked up by major search engines when typing "thrombophilia" or "factor V Leiden." Prior to analysis, the moderator and medical advisor of the group were contacted, and an e-mail was sent to the group about the project.

Based on an analysis of 6 months of traffic on the online group in 2003, I discovered that of the 3,600 messages exchanged, which belonged to a thread of three or more posts, approximately one-fourth (900) focused on anticoagulants, making drugs the most prominent topic on the list. This chapter does not focus on anticoagulant use, which I have discussed elsewhere (Saukko, 2009). This chapter focuses on the gendered dimensions of the discussion. Most of the participants on the online group were women, which is explained by the fact that women are referred to the test in greater numbers due to the gendered nature of the risk; online health groups also attract women more than men. Gender does not feature as a topic in the online forum (nobody discusses "gender"), but it structures both the content—topics—and form of communication—a "caring" mode of discussing and relating to thrombophilia (on the feminine mode of communication in online health groups see Seale et al., 2006; Sharf, 1997, Sullivan, 2002). The following analyzes three gendered themes that emerge from the discussion: the use of the contraceptive pill, the management of pregnancy, and taking care of others, such as family members. By focusing on these three topics the goal is to understand the gendered nature and implications of the online discussion better.

Importantly, however, the online discussion is not necessarily representative of the concerns of individuals or women with thrombophilia in general. Together with colleagues I have conducted an offline interview study with individuals tested for thrombophilia in South West England (Saukko, Richards, Shepherd, & Campbell, 2006). These individuals often had a rather disengaged attitude toward thrombophilia, describing themselves as "not too anxious" or "blasé" about the condition. The offline interviewees rarely discussed or were on anticoagulant medications. The differences between the views of the two groups reflected the fact that the most frequent participants on the online group were much "sicker" than the offline interviewees, who were mostly healthy people vaguely aware of a genetic risk. These findings highlight that treating online groups as if "representing" a certain patient group is problematic.

Beyond Pill Scares?

Even if thrombophilia is often discussed in relation to contraception in the clinical literature, the Pill was rarely discussed in the group: only 40 messages were exchanged on this topic during the 6-month observation period. Because most of the traffic focuses on problems to do with anticoagulant medications experienced by people who have recently had a DVT or who are permanently on medications due to multiple clotting episodes, the less dramatic issue of contraception may be left out of the conversation.

Contraception was nearly always raised by a newcomer to the list, who had been tested recently and wanted advice on what contraception was safe. The new participants could ask about a variety of contraceptive options, such as, "Is it safe for me to get the needle form of birth control?" referring to DepoProvera injections. The most often asked about option was Mini Pills, "I have seen on some sites that it is ok for FVL people to take 'mini pills.' . . . I am wondering how true this is."

Some participants had specific concerns, such as a woman who had experienced a DVT and was asking the list about the safety of the Mirena Coil—which has progesterone, not estrogen—but was wondering if she could take it when not anticoagulated: "My gynecologist has a concern about the progesterone since I am presently not on [anticoagulants] and will not be going on unless I have another event (DVT). Is there anyone who is using this and at present is not on anticoagulants?" For others birth control was an ongoing story on the list, communicating anxieties about differing advice and changing options:

Well to those who remember me talking about my monthly friend visiting and how heavy it was. My doctors decided to put me on Depo. I told her I was concerned because some of you told me not to take [Depo], and she said that we needed to stop my periods completely. Now I am scared, because I have 2 injections of Depo in my system, and they are wanting me to try this low dose progestin, Micronor. A BCP [birth control pill]!

The responses the new members received varied. Some were reassuring, stating that the Mini Pill is "okay for us FVLers." Other reassured, sometimes with caveats, based on personal experiences:

I tried the depo shot. . . . Hated it! I spotted on and off for 3 months. I also emotionally never felt like myself. I now have been taking the progestin-Micronor for 4 months it has been much better[,] no period, thus far. . . . [or] My daughter has an IUD. She is hetero FVL. She has never had a clot and has only had to take Lovenox during her pregnancy. She does have some severe pain that she thinks is caused by the IUD.

Others shared different experiences, "[My doctor] advised me that although he advises I do not take ANY kind of hormone therapy, that if they really felt I had to so, I absolutely had to be on Coumidin [sic]." Some gave more general advice, "You don't want anything with hormones in them—that's the clotting risk factor" or equaled taking hormones to "play[ing] in traffic or refus[ing to wear] bike helmets." Still others shared more dramatic experiences: "A 41-year-old teacher at my daughter's school started birth control pills last week to help with female concerns. She died of a PE [pulmonary embolism, clot in the lungs] Tuesday, funeral was yesterday."

Some concluded that everyone had to weigh their personal risks and preferences, "Basically, if you are using a hormonal method you are adding risk. You have to figure out what method is right for you, and whether or not the risk is worth it." Some suggested entirely new approaches:

> My husband and I use Natural Family Planning. I couldn't be on the pill (the estrogen pill was out because of the clotting and I had horrible side effects, though no DVTs, with the progesterone-only pill) and we hated using a condom or diaphragm.

The posts on contraception also included a message by one of the participants who had become pregnant without contraception (because of a fear of DVT) and was concerned not only about unplanned pregnancy but also about the potential harmful effects of taking Warfarin while pregnant:

> I just got back from the doctor's and found out that I am indeed pregnant. Now I have to see the doctor first thing in the morning to discuss this with him because I have been taking my Warfarin all along, unaware that I was pregnant. I am soooooo confused and sooooooo scared right now.

As Briggs discusses in this volume (also Marks, 2001), scientific and public health authorities have traditionally attempted to suppress the discussion about the association between the Pill and DVT, because the Pill was perceived a superior form of birth control, particularly for poor, ethnic minority, and Third World women. Against this background the discussion on the online list offers women a space to openly air and debate their doubts and experiences about the Pill and contraceptive alternatives. As such, the discussion can be seen as an instance of lay empowerment, of ordinary women getting together to produce alternative knowledge, or bringing to the fore more choices, that may go against the medical perspective. The blending of medical information and evocative personal accounts is also typical of women's online health groups, which can be seen to have developed new modes of peer-to-peer support (e.g., Sharf, 1997).

However, the discussion also brings into relief the double-edged nature of "choice." The online exchanges offer women following the threads myriad views, experiences, and ideas about contraception interspersed with often frightening stories of life-threatening illness. While these stories can be interpreted as empowering women by offering them different perspectives and choices, they also illustrate the difficulties women face when making decisions about contraception, possibly dangerous medications, illness, and sexual activities amid contradiction, confusion, and emotionally laden appeals. The conversation also illustrates the broader political zeitgeist embedded in this form of communication in that it shifts responsibility for making the right choice from the health-care establishment onto the women themselves. Whatever the outcome, including DVT or pregnancy, it presumably reflects the woman's choice.

Caring for Life

Pregnancy was another gendered topic frequently discussed on the list being discussed in 330 posts, making it one of the most popular topics in the group. Why pregnancy was discussed so frequently while contraception was not is difficult to ascertain. Perhaps pregnancy raises a more acute issue of medications and miscarriage/stillbirth, making women more likely to seek information online on such a sensitive issue.

The pregnancy discussion on the list focused mostly on the use of medications to prevent miscarriage and DVTs. Most of the threads were initiated by newcomers, newly pregnant, querying whether they should take prophylactic medications during pregnancy or whether they should take aspirin or a "proper" anticoagulant (such as Heparin/Lovenox). Other members of the list typically encouraged pregnant women to go on "proper" anticoagulants. Participants were more likely to be unanimous in this respect than they were in relation to contraception, although a few disputes arose. Queries on prophylaxis were frequently responded to by women who had experienced a traumatizing miscarriage or a stillbirth:

> Just from my own personal experience, I had 3 pregnancies. I took baby aspirin thru [sic] all of them. My sister had a full-term stillbirth and at the time, there was no test for FVL. My first 2 babies were fine. But with the last one, born 10 months ago, I had a complete placental abruption at 38 weeks. The baby died, and I almost did as well from the massive blood loss. The physical recovery took 5 or 6 months and I still have some female problems from this. The emotional scars may never heal for my family.
>
> If I were to get pregnant again, I'd be on Lovenox shots and induction at 36 weeks. To me, I wouldn't chance it with just the baby aspirin. The mother and baby's life [sic] is much too important to play around with. If I were you, I'd get another opinion and do the lovenox [sic] shots with early induction. You have to be so forceful with your medical care sometimes, the drs just want to do things their way.

This post is a classic example of lay health advice that mixes medical knowledge, critical commentary on doctors, and intense personal experience. It can be read as offering important and compassionate peer advice to other women on the Internet on how to take care of their health and negotiate with their possibly reluctant health-care providers to avoid the tragedy of stillbirth. Still, the message can also be read as drawing general conclusions from a specific sad case and fueling an interventionist approach recommending the more potent, prophylactic treatment in a situation of uncertainty. Both readings are valid, and illustrate the difficult and highly emotional decisions women need to make against new and uncertain medical knowledge when they are pregnant.

However, what is unusual but interesting about the participant's post is that it contained a link to a web page her family had constructed in memory of Thomas, her stillborn baby. The pages display scanned images from the participant's sonograms at several stages of gestation, striking baby pictures of Thomas, dressed-up in a cute baby outfit, appearing as a beautiful newborn albeit with a bluish hue. There are also pictures of mother and father holding him and pictures of family members, including the other children of the family at the funeral. The web pages contain a link to the list server's information pages so that "other tragedies will be avoided" as well as a link to an organization that campaigns for issuing birth certificates for stillborn babies, legally acknowledging the "birth" and individuality of the "beloved baby" (also Layne, 2003).

The web pages on Thomas evoke many, partly contradictory, discourses. When I initially analyzed Thomas's web pages, I was reminded of a presentation by a clinical geneticist. The presentation was constructed around a series of slides depicting fetuses with genetic "defects." Each of the images focused on a "defective" part of the bodies of the fetuses, such as missing limbs or extra fingers. They also constructed the fetuses as clinical objects, de-individualizing them so that, for example, the head and face of the fetus were in often covered with a white cloth. Much has been written about the "ocular" fixation of medicine, which defines truth as something that is seen from a universal, objective point of view (e.g., Haraway, 1988). The practice of looking for difference still applies to clinical genetics, this time supported by biomolecular evidence of a correspondence between physical appearance and DNA markers.

The images of Thomas are also visually powerful. However, in them genetics and unborn fetuses/babies come together in a different way. Rather than genetics being evoked as having identified a defective fetus to be eliminated; the picture of Thomas's small dead body carries the message that genetics could have "saved" him. Twentieth-century genetics had been harnessed to execute large-scale prenatal screening programs, such as Down's syndrome screening, which sought to detect chromosomal or genetic defects in the fetus, typically to eliminate the fetus's falling short of "normal." This idea is still very much alive and well today, as witnessed by extensive prenatal screening programs, and the aberrant post on the list, querying about terminating a fetus homozygous for FVL. The exchanges on the list, on the contrary, do not see genes as destiny but, as Rabinow (1996) discussed, biological nature is seen as malleable, to be modified with taking care of one's self with drugs, information, behavior, and so on. While this "biomedicalization" has been criticized (e.g., Clarke et al., 2003), it is benevolent in comparison with eugenistic stances. This became into particularly sharp relief in relation to a query on the list, which asked whether fetuses, who were homozygous for FVL,[1] should be terminated (see Saukko, 2004). All who responded to this query—many were homozygous themselves—were strongly against and appalled by the suggestion, noting they had lived a fulfilling life and were now age 63.

However, Thomas's pictures can also be interpreted differently. Feminists have written extensively on the use of fetal imagery in pro-life and health campaigns, which underline women's responsibility for the fetus and obligation not to harm it via smoking, termination, and so on (e.g. Franklin, 1997; Stabile, 1993). Thomas's pages also constitute him as an object of the medical discourse or the baby, who could have been saved via new technologies with the aid of the mother, who subjects herself to a regime of daily injections of anticoagulants, close surveillance, induction, and so on. This discourse frames the woman as responsible for doing everything within her means to guarantee the health and well-being of the unborn child. In the case of genetic thrombophilia this means presenting the woman with a "choice" to make in the face of complicated and uncertain knowledge about risks and benefits of tests and medications in a situation where women often feel particularly vulnerable.

The difficulty and sensitivity of the situation explains the aggressively interventionist stance on the list, which advocates doing everything possible to "save" the baby and the mother. Because many of the most active participants in these discussions had experienced a miscarriage, their stance is understandable from a personal perspective, but it neglects that saving babies with potent and expensive medications also has its side effects and cost. Just like in the case of the Pill, the online discussion on pregnancy, thrombophilia, and anticoagulants can be interpreted as either women's empowerment through new technologies to have safer pregnancies or as an act of self-medicalization. This contradiction reflects the promises and perils embedded in both new genomic technologies and new communication technologies, which offer individuals more choices.

Care for the Self and Others

Women's "caring" in relation to thrombophilia, however, did not stop at the end of pregnancy. The conversations on the list illustrated that caring for family in relation to thrombophilia was a continuous project for the women on the list. This caring attitude permeated the list and manifested in a specific gendered rhetoric of care for others (Gilligan, 1993). Similar gendered rhetoric of care has also been observed in women's online self-help lists more generally (see Sharf, 1997), but it was probably accentuated on the thrombophilia list by the genetic focus on families (also Franklin & McKinnon, 2002; Hallowell, 1999).

An issue participants frequently discussed in their role as mothers was whether to test children for thrombophilia. If the decision was to test, then the question often was at what age to test:

My hematologist told me that they wouldn't test my daughter until she was 13 or so, as children weren't at risk. But I see from reading your messages that some of your kids have had problems at quite a young age. Do you think I should press the doctor to get my daughter tested?

As with the pregnancy, the list members typically erred on the side of prevention above all else recommending testing children so as to best protect them:

I have four children ages 21,18,13 and 11. I had all of them tested because I believe it is important to have as much medical information on your children as you can. What if your child breaks a bone and needs emergency surgery. You will need to know immediately that your child is in jeopardy of developing clots from the surgery and the . immobilization.

Occasionally a member of the group suggested waiting, which would allow the child a "normal" childhood:

I probably would not have them tested before the teenage years out of one simple reason: even if you swear you will let your child live a normal life, if you know the child is FVL+, you will not be able to do that . . . so he/she should not be doing this because of the possibility of injury.

Occasional posts illustrated the sensitivity of disclosing information to children:

I had my daughter tested for exactly the reasons Jane listed—she is age 13, a cheerleader, into gymnastics, etc. so is a potential risk for injury. The issue I ran into with my daughter was that she doesn't want to know her own test results. The pediatrician's office called me on her 13th birthday (ironically) to give me the test results.

The most frequent questions in relation to older children were contraception and pregnancy, sometimes grandmothers posting asking about what to recommend the granddaughter to do. The worries about "female issues" later in life could concern already in relation to very young girls:

My youngest son has a 7 month old daughter. I am concerned for her. My older brother just found out he has FVL hetero too. He has never had problems either, but is concerned for his 6 year old granddaughter.

With younger children the discussion frequently focused on sports and exercises. One mother asked, "I have a son (12) that hasn't been tested (insurance reasons). He wants to go play paintball with his friends. I've heard that paintball tends to leave lots of bruises. . . . Anyone know anything about this?" She received mainly reassuring answers:

There's a group of guys from my work that play. They always come back covered in bruises. But since your son is not on anticoagulants, he may just come home with some black and blue marks or perhaps he'll win and won't have any!

However, in relation to contact sports, most participants on the list advised parents (and in this issue more fathers posted) to not allow their children to play them: "Remind your son that there are a lot of great non-contact sports out there—cycling, running, etc. To everyone, make sure you stay active and keep the blood flowing."

But the care was not limited to taking care of children's health but also extended to, in particular, to other frail members of the family, such as the elderly. A long story evolved on the list when the father, who had thrombophilia, of one of the frequent participants had heart surgery in Austria:

My dad (FVL+; 69 years old) will undergo triple bypass surgery tomorrow in Austria. He is on Coumadin and was not able to go down enough with his INR, so I guess they will give him vit K shot, and he also has other health problems.

The father developed complications, and the participant flew to be by his side for weeks to double-check that he received adequate care, remembering her own days at the hospital:

As to being your own advocate: with my DVTs, I learned fast to watch out for myself! When the IV was almost empty, I would call the nurse (quite often they would tell me it wouldn't really hurt me if it ran dry . . .), I would watch and make sure I got the meds I was supposed to get, and then I would remind the nurses when it was time for them, because quite often they would forget.

Overall, the list was rife with advice about how to take care of family health matters in terms of insurance, vacationing (taking care of long flights, avoiding high altitudes), breaking the news of a genetic susceptibility to family members, and diets to eat in general and in particular when taking Coumadin.

The way in which the participants on the list, most of them women, worked on seeking information, managing everyday life and health care and giving emotional support for their family members and to other participants on the list can be interpreted in two ways. First, the exchanges provided the women an opportunity to both get practical information about how to best care for their children and other relatives in relation to thrombophilia; the list also offered emotional support and encouragement for the women in their everyday care work. As observed by others (Drentea & Moren-Cross, 2005) online support groups may provide mothers, often isolated in their caring, "social capital" understood in terms of both instrumental and emotional support. Second, however, the group also bolstered an ethos of caring, which consolidated the idea that health and well-being is the responsibility of the private sphere of selfless female nurturance. The ethos of both preventive genomics and online health groups is that individuals should take a greater responsibility for their health, which not only democraticizes medicine but also shifts the burden for public health on private individuals. The individuals typically in charge of the health and well-being of families are women, and the privatization and democratization of medicine both empowers them in this labor of love as well as adds to the already unequally distributed burden of care.

Conclusion

The online discussion on thrombophilia illustrates the contradictions embedded in the shift from governing through normalization toward governing through individualization in contemporary medicine. Twentieth-century medicine was characterized by paternalistic public health programs, such as the push toward hormonal contraception and prenatal screening, which often suppressed dissenting views and imposed the same normative agenda on everyone. Contemporary medicine is becoming more sensitive to both biological and cultural or value differences between individuals.

Preventive genomics and online health groups are both manifestations of the new interest in individuality in medicine and health, in that while the former seeks to individualize medical treatments, the latter fosters a culture of respect of ordinary individuals' views about their health and treatment. The online discussion on thrombophilia illustrates the contradictions of this new sensibility in health.

The online discussion on side effects of oral contraceptives illustrates how airing multiple lay and expert views (many of the lay views were indirect expert views, provided by the participants' doctors) and "choices" is not only empowering but also can be confusing, and occasionally frightening, particularly in a situation of scientific uncertainty and controversy. The proliferation of alternatives not only enhances a democratic pluralism of view but also subtly shifts responsibility for health and illness to the individual, making it seem that the outcomes of our choices—in this case the possible worst case scenarios include a DVT or an unplanned pregnancy—are our individual responsibility.

The discussion on pregnancy raises both similar and different issues. The exchanges on how to secure a full-term, healthy pregnancy using genetic information and drugs reflects a move away from eugenistic ideas about prenatal genetic testing to eliminate abnormal fetuses and toward a biosocial understanding (Rabinow, 1996), which views nature, including genes, not as a fate but as malleable and amenable to intervention. The case of pregnancy was slightly different in that rather than offering many views, the online conversation cohered in suggesting that all pregnant women with thrombophilia should go on anticoagulants to prevent miscarriage and stillbirth. The scientific opinion on this matter is, again, uncertain, illustrating the difficult situation facing women having to make decisions about serious medications while pregnant. Furthermore, the converging advice given by the group members also complicates the notion of innocent "lay" views, bringing to the fore their invested nature. In research on online health groups, the status of the opinions as representing individuals with a health condition is often, at least indirectly, taken for granted. The exchanges on the online group were mainly produced by individuals who had developed a serious medical condition, rather than having a mere genetic susceptibility. The conversation raises the question of whether the discussion on pregnancy and anticoagulants represents self-empowerment or self-medicalization or both.

The last topic, exchanges focused on tips to care for relatives and family members, mostly posted by women, bring to the fore yet another dilemma. Research on online groups (e.g., Sharf, 1997 has noted their often gendered nature, or the way in which they provide forums in which to developed specific female modes of communication based on reciprocity, addressing emotions and caring responsibilities. The thrombophilia group is a decidedly feminine space, addressing all the issues Sharf described. However, it may also work to naturalize the state of affairs where taking care of families' health belongs to the private, female sphere of nurturance and does not address the inequalities of this gendered division of labor or the fact that private individuals are decreasingly able to count on public services to help them with their caring activities.

In conclusion, the online discussion on thrombophilia illustrates the contradictions embedded in contemporary personalized medicine. Optimists have argued that preventive genetics will lead to a new era of public health, where common disease, including cardiovascular disease, can increasingly be prevented through advice on lifestyle and prophylactic medications (Department of Health, 2003). Critical commentators have argued that this will lead to individualization and geneticization (Petersen & Bunton, 2002), which directs attention away from social causes of disease and shoulders individuals with the responsibility of their health and sickness. The discussion on thrombophilia illustrates how lay communication about preventive genetics may both democratize conversations about medicine and shift the responsibility for health to individuals in a difficult situation of uncertainty; it can also challenge deterministic views about genes, while promoting self-medicalization through potent drugs for pregnant women; finally, it may also enhance new, gendered modes of conversation while also running the risk of naturalizing those modes of communication and their private structures of care that they consolidate. Lay communication about preventive genetics does not seem to warrant straightforward celebration or despair.

Rather, the conversation in the online community draws attention to several tensions, which characterize contemporary health and medicine more generally and call for more nuanced analysis of their contradictions to balance out the often black-and-white public pronouncements.

Notes

1. Most individuals with FVL are heterozygous (inherited the allele from one parent), those who are homozygous (inherited the allele from both parents) have a more significant risk of clotting.

References

Bauer, K. (2001). The thrombophilias: Well-defined risk-factors with uncertain therapeutic implications, *Annals of Internal Medicine, 135*, 5, 367–373.

Bertina, R. M., Koleman, B. P., Koster, T., Rosendaal, F. R., Dirven, R. J., de Ronde, H., van der Velden, P. A., & Reitsma, P. H. (1994 May 5). Mutation in blood coagulation factor V associated with resistance to activated protein C. *Nature, 369*, 64.

Clarke, A. E., Shim, J. K., Mamo, L., Fosket, J. R., & Fishman, J. R. (2003). Biomedicalization: Technoscientific Transformations of Health, Illness, and U.S. Biomedicine. *American Sociological Review, 68*, 161–194.

Collins, F., Green, E., Guttmacher, A., & Guyer, M. (2003). A vision for the future of genomic research: A blueprint for the genomic era. *Nature, 422*, 835–847.

Deleuze, G. (1992, October). Postscript on the societies of control. *Winter*, 3–7.

Department of Health. (2003). *Our inheritance, our future: Realising the potential of genetics in the NHS*. London: Stationary Office.

Drentea, P., & Moren-Cross, J. (2005). Social capital and support on the web: The case of an Internet mother site. *Sociology of Health and Illness, 27*, 920–943.

Drife, J. O. (1996). Old men and young girls. *British Medical Journal, 313*, 368.

Foucault, M. (1991). Governmentality. In G. Burchell, C. Gordon, & P. Miller (Eds.). *The Foucault effect: Studies in governmentality* (pp. 87–104). Chicago: University of Chicago Press.

Franklin, S. (1997). *Embodied progress: A cultural account of assisted conception*. London: Routledge.

Franklin, S., & McKinnon, S. (Eds). (2002). *Relative values: Reconfiguring kinship*. Durham, NC: Duke University Press.

GeneWatch/U.K. (2002, May). *Genetics and "predictive medicine": Selling pills, ignoring causes*. Briefing Number 18. Retrieved November 32, 2007 from: http://www. genewatch.org/uploads/f03c6d66a9b3545357384831c3d49e4/Brief18.pdf

Gilligan, C. (1993). *In a different voice: Psychological theory and women's development*. Cambridge, MA: Harvard University Press.

Hallowell, N. (1999). Doing the right thing: Genetic risk and responsibility. *Sociology of Health and Illness, 21*(5), 597–621.

Haraway, D. (1988). Situated knowledges: The science question in feminism and the privilege of partial perspective. *Feminist Studies, 14*, 575–599.

Hellmann, E., Leslie, N., & Moll, S. (2003). Knowledge and educational needs of individuals with the factor V Leiden mutation. *Journal of Thrombosis and Haemostasis, 1*, 2335–2339.

Jordan, W. M. (1961, November 18). Letter to editor. *Lancet*, 1146–1147.

Layne, L. (2003). *Motherhood lost: A feminist account of pregnancy loss in America*. New York: Routledge.

Marks, L. (2001). *Sexual chemistry: History of the contraceptive pill*. New Heaven, CT: Yale University Press.

Melzer, D., & Zimmern, R. (2002). Genetics and medicalisation, *BMJ*, *324*, 863–864.

Middeldorp, S., Meinardi, J., Koopman, M., Van Pampus, E., Hamulyak, K, van der Meer, J., Prins, M., & Büller, H. (2001). A prospective study of asymptomatic carriers of the Factor V Leiden mutation to determine the incidence of venuous thromboembolism, *Annals of Internal Medicine*, *135*, 322–327.

Novas, C., & Rose, N. (2000). Genetic risks and the birth of the somatic individual. *Economy and Society*, *29*, 485–513.

Petersen, A. (2003). *The new genetics and "citizenship."* Retrieved September 16, 2004, from http://www.lse.ac.uk/collections/BIOS/docs/AlanPetersen.pdf

Petersen, A., & Bunton, R. (2002). *The new genetics and the public's health*. London: Routledge.

Rabinow, P. (1996). Artificiality and enlightenment: From socio-biology to biosociality. In P. Rabinow, *Essays on the anthropology of reason* (pp. 91–111). Princeton, NJ: Princeton University Press.

Rapp. R., Heath, D., & Taussig, K.-S. (2001). Genealogical dis-ease: Where hereditary abnormality, biomedical explanation and family responsibility meet. In S. Franklin & S. McKinnon (Eds.), *Relative values: Reconfiguring kinship studies* (pp. 384–412). Durham, NC: Duke University Press.

Richardson, K. (2003). Health risks on the Internet: Establishing credibility on line, *Health, Risk and Society*, *5*, 171–184.

Saukko, P. (2004). Genomic susceptibility-testing and pregnancy: Something old, something new. *New Genetics and Society*, *23*, 313–325.

Saukko, P. (2009). Genetic risk online: Two ways of being susceptible to blood clots. *Health, Risk and Society*, *11*, 1–16.

Saukko, P., Richards, S., Shepherd, M., & Campbell, J. (2006). Are genetic tests exceptional? Lessons from a qualitative study on thrombophilia. *Social Science and Medicine*, *63*, 1947–1959.

Seale, C., Ziebland, S., & Charteris-Black, J. (2006). Gender, cancer experience and Internet use: A comparative keyword analysis of interviews and online cancer support groups. *Social Science and Medicine*, *62*, 2577–2590.

Sharf, B. (1997). Communicating breast-cancer on-line: Support and empowerment on the Internet. *Women and Health*, *26*, 65–84.

Smith, J., Michie, S., Stephenson, M., & Quarrel, O. (2002). Risk perception and decision-making in candidates for genetic testing for Huntington's disease: An interpretative phenomenological analysis. *Journal of Health Psychology*, *7*, 131–144.

Stabile, C. (1993). Shooting the mother: Fetal photography and the politics of disappearance. *Camera Obscura*, *28*, 179–206.

Sullivan, C. (2003). Gendered cybersupport: A thematic analysis of two online cancer support groups, *Journal of Health Psychology*, 8, 1, 83-103.

Timmermans, S., & Berg, M. (2003). *The gold standard. The challenge of evidence-based medicine and standardization in health care*. Philadelphia: Temple University Press.

Weinshilboum, R. (2003). Inheritance and drug response. *New England Journal of Medicine*, *348*, 529–537.

3

Gender, Pathology, Spectacle

Internet Addiction and the Cultural Organization of
"Healthy" Computer Use

LORI REED

IN THE LATE 1990s, a barrage of media reports declared that women
were becoming uncontrollably addicted to the Internet and some were
neglecting—or even leaving—their husbands and children as a result of
their online obsession. Headlines described the strange phenomenon:
"Internet Blamed for Neglect: Police Say Mother Addicted to Web"
(Bricking, 1997), "'Net-addicted Mother Loses Custody of Her Children"
(1997), and "Net Addiction Like Drugs or Alcohol: Woman Left Husband
for Computer" (Snodgrass, 1997). When psychologist and professor
Kimberly Young (1996a, 1996b) concluded in her academic study that
women were more likely than men to self-report an addiction to the
Internet (see also, American Psychological Association, 1996, 1997;
Young, 1998), the popular media reported that women were particularly
at risk for the condition. For example, Snodgrass reported that "women
are nearly twice as likely to suffer from Internet Addiction." And the examples of female Internet addicts were, indeed, quite striking: One woman,
for example, was reported to have been so involved in the Internet that
she neglected to provide food and health care for her children, and she
forgot to buy heating oil for the house (Bricking, 1997). It was reported
that when Pam Albridge's husband demanded that she choose him or
the computer, she chose the computer (Snodgrass, 1997). In yet another
spectacular case, news media described that, while she was online, Sandra
Hacker would lock her children in a "playroom" that had "broken glass,
debris, and child handprints of feces on the wall." Police described, "The
place was in a shambles, but the computer area was clean—completely
immaculate" (Bricking, 1997). These and other cases of child neglect
circulated in the popular media became emblematic of Internet Addiction Disorder (IAD) or Pathological Internet Use (PIU).

If the popular and psychological discourses surrounding Internet addiction are approached through the lens of feminist and cultural studies of science and technology, then the cultural formation of computer technologies *and* definitions of "health" and "illness" must be viewed as historically situated and as implicated in cultural, economic, and political relationships. Foucault (1972, 1978, 1991) provides a useful framework for analysis: He is interested in the historical production of truth, and he works to understand the processes by which certain concepts become accepted as true and the effects these truths have on people's lives. Foucault assumes that knowledge practices cannot exist outside of power and politics, and he works to describe knowledge practices that organize human behaviors into the "appropriate" and "inappropriate," "normal" and "abnormal." Related feminist analyses regarding the "sexual politics of sickness" such as definitions and diagnoses of "hysteria" or brain disease (cf. Ehrenreich & English, 1979; Gilman, 1899/1973) or addiction (Cole, 1998; Rapping, 1996; Schor & Weed, 1993; Sedgwick, 1992) have also been examined as social products of particular and historically situated gendered perspectives and ideals. From these perspectives, denaturalizing such seemingly natural and bounded truths is necessary by foregrounding the procedures, assumptions, and institutional arrangements that produce such objects of knowledge.

Thus, in the case of Internet addiction, it is important to look at the knowledge practices surrounding the condition as being implicated in how people negotiate the "conduct of conduct"—how people regulate and govern others (and regulate and govern themselves) through the production of truth (Rose, 1998, p. 11). Umiker-Sebeok (2001), for example, draws on this framework to explore Internet addiction as a disciplinary technology. She draws on psychological and popular discourses surrounding Internet addiction, as well as the voices of Internet addicts, to investigate critically how Internet addiction functions to produce and regulate particular behaviors and selves (see also Reed, 2002). Toward similar ends, this chapter seeks to describe some of the significant ways in which Internet addiction functions as an apparatus of governance by mapping the "correlation between fields of knowledge, types of normativity, and forms of subjectivity" in a particular context (Foucault quoted in Rose, 1998, p. 11). It pays particular attention to the ways in which Internet addiction functions as a "technology of gender" (Balsamo, 1996; de Lauretis, 1987), as an apparatus that functions contextually toward the production, definition, negotiation, and management of people's developing relations with this new media technology even while it produces and manages—or governs—related definitions of "appropriate" and "normal" social practices surrounding gender and family.

Indeed, the formation of female Internet addiction as a "disorderly" sociotechnological practice has become the entry point for many psychologists' assessments about the "appropriate" use of computer networking technologies, as well as for definitions of "appropriate" femininity, motherhood, and arrangements of, and within, the idealized nuclear family. Rose (1999) contends that, at least since the 1950s, psychologists and sociologists have viewed "family to be the central mechanism in modern societies for the transmission of values and standards of conduct" (p. 175). He discusses the family as a "governed" institution that, at the same time, functions to "govern" the values, conducts, and skills of citizenship of the individuals who make up the family (e.g., father, mother, child, husband, wife; p. 177). In other words, as Rose (1999) and Reid (1995) both assert, individuals are educated as to the appropriate ways to function in the conduct of personal, social, and political life through particular familial relation, and the desire for such family relations must be continuously (re)produced and encouraged. Historically, according to Reid, "handwringing and expressions of alarm over the decline or death of The Family have always been a tactic for reinscribing and protecting the so-called normative" (p. 185). He describes the contemporary proliferation of stories about "Toxic parents" and other threats to the family as a continuation of a longer history of social management through discourses on the family. Drawing on Reid's observations about "family," with regard to Internet addiction, statements that are "ostensibly about health turn out to be always already" about gender in the form of "family" (p. 185). "Family" is perceived to be the institution that ensures social order, and it is perceived to be "the sole barrier standing between social order and anarchy" (p. 189). Thus, social subjects who do not conform to such familial ideals, whether it manifests itself in child or spousal neglect, sexual promiscuity, or another "antifamily" practice, may be deemed "pathological," as is the case with IAD and (quite literally) with PIU.

At the same time, and relatedly, feminists raise questions about the increased and particular "diseasing of everyday life" (Cole, 1998; Rapping, 1996; Schor & Weed, 1993; Sedgwick, 1992). Rapping traces changes in the discourse on addiction throughout the 1980s and into the 1990s, and she argues that a significant shift takes place from the Alcoholics Anonymous discourse of the 1950s which sees chemical dependencies as "allergies" that randomly affect particular bodies, to a more problematic discourse that works to "disease" increasing aspects of everyday life. She describes the 1980s and 1990s discourse on addiction as transforming itself to include what has come to be called "emotional" or "behavioral" addictions, such as shopping, eating, or computer use. An essential component to this shift, according to Rapping, is a psychologization or individualization of addiction; that is to say that, "addiction" is seen as a problem "within" the individual rather than a social problem affecting the person. Rapping investigates the gendered politics of the "culture of recovery" and interrogates therapeutic practice as an ambivalent one that addresses women's needs and gives them important voice, even while it offers an unproductive and "simplistic narrative pattern to explain our lives" (p. 9). She suggests that self-help practices and the language of disease often work in a variety of complex ways toward the debilitation of a feminist politics and toward the maintenance of unequal gendered and family relations. For example, behaviors such as male sexual assault may be seen as an individualized "disease" rather than a broader social problem that demands social change (p. 107). Or, women's struggle with, or rejection of, traditionally feminine behavior may be viewed as individualized "dysfunction" to be managed rather than a call for change regarding rigid and unequal social roles. Ultimately, Rapping argues that such translations can be debilitating for a feminist politics. As Schor and Weed (1993) describe the culture of addiction, it renders particular (gendered and classed) subjectivities "as always on the edge and yet somehow susceptible to management" (Front page, "Editor's Note"). With this in mind, we need to investigate the discourse on computer addiction as simultaneously a prescriptive, moral, and "normalizing" discourse on gender, sexuality, and the family. "Disorderly" social arrangements are strategically managed, and public, professional, and medico-psychological discursive practices are deployed and "work" to put such idealized relations (back) into place.

New Social Technologies and the Panic Over Gender

Throughout the history of "new" media similar fears and panics have emerged regarding how the technology may cause mental abnormality or may disrupt or overturn accepted gender and family roles (Cassidy, 2001; Reed, 2000). The telegraph, for example, was perceived as dangerous for its causing of insanity (Garland, 1901), as well as for the ways it could disrupt gender, class, and sexual behaviors that could result from communication that did not require face-to-face contact (Marvin, 1988, p. 88). Fears surrounding the telephone, radio, and television also included biotechnical fears such as worries about contracting a disease from the telephone apparatus (Marvin, 1988), nervous disorders from radio (Douglas, 1991), and psychological effects of television on children (Spigel, 1992). Public discussion about the telephone addressed appropriate and inappropriate uses of the phone in gendered terms: women were said to waste the technology with gossip whereas men used it for serious business (Fischer, 1992, p. 231; Lubar, 1992, p. 32; Marvin, 1988, p. 23). Disease and drug metaphors were attached to radio (Douglas, 1991, p. xv), and Spigel (1992) describes how the incorporation of the radio into the space of the home was met with an astute concentration on how it could be used without distracting women from their necessary domestic responsibilities or disrupting accepted gender roles (see also Wilkins, 1931). Later, similar fears arose with television. Spigel describes the particularly gendered narratives through which television was installed into the home, and pays particular attention to the public discourse surrounding, and management of, concerns regarding television's potential to disrupt the gendered order of the home. NBC, for example, managed gender by suggesting that women could make their domestic chores more pleasant by organizing and performing their tasks around their favorite television programs (p. 86).

Similarly, worries about computer technologies focused, at least in part, on concerns about how the new machine might disrupt or overturn traditional gender and family ideals. Faflick (1982), for example, described "how families come apart in the face of the micro invasion" (p. 80). It is well-known that the introduction of computers into U.S. culture did not occur without struggle, that it required much work to rearticulate computers from being feared (masculine) war machines into "friendly" household appliances (Reed, 2000). Early in the history of computing, the "friendship" between people and computers was largely a friendship between men and their computers, and it was during this time that the term "computer widow" emerged (cf. Van Dusen, 1983). Articles such as "My Husband's Computer Was My Competition" (Scott, 1982) counseled women about how to cope with their husbands' neglect as a result of his "computer enthusiasm" (Hollands, 1985). Other books and articles similarly "guided" families about how to bring the computer into the home with minimal interruption (Levine, 1983; Joan & Levine et al., 1984; Wollman, 1984). A 1982 issue of the *Saturday Evening Post*, for example, included, "A Family Computer Album" and declared, "When in need of answers or entertainment, families in this Midwest community are finding their computer a friend indeed" (Olsen, 1982, p. 71). Photo captions throughout Olsen's essay emphasized the computer as friend of the family, both in terms of friendly interactions with individuals, as well as being a friend to the notion or concept of the "family" as a social institution.

In time, computer manufacturers and marketers realized that in order to move the computer into the home successfully, they had to encourage the comfortable and proficient female computer user. Advertisers began to market the computer to the female user in ways it had not previously (Lewyn, 1990), and women's magazines such as *Ladies Home Journal* (Asimov, 1983; Hait, 1983) and *Good Housekeeping* ("I Couldn't Learn," 1987) included advice regarding how women could overcome computer fear to use computers confidently. Women were advised to stop viewing their computers as tools and to, instead, view them as "appliances," just like a toaster, washing machine, or any other household convenience (Van Gelder, 1983, 1985, pp. 89–91). Computer classes especially for women helped to produce confident computer users ("A Computer Lesson," 1984). As women became increasingly competent computer users during the 1970s and 1980s, the discourse on computers converged with contemporaneous and emergent debates regarding "women's rights" and a woman's "correct" place in the family and society. Isaac Asimov, for example, advocated that "one of the most significant uses for computers [will be], that of finally raising the role of women in the world to full equality with that of men" (p. 66). On the other hand, a prominent conservative figure announced, "We are against the women's rights movement . . . and we are very concerned about the growing menace of home computers" (quoted in Van Gelder, p. 36). And it made perfect sense when *Ms. Magazine* provided guidance and instruction on how a woman could find herself "falling in love with [her] computer" (p. 36). So while the manufacture of female computerphilia was necessary and beneficial to the computer industry, it simultaneously raised cultural anxieties about how the machine might threaten traditional gender and family roles. As a result, much of the 1990s discourse on computer can also be seen as a prescriptive and mediating discourse on gender, the family, and the politics of domestic space (cf. Cassidy, 2001).

When Love Turns to Obsession: Assembling Healthy Women and Healthy Families

Into the 1990s, women increasingly used computers at home and questions continued about just how computer technologies could and should be incorporated into people's lives. Who should use computers? For what purpose? Where should they use them? How should they use them? What are the dangers pertaining to computer use? As Marvin (1988) describes in her history of "new" media, "new media intrude on existing habits and organizations and new media provide new platforms on which old groups confront one another. Old habits of transacting between groups

are projected onto new technologies that alter, or seem to alter," existing
social organization. . . . "Efforts are launched to restore social equilibrium, and these efforts have significant social risks" (p. 5). She further
explains that the history of electronic media can be seen as a "series
of arenas for negotiating issues crucial to the conduct of social life,
among them, who is inside and outside, who may speak, who may not,
and who has authority and may be believed" (p. 4). Not insignificantly,
the popular acceptance of the Internet and the World Wide Web was
contemporaneous with the "culture of recovery" (Rapping, 1996) in the
1990s, and women's love for the machine was said to, in some cases, turn
to obsession, and several cases of female child neglect due to Internet
addiction received wide public attention. In addition to the proliferation
of newspaper reports, television profiles about Internet addiction and
Internet-induced family and gender disruptions appeared on shows such
as *Dateline NBC* (1997), *Inside Edition* (1996), *The Maury Povich Show*
(1998), and *NBC Nightly News* (1997), among others. Psychological and
psychiatric discourses continued with the warnings first seen throughout
the 1970s and 1980s, that home computers constituted a looming threat
to the family and, as mentioned, it was declared in the 1990s that women
were particularly "at risk" for computer addiction (Snodgrass, 1997).
And while men were and still are at times designated as computer or
Internet addicts, focusing on the specificity of the designation as it
forms in relation to women it is useful because the intelligibility of the
designation depends on and reproduces a normative femininity as it
governs and regulates the female body.

**Glenda's Story: The Talking Cure
and Technologies of Presence**

These processes and dynamics regarding contests over proper Internet
use, gender, and family practices, and Internet addiction as both an
apparatus through which a new, normative media "technohabitus" is
produced and managed through the governing or regulation of the
nuclear family are illustrated in two cases of the condition as they were
chronicled separately on *Dateline NBC* (1997) and the *Maury Povich Show*
(1998). The first segment, from *Dateline NBC*, presents a report on the
recovery of Glenda Farrell, a self-described Internet addict. The segment
begins by describing the ominous threat of an emerging epidemic:

> Drugs, alcohol, sex. As we enter the twenty-first century we're getting a
> little better at recognizing and treating addictions that have haunted
> humanity for centuries. But with this new age also comes a strange new

kind of addiction. It can cause people to abandon their work, their spouses, their children, while they sit alone for hours on end talking to strangers. (*Dateline*, 1997)

The segment presents a report on the new disorder and emphasizes the trials and tribulations of Glenda's story. Introduced as "Tammy's mother," Glenda Farrell is said to have been "the perfect model of the perfect mother." She was a Cub Scout den mother, an assistant Brownie leader, and Booster Club secretary. As her daughter Tammy explains, "It seemed like we had the perfect life . . ..[until] . . . the computer. . . .Until the computer. And then that's when everything just . . . it just seemed to go bad." Glenda herself admitted that in only a couple of months she was "hooked" on the Internet. Prior to the acquisition of the computer Glenda's marriage was "a very good marriage." She remembers, "I was very happy, or I thought I was very happy until I found the—the computer." When away from the computer, Glenda suffered symptoms of withdrawal, "I would get very nervous, very upset, very short with, you know, with people, you know because I was wanting to be on the box."

Glenda's online persona, "Jeepers," was said to have an identity that was quite different from the one Glenda lived off line. As Keith Morrison narrates:

Glenda was a full-time mom and wife, probably quiet, involved in homey things. And Jeepers talked a lot, very outgoing personality. . . . The person I felt I was inside, that maybe didn't always show in my everyday life, the young person that I was, that I'd been.

The report explains that Glenda stopped cooking dinner, stopped helping the kids with their homework, and stopped her other domestic chores. While leading the life of Jeepers, Glenda lost more than 60 pounds, became more outgoing, made friends, and describes this as a time when she felt generally good about herself and her life. In time, Glenda left her husband of 19 years and her three teenage children. Morrison asks what caused Glenda's betrayal of her family. Tammy, Glenda's daughter, offers an explanation. "To me it was the computer. It was just like a drug, I think. Because it was like a little fantasy you can make up your own little world, and everything, instead of just facing reality about everything."

Glenda also appeals to a higher authority for an explanation, "I don't know how to explain the power that the box has over people! And it wasn't just me, it was several others leaving their husbands or their wives." Indeed, the concept of "addiction" makes Glenda's behavior intelligible in that it could only be an outside (and uncontrollable) force that could drive Glenda away from her familial responsibilities. After all, she was "happy" before the computer entered her life. Eventually, Glenda came to realize that Jeepers was "not real," not her "true" self, and as Glenda is depicted performing the "appropriately" feminine substitute activity of knitting, the segment concludes with commentary by reporter Keith Morrison: "[Glenda] still sees the man she met online . . . [but they have their problems]. . . .She's gotten a job and lives alone. She still has a computer. . . .But she works now and has little time to chat." It is reported that, eventually, Glenda saw the errors of her ways and was brought back to "normality" to be, according to Morrison, "like the vast majority of the over 10 million Americans online." And Glenda's televised confession functions as part of the therapeutic return to her "true" self, and as a "cautionary tale" to help other people avoid the dangerous lure of the Internet.[1]

If Glenda's therapeutic recovery and eventual truth-telling of her "cautionary tale" is considered through the lens of Foucault's notion of "confession," we can explore Glenda's story as a product and apparatus of power, and as implicated in the broader governing of the social body. Foucault (1978) describes Western society as "a singularly confessing society" (p. 62). He posits that the modern "obligation to confess is now related through so many different points, is so deeply ingrained in us, that we no longer perceive it as the effect of a power that constrains us" (p. 62). Foucault insists that truth is not simply "free" and waiting to be released from repression but, rather, its production is thoroughly imbued with relations of power. The practice of confession is an emblematic example of this dynamic (p. 60). Yet, significantly, the confession is not coerced from a power located "above" but is formed from below "as an obligatory act of speech. . . . And this discourse of truth finally takes effect, not in the one who receives it, but in the one from whom it is wrested" (p. 62). One confesses—or is forced to confess:

> The confession is a ritual of discourse in which the speaking subject is also the subject of the statement; it is also a ritual that unfolds within a power relationship, for one does not confess without the presence (or virtual presence) of a partner who is not simply the interlocutor but the authority who requires the confession, prescribes, and appreciates it, and intervenes in order to judge, punish, forgive, console, and reconcile; a ritual in which the truth is corroborated by the obstacles and resistances it has had to surmount in order to be formulated; and finally, a ritual in which the expression alone, independently of its external consequences, produces intrinsic modifications in the

person who articulates it: it exonerates, redeems, and purifies him;
it unburdens him of his wrongs, liberates him, and promises him
salvation. (p. 62)

Cole (1998) specifically addresses confession in the context of 12-step
recovery programs as she argues that the recovering addict turns over his
or her authority to a higher power, thus acknowledging the lack of free
will and moral failure (p. 269). Yet, rather than view Glenda's situation
as either the acquisition or lack of free will, addressing the particular
activation of Glenda's participation toward her own subjectification
and toward the production and formation of particular legitimations of
computer use—toward a particular (and interested) Internet "temper-
ance—is useful." (See Miller, 1996, for a discussion of cultural citizenship
and the "tempered" self.) Foucault (1978) outlines several delineations
through which the ritual of confession is imbued with relations of power,
including "through a clinical codification of the inducement to speak,"
"through the method of interpretation," and "through the medicalization of the effects of confession" (pp. 65–67). In Glenda it becomes
apparent how the inducement to speak, the subjection to an authoritative
interpretant, and the medicalization of the effects of confession (translation of computer use through the med-psych apparatus of addiction)
functions toward managing individual and social bodies. Glenda is
both physically and internally separated—and separates herself—from
others ("normal" computer users, "healthy" women) even while her new
knowledge about her own irresponsibility and deviation from her true
self heightens her susceptibility to a prescriptive normativity. Glenda's
"crisis" of identity is further reinforced through a close-up of a computer
screen which displays the question, "Who Am I?" She is encouraged to
draw on an authoritative psychological vocabulary of which she is both
the subject and the object. (See Nadeson, 1997, for a discussion of
these issues surrounding personality testing.) The addiction apparatus
successfully transforms Glenda—and Glenda transforms herself—into a
normal computer user and healthy woman/mother: a responsible cyborg
citizen amid the threat of myriad alternatives.

   At the same time, Glenda's narrative represents and manages a
broader cultural crisis surrounding issues of "presence" as has been
activated by technological change, and functions toward the production
and eventually "stabilized" technohabitus that includes particularly structured relation among computers, bodies, identities, and selves. Stone
(1996) and Derrida (1993), respectively, posit that "technosociality,"
and "the technological condition," including chemical and medical
(re)constitutions of bodies, computer technologies, and formations of

virtual identities and bodies, participate in a cultural crisis as various configurations of technobodies challenge cultural assumptions about realities of bodies and "presence," relations between bodies and selves. More specifically, Stone addresses particular boundary crossings that challenge assumptions about what bodies should be or do, what forms bodies should take, and prescribed relations between bodies and selves (p. 89). Toward this end, she investigates two contests surrounding multiple personality: (1) the case of a physical rape of a female with multiple personalities, and the cultural and legal struggle over which identity was authorized to provide consent for the actions of the physical body; and (2) the construction of a virtual identity in which the online gendered persona is not what one might first expect, given the physical sex of the body at the keyboard—the case of the cross-dressing psychiatrist. Stone strategically juxtaposes these two cases of multiple identity to raise questions about the production of the modern unitary individual, relations between bodies and selves. She suggests that instances of multiple identities online raise questions about the cultural imperative that a body carries one primary persona, one "true identity" against which other quasi-identities are judged, and by which our social being is judged, authorized, and grounded (p. 171). For Glenda/Jeepers, Glenda is ultimately legitimized as the real bodily inhabitant. Jeepers is dismissed as "not real," as a "quasi-identity" (Stone) forged through a temporary lapse in judgment. Glenda's case illustrates Stone's proposition that in a technosocial environment such as cyberspace—where boundaries between technology and nature are blurred—productive possibilities emerge when traditional boundaries are blurred and conditions are created for "non-traumatic multiplicity" (p. 36). Yet, at the same time, Glenda's case demonstrates how implicit assumptions about bodies and selves are mobilized toward a technohabitus that both conditions and is conditioned by the redirection or management of multiplicity into familiar unitary subjectivity and binary structure. Thus, as Stone also described, if the modern is structured through mutually exclusive binary oppositions (e.g., body/mind, self/society, male/female), then various practices that disrupt, blend, or challenge this social architecture must be managed. Indeed, as Jeepers disrupts the gendered order of the Farrell household, bodies and selves are reconfigured and managed to restore social and corporeal equilibrium.

Stone (1996) addresses this crisis of "presence" as it has been negotiated by and through computer networking technologies but also points to broader reconfigurations in technosocial space. Her illustrations are particularly useful for an investigation into the cultural politics of Internet addiction in that the Internet addiction apparatus is doubly imbricated in this technologically aided crisis surrounding issues of "presence." Derrida's (1993) and Sedgwick's (1992) perspectives about the cultural formation of addiction converge around questions regarding issues of "presence," of how technological practices—chemical or otherwise—challenge accepted notions of the natural body (in Cole, 1998). As such, the deployment of the addiction apparatus as a classificatory scheme functions to organize and govern related crises and disruptions of modern logic surrounding the body (Cole, 1998). For Sedgwick, the postmodern condition of the body is emblematized in the notion of steroid man. Like the cyborg, steroid man "destabilizes binaries along multiple axes: body machine; human/animal; healthy/unhealthy body . . . natural/prosthetic" (in Cole, 1998, p. 272). For Derrida, the emblematic technosocial figure is the drug addict—body and experience as chemically-technologically reconfigured, and for Stone it is the technosocial nontraumatic multiple.

Derrida (1993) asserts that "addiction appears to be governed by a subject-object relation in which a diseased-self relies or becomes dependent upon an object inscribed with mystical qualities" (Cole, 1998, p. 270). As Glenda's daughter states, the computer is "like a drug," and life online is a life of fantasy—it is "not real." Historically, what may lend computer technologies to the relatively ready and intelligible link to addiction is the historical association of the technology with the 1960s drug counterculture, a powerful aura surrounding computers as mysterious (even mystical; see Sconce, 2000, for a discussion of the history of media and its connections to "mysticism"), as linked to alternate realities, and the contemporaneous formation of computer technologies and the formation of the "culture of addiction" or the "culture of recovery" (Rapping, 1996). Gibson's famous description of cyberspace as a collective consensual hallucination both draws on and connects the computer "elsewhere" to the alternate reality of a drug trip. Derrida (1993) describes the drug addict as one who "cuts himself off from the world, in exile from reality, far from objective reality and the real life of the city and the community; that he escapes into a world of simulacrum and fiction. We disapprove of his taste for something like hallucinations." He suggests that the escape to fantasy, to an alternate reality, is at the root of any prohibition of drugs (or the Internet; p. 7). This description is also appropriate to the Internet "addict," and likewise, the drug/Internet users'"trip" takes place in the "in between," in a "place" that does not fit neatly into usual oppositions of natural/artificial. Thus, Derrida argues that in the case of drugs (and to extend to cyberspace), it is in the name of an organized and originary "naturalness" of the body that the "war on drugs" is waged as a war against artificiality, and as a desire to reconstitute the "ideal [natural] body" (p. 7).

Derrida (1993) argues that this "modern logic of technological supplementarity" undergirds the addiction apparatus, as the main positions in the drug addiction discourse (prohibitionist and "pro" drugs) neglect to take into account what Derrida calls "the technological condition." (See Cole, 1998, for an extended discussion of Derrida's position and the cyborg.) Similar to Stone's (1996) "technosociality," Derrida argues that in the context of the technological condition, there is no natural, originary body. A modern logic of technological supplementarity suggests that technology has:

> simply added itself, from outside or after the fact, as a foreign body. Certainly, this foreign or dangerous supplement is "originarily" at work and in place in the supposedly ideal interiority of the "body and soul." . . . Without being absolutely new, now takes on particular and macroscopic forms, is this paradox of a "crisis," as we superficially call it, of naturalness. This alleged "crisis" also comes up, for example, throughout the problems of biotechnology and throughout the new and so-called artificial possibilities for dealing with life, from the womb to the grave. . . . The recourse to dangerous experimentation with what we call "drugs" may be guided by a desire to consider this alleged boundary from both sides at once. (p. 15)

Similarly, Stone (1996) suggests that the crisis over naturalness, or the War of Transformation, is:

> about negotiating realities and demarcating experiences. For example, questions arise over the organization of bodies and selves: many persons in a single body (multiple personality); many persons outside a single body (personae within cyberspace); a single person in/outside many bodies (institutional social behavior). (p. 87)

And, it is significant to emphasize that such reconfigurations of presence refer not only to a human-machine interface, but also to more specific and situated presences such as those addressed here surrounding what we might call "gendered presences" in a technosocial environment. If Glenda's "cautionary tale" is useful for how it reveals struggles over multiplicity, over possibilities of technosociality in an age of limits, a second case of Internet addiction also engages with larger reconfigurations and stabilizations surrounding presence, technosociality, bodies, and selves—technologies of presence. As a situated and social technology

active in the constitution of gender and family, the formation of Internet
addiction, as it traverses through the bodily presence of Sandra Hacker,
displays the "public response to a visible transgression of cultural norms
of unitary subjectivity" (Stone, p. 29). Thus, in a broader sense, the
formation and mobilization of Internet addiction can be viewed as
implicated in current debates and tensions surrounding individual
and collective selves, (virtual) communities, and physical bodies, in
the negotiation of a perpetually forming and transforming Internet
technohabitus.

Technologies of Dis-Location:
Subjectivity, Resistance, the Unruly Woman

Sandra Hacker's situation offers a slightly different perspective on
the process of "becoming an addict," the cultural materialization of
Internet addiction, and the ways in which definitions of "normal" and
"appropriate" Internet use are imbued with traditional gender ideals. In
spite of much outside encouragement, Hacker refuses to call herself an
"addict." Instead, she demands that her behavior be seen as a rejection
of the traditionally feminine domestic role, and as a statement that
child care and housework are not solely the responsibility of women.
Hacker's spectacular "case" provides the tantalizing opening for *The
Maury Povich Show*:

> POVICH: Today we are going to meet people who admit they are
> addicted to their computers. . . . They neglect their housework and
> jobs, drive their spouses away, or lose custody of their children. Take
> Sandra Hacker. She spent hours in chat rooms while her family lived
> in squalor and her children played in their own excrement. . . . [She]
> got her reality check when she was accused of being addicted to the
> Internet. . . . She was arrested, put in jail, and she's currently on
> probation for child neglect.

When asked, Hacker tries to explain that her husband shares equal or
more responsibility for the household mess and unsanitary conditions
the children lived in:

> HACKER: We were separated. I was gonna go out of town and ask
> him if it was okay. I've never been away from the family. . . . And
> he said okay. I went to Chicago. . . . I was there for a day. He called
> me . . . and said that if I didn't come back home he was gonna call the
> police for child abandonment because I left the state. So I drive

right back home. He had the locks changed on my apartment. The only way he would agree to give me a key to my apartment is if I agreed to work on the marriage. So I told him I would in order to be able to get into my home. When I get into my home, my house in a shambles.

But Povich directs the discussion elsewhere:

> POVICH: You're talking about him, and you're the one on probation, you're the one who lost the kids. . . . And the reason, according to many, is that you got addicted to the Internet.
> HACKER: The reasoning is because my husband told the news that.
> POVICH: Were you addicted to the Internet?
> HACKER: I don't believe I was addicted. I've only been online since, like, April. There are time[s] when, you know, I'm probably . . . shouldn't been. . . . This was my day schedule. I would get up at 5 a.m., get the kids ready for day care, take the kids to day care, take my husband to work, drive myself to work, then I would go and pick the kids up from day care, wait an hour to pick him up, then come home, make dinner, get the kids ready for bed.

Povich finds this to be implausible, given the reported conditions of the household. After all, Hacker's description of her own behavior sounds quite "normal."

> POVICH: . . . You were never online until after dinner?
> HACKER: Yeah, because I wasn't home 'til after dinner. . . . And then the kids went to bed at 8:00. . . .

Povich then moves to locate the cause of Hacker's behavior in the Internet. Hacker avoids this interpretation and, instead, describes a general problem with the marital arrangements:

> POVICH: But this Internet according to the authorities, and your ex-husband. . . . this Internet caused all your problems
> HACKER: No, we had problems before I even know [sic] what AOL was. . . . Our whole marriage, he was never working at home. I went to school.
> POVICH: Your attitude now is you're not going to blame the Internet for any of your problems. . . . You're gonna blame your husband, you're gonna blame other things, you're not gonna blame the Internet, and your use of it.

HACKER: Not . . . not really because he was on it, you know, all the
   time, too. . . . And, I didn't, you know, say he was addicted.
POVICH: So in a way, you're in denial?
HACKER: I wouldn't say that.

When Hacker refuses to subject herself to the position of "addict,"
Povich continues to impose the addiction discourse onto translations of
Hacker's computer use. When she further rejects this interpretation, he
delves deeper into the discourse to delegitimize her resistance, "So in a
way, you're in denial?" At this point, within the discourse on addiction,
her further rejection of the designation becomes further evidence of
her "addiction" and need for authoritative intervention.

As the discussion continues, a frustrated Povich, who becomes
impatient with Hacker's refusal to speak her "addiction," turns to the
teleprompter to preview the next segments of the show. Hacker's story
is only briefly addressed again when Povich asks psychological expert,
Dr. Greenfield, for a diagnosis of Hacker's condition. But Greenfield
abstains from coming to the conclusion that Hacker is clinically
addicted, "I don't know whether she's addicted. And based on her
story today, I would say it's inconclusive, but certainly, based on the
media's coverage, I would say she is." Later, however, Greenfield offers
that the Internet is "a very powerful, powerful medium. And everybody
that gets online reports this phenomenon of being overwhelmed by it
and taken over by it." In this instance, through Povich's prodding, the
audience's reactions, the expert diagnoses, Hacker is not encouraged
to be the subject of her own perceptions. Rather, following Sedgwick's
(1992) analysis of the politics of addiction and confession culture, it
can be said that Hacker "is installed as the proper object of compulsory
institutional disciplines, legal and medical, which, without actually
being able to do anything to 'help' her, nonetheless presume to know
her better than she can know herself" (p. 582). The addiction discourse
offers Hacker a vehicle for self-knowledge and self-transformation, a
"symbolic and normative vocabulary for identifying and transcending
individual 'failing'" (Nadeson, 1997, p. 208). Hacker refuses to be
spoken of in this way. Yet, her willful rejection of the "addict" designation, her option to be nonaddicted becomes suspect and is mobilized
as further "proof" of her pathology. As Nadeson describes the process
of subjectification, "the individual's capacity for maintaining and
achieving 'health' is viewed as being structured around his or her use
of the discourse and techniques of psychology for self-knowledge and
self-transformation." Furthermore, the discursive equation between
disease and psychological 'pathology' introduces a moral compulsion

for the individual to take care of himself or herself. Indeed, "a failure of the self to take care of itself constitutes irrationality and a moral failure" (p. 210). Thus, Hacker's refusal to become an "addict" is even more problematic in that it suggests that she "willfully" neglected her children. In turn, this willful act reveals the "work" necessary toward the attainment of "natural" gender and familial arrangements.

The spectacle of Sandra Hacker at the moment of confession (internalization of the discourse) and resistance is a useful illustration of what Stone (1996) describes as the violence waged at the formation of subjectivity. Stone describes a courtroom audience as intent on the moment of rupture and the revelation of the construction of reality during arguments about the rape of a female, Sara, who was diagnosed with multiple personality disorder. Like Sara, Sandra Hacker is a liminal figure, a "technosocial actant" who struggles within a historically specific sociotechnological matrix. Hacker's struggle functions at an individual level yet it is emblematic of a broader struggle of the time surrounding the assemblage and organization of new media into the existing (albeit continually forming) social context. At the same time, the spectacle-ization of Hacker's Internet use placed her story into the position of cultural symbol through which the broader technohabitus became negotiated, structured, and formed (even while it also structured Hacker's push into the limelight). Also like Sara, Hacker disrupts boundaries of body, gender, location, and family. In Hacker's case, the practices of norm and prohibition function both spatially and internally as she exceeds both geographical and subjective limits. Sandra Hacker left her family in Cincinnati for a trip to Chicago. The question of her physical location is directly connected to the question of her psychological location or normality. Where was she? Where *should* she have been? Stone discusses subjectivity as tied to being *in place*, wherein "the individual societal actor becomes fixed in respect to geographical coordinates" (p. 91). Social order, then, requires spatial accountability—knowing where the subject under the law is. In other words, "accountability traditionally referred to the physical body and most visibly took the form of laws that fixed the physical body within a juridical field whose fiduciary characteristics were precisely determined—the census, the introduction of street addresses, passports, telephone numbers—the invention and deployment of documentations of citizenship in all their forms, which is to say, fine-tuning surveillance and control in the interests of producing a more 'stable,' manageable citizen" (Stone, p. 90). In this way, both Sandra Hacker and Glenda Farrell, each differently challenge notions of the body, self, and place because they are "unstable"—they move physically and virtually in such a way as to remain inapprehensible. Yet, in an increasingly mobile and networked social space, the mobilization of the psy-disciplines toward individual self-regulation and self-modulation functions as a traveling mode of discipline that exceeds confinement—what Deleuze (1992) terms as a move from discipline as confinement to the control society wherein regulation is transformed to matters of self-modulation, and to what Grossberg (1992) in another context describes as "mobile discipinarity."

Yet, and relatedly, Stone (1996) posits that the imperative exists that a given body carries "within" it one socially articulated and intelligible (and regulatable) self that is the true site of agency. Significantly, this articulation of body and self—and not simply the body on its own—privileges the body as the site of "political authentication and political action" (p. 91). Toward this end, the "fiduciary subject is fixed and stabilized within a grid of coordinates that implicates virtual location technologies—making the boundaries between the jurisdictions of the physical and those of the symbolic extremely permeable—by techniques such as psychological testing" (p. 91). Stone's notion of a warranting technology is useful here: The practice of warranting refers to the implied link between the virtual body and the convergence of discourses that constitute the body in physical space—ensuring that a physical human body is involved in an interaction (p. 87).

> By means of warranting, this discursive entity is tied to an association with a particular physical body, and the two together, the physical and the discursive, constitute the socially apprehensible citizen. Within a political framework, the discursive entity—including the meaning associated with the physical body—is produced by means of texts, such as legal, medical, and psychological description. (p. 90)

If a warranting technology functions as an apparatus toward the (dis)articulation of virtual and physical bodies, the mobilization of Internet addiction through the *Diagnostic and Statistical Manual of Mental Disorders (DSM)* functions also as a "location technology" (p. 90). The *DSM* functions as an apparatus of location in that:

> in the process of defining a psychological disorder it simultaneously produces, organizes, and legitimizes a discursive space. . . . The inhabitant proper to this space is the virtual entity of psychological testing, census taking, legal documentation, telephone numbers, street addresses—in brief, a collection of virtual elements that, taken together, for a *materialized discursivity* of their own . . . the *fiduciary*

subject. (p. 40; see also Figert, 1996, for a discussion of the *DSM* and premenstrual syndrome; Kirk and Kutchins, 1992, for a general discussion of the politics of the *DSM* and surrounding the *DSM* and homosexuality)

As Stone argues, this notion of a location technology is useful toward analyzing these two cases of Internet addiction because they link to cultural struggles surrounding definitions of a proper single physical body, a proper single awareness of self, proper geography through techniques of psychological testing, and classification within a "grid of coordinates," all of which become internalized by and through a specific technohabitus even as they participate in the formation of that same technohabitus. And, again, this "location" is internalized and therefore mobile and functions as one instance of the materialization of the new media technohabitus as particular modes of technological being, habits and lifestyles become assembled, naturalized, and internalized.

Conclusion: On Healthy Computer Use as a Technology of Gender, Communication, Family, and Home

In conclusion, the discourses and practices around computer addiction can be seen as the structuring structure of sociotechnological relations that become organized, stabilized, and internalized as the "proper" set of dispositions and relations between humans and new technological prostheses, of body, self, and identities. In this sense, Internet addiction functions toward the organization of a specific technohabitus through its articulation to this extended history surrounding the "hystericization" of female bodies, women's historical struggles and strategies to elude authorities (psychomedical, discursive, and material), and related prescriptions and containments of gendered bodies and behaviors.

Thus, amid myriad possibilities, as Balsamo (1996), Nakamura (1999)—and the cases of Sandra Hacker and Glenda Farrell described here—demonstrate, cyberspace and other technosocial environments are not simply spaces of unlimited—or, rather, unorganized—formations. Rather, many familiar social codes have been, and are in the process of becoming renaturalized in technosocial spaces. In turn, new media technological practices become normalized through their produced attachment to existing cultural values and practices. Nakamura, for example, suggests that, while escaping racial categories and boundaries is technologically possible, the culturally intelligible body online still remains fixed in a modern logic of racial boundaries. Balsamo (1996) similarly argues that even while the "natural" human body and gender may be technologically open to reconfiguration, it appears that they are "vigilantly guarded" by a culture that is highly invested in a particularly gendered "proper order of things" (p. 10). Research on the construction of technosocial selves, both online and offline, has been key toward the formation of digital and virtual cultures, and toward an understanding of the ways in which computer networks and the virtual socialities they embody function to reveal the interworkings and internalizations of "appropriate" sociality in physical space, be it in relation to gender, family, or other constitutions of bodies and selves.

This chapter has delineated some ways through which notions of "appropriate" and "inappropriate" communication, interactivity, sociality, bodies, and selves are struggled over through definitions of proper uses of new media, specifically related to treatments for various forms of online addiction. Most certainly, the formation and mobilization of "pathological" Internet use, including "addiction" is tied to cultural notions surrounding the organization and assemblage of bodies and identities. Indeed, both Glenda Farrell and Sandra Hacker, each in their own specific ways, push the boundaries and exceed "acceptable" limits of body, gender, and self. Similar to historical notions of women's excess such as "hysteria" or "madness," the concept of Internet addiction functions as an apparatus or technology of gender that collects and organizes such excess, and reassembles and reorganizes social practices in line with (a binary and) culturally acceptable structure of gender/femininity. Glenda Farrell functions as an exemplary subject as she readily speaks of her gender transgressions in terms of computer use, and her computer use through the addiction apparatus. Ultimately, she constitutes her transgressions as inappropriate acts of irresponsibility and lapses in judgment. She accepts a singular self (Jeepers was "not real") and that Glenda's life prior to her Internet addiction is/was her real life. Glenda expresses regret for her "antifamily" practices as she self-mobilizes the addiction apparatus as a means to gain (and to speak) her "freedom" to choose her own behavior and to return to her "true" self. Sandra Hacker, on the other hand, is an "unruly" subject who rejects the addiction apparatus as an organizing device and explanatory framework for her gender transgressions. She refuses the "addict" designation and the notion that she is an "unhealthy" *woman*. Instead, she argues that her behavior be viewed as commentary on the gendered division of domestic labor. As Rapping (1996) argues regarding the politics of "recovery," translating Hacker's behavior into the discourse on addiction both defuses the social commentary and delegitimizes her oppositional voice.

Together, the cases of Glenda Farrell and Sandra Hacker offer a useful illustration of technologies as "crystallizations of social networks" (Stone, 1996). At the same time, and relatedly, they demonstrate how the dual process of subjectification operates in two important ways to enhance the governability of populations:

> First, they operated as dividing practices which partition the individual internally or separate him or her from others. Second, they operated as a technique of subjectification by transforming individuals into particular kinds of subjects by heightening their existential insecurity and their sensitivity to normativity. In their efforts to secure their identities, individuals drew on the very same psychological vocabulary that effected their objectification. (Nadeson, 1997, p. 202)

Insofar as IAD and PIU are actively mobilized toward reordering individual and social arrangements, they can be viewed as a normalizing practices that advocate, prescribe, and even activate particular notions of "normal" and "healthy" gender, sexuality, and family. The (attempted) restoration of "health" and "freedom from addiction/compulsion" is also the (attempted) restoration of "appropriate" femininity and "appropriate" motherhood. Rose (1995) describes this as the process of relocating questions about the conduct of life within the field of expertise such that a specific knowledge is activated through the subject as a seemingly autonomous quest for the true self—it appears as a matter of freedom. Thus, the diagnosis and identification of Internet addiction, importantly, cannot be viewed as a mere technical byproduct or result of scientifically pure psychological discourses on addiction, or as simply a means of regaining lost control or of attaining "freedom" over one's life. Rather, the medicalization of Internet use and the culturally specific definitions and formations of Internet addiction are significantly implicated in competing, contested, and political notions of gender, familial, and technological practices. An exploration into gendered dynamics surrounding the definition and management of computer and Internet addiction make present the governing logics surrounding the forming technohabitus surrounding computer networks and the organization of their uses and users.

Marvin (1988) and Stone (1996) envision the history of technology as a complex assemblage of sociotechnological forces are useful for understanding "technologies as crystallizations of social networks [with] the technologies and the networks co-creating each other in an overlapping multiplicity of complex interactions" (Stone, p. 88) In this way, technologies can be seen "simultaneously [as] causes of and responses to social crisis." The history of communication technologies can be viewed as a process whereby "social groups search for ways to enact and stabilize a sense of *presence* in increasingly diffuse and distributed network of electronically mediated interaction, and thus also for ways to stabilize self-selves in shifting and unstable fields of power" (p. 89). By extension, Internet addiction can been viewed as being actively mobilized toward the production of a historically specific structuring structure of technological relations, toward the organization of particular and contested "selves," and toward the (interested) regulation of social conduct—in this case, toward specific practices of technosociality: communication, identity formation, body, gender, family, and home.

Notes

1. Significantly, this moral and cultural panic over female Internet addiction in Glenda and other women disrupting or leaving their families took place during a historical moment when state authorities became especially concerned about the rising divorce rate and positioned itself to reinstall women into marriage via policies such as welfare reform and other policies; thanks to Maria Mastronardi, personal communication, for pointing this out).

References

American Psychological Association. (1996, August 10). Internet can be as addicting as alcohol, drugs and gambling, says new research. [News Release]. Washington, DC: APA Public Affairs Office.

American Psychological Association. (1997, August 14). Pathological Internet use: Psychologists examine who is hooked on the Net and why. [News Release]. Washington, DC: APA Public Affairs Office.

Asimov, Isaac. (1983, September). How to get smart about computers. *Ladies Home Journal*, 66–69.

Balsamo, A. (1996). *Technologies of the gendered body: Reading cyborg women.* Chapel Hill, NC: Duke University Press.

Bricking T. (1997, June 16). Internet blamed for neglect. *Cincinnati Enquirer.* Retrieved April 11, 2003 from http://enquirer.com/editions/1997/06/16/loc_hacker.html

Cassidy, M. F. (2001). Cyberspace meets domestic space: Personal computers, women's work, and the gendered territories of the family home. *Critical Studies in Media Communication, 18,* 44–65.

Cole, C. L. (1998). Addiction, exercise, and cyborgs: Technologies of deviant bodies. In G. Rail (Ed.), *Sport and postmodern time* (pp. 261–276). Albany: State University of New York Press.

A computer lesson in a party atmosphere. (1984, October). *Personal Computing,* pp. 65–66.

De Lauretis, T. (1987). *Technologies of gender: Essays on theory, film and fiction.* Bloomington: Indiana University Press.

Deleuze, G. (1992). Postscript on the societies of control. *October,* Winter, 3–7.

Derrida, J. (1993). The rhetoric of drugs. *differences: A Journal of Feminist Cultural Studies, 5*, 1–25.

Douglas, S. (1991). *Inventing American broadcasting.* Baltimore, MD: Johns Hopkins University Press.

Ehrenreich, B., & English, D. (1979). *For her own good: 150 years of doctors' advice to women.* New York: Doubleday.

Faflick, P. (1982, August 30). The real apple of his eye: How families come apart in the face of the micro invasion. *Time,* p. 80.

Figert, A. (1996). *Women and the ownership of PMS: The structuring of a psychiatric disorder.* London: de Gruyter.

Fischer, C. (1992). *America calling: A social history of the telephone to 1940.* Berkeley: University of California Press.

Foucault, M. (1972). *The archaeology of knowledge.* New York: Pantheon.

Foucault, M. (1978). *The history of sexuality. Vol. 1: An introduction.* New York: Random House.

Foucault, M. (1991). Politics and the study of discourse. In G. Burchell, C. Gordon, & P. Miller (Eds.), *The Foucault effect: Studies in governmentality.* Chicago: University of Chicago Press.

Garland, C. H. (1901, September). Insanity and telegraphists: A case for inquiry in the post office. *Westminster Review, 156,* 332–4.

Gilman, C. P. (1899/1973). *The yellow wallpaper.* New York: Feminist Press.

Grossberg, L. (1992). *We gotta get out of this place.* New York: Routledge.

Hait, P. (1983, September). How I learned to love my computer. *Ladies Home Journal,* p. 72.

Hollands, Jean. (1985). *Silicon syndrome: How to survive a high-tech relationship* New York: Bantam.

I couldn't learn to use a computer at work. (1987, June). *Good Housekeeping,* pp. 28+.

Joan, J., & Levine, J. A., et al. (1984). A family computer diary. In S. Ditlea (Ed.), *Digital deli* (pp. 117–120). New York: Workman.

Kirk, S. A., & Kutchins, H. (1992). *The selling of DSM: The rhetoric of science in psychiatry.* New York: de Gruyter.

Levine, J. A. (1983, July). A computer in the family. *Parents,* pp. 53–58.

Lewyn, M. (1990, January 15). PC makers, palms sweating, try talking to women. *BusinessWeek,* p. 48.

Lubar, S. (1992). *Infoculture: The Smithsonian book of the inventions of the information age.* Boston: Houghton Mifflin.

Marvin, C. (1988). *When old technologies were new.* New York: Oxford University Press.

Miller, Toby. (1996). *The well-tempered self.* Philadelphia: Temple University Press.

Nadeson, M. H. (1997, August). Constructing paper dolls: The discourse of personality testing in organizational practice. *Communication Theory, 7*(3), 189–218.

Nakamura, L. (1999). Race and/In cyberspace: Identity tourism on the Internet. Retrieved October 3, 2007 at: http://www.humanities.uci.edu/mposter/syllabi/readings/nakamura.html

Net-addicted mother loses custody of her children. (1997, October 23). *Champaign-Urbana News-Gazette,* pp. 25.

Olsen, G. (1982, April). A family computer album. *Saturday Evening Post,* pp. 70–77ff.

Rapping, E. (1996). *The culture of recovery: Making sense of the self-help movement in women's lives.* Boston: Beacon.

Reed, L (2000). Domesticating the personal computer: The mainstreaming of a new technology and the cultural management of a widespread technophobia. *Critical Studies in Media Communication, 17*(2), 159–185.

Reed, L (2002). Governing (through) the Internet: The discourse on pathological computer use as mobilized knowledge. *European Journal of Cultural Studies, 5*(2), 131–153.

Reid, R. (1995). Death of the family. In J. Halberstam & S. Livingstone (Eds.), *Post human bodies* (pp. 177–202). Bloomington: Indiana University Press.

Rose, N. (1999). *Governing the soul: The shaping of the private self* (2nd ed.). London: Free Association.

Rose, N. (1998). *Inventing ourselves: Psychology, power, and personhood.* New York: Cambridge University Press.

Schor, N., & Weed, E. (1993, Spring). Editor's note. In N. Schor & E. Weed (Eds.), *differences: A Journal of Feminist Cultural Studies, 5* , 1–3.

Sconce, J. (2000). *Haunted media: Electronic presence from telegraphy to television.* Chapel Hill, NC: Duke University Press.

Scott, S. (1982, January). My husband's computer was my competition. *Good Housekeeping,* pp. 14–15.

Sedgwick, E. K. (1992). Epidemics of the will. In J. Crary & S. Kwinter (Eds.), *Incorporations* (pp. 582–595). New York: Urzone.

Snodgrass, J. (1997). Net addiction may be like drugs or alcohol: Woman left husband for computer. *Cyberia Magazine.* Retrieved June 15, 2003, from http://magazine.cyberiacafe.net/issue6/news/news14.html

Spigel, L. (1992). *Make room for TV: Television and the family ideal in postwar America.* Chicago: University of Chicago Press.

Stone, A. R. (1996). *The war of desire and technology at the close of the mechanical age.* Cambridge, MA: MIT Press.

Umiker-Sebeok, J. (2001). The semiotic swarm of cyberspace: Cybergluttony and Internet addiction in the global village. Retrieved October 20, 2005, from http://www.slis.indiana.edu/faculty/umikerse/papers/cgsec1.html

Van Dusen, J. (1983, September 26). The computer widows. *Maclean's,* p. 57.

Van Gelder, L. (1983, February). Falling in love with your computer. *Ms.,* pp. 36–40.

Van Gelder, L. (1985, January). Help for technophobes: Think of your computer as just another appliance. *Ms.,* pp. 89–91.

Wilkins, M. E. (1931, November). Women, radio and the home. *Canadian Magazine,* pp. 32–33.

Wollman, J. (1984, April). The plugged in family. *Working Woman,* pp. 129–133.

Young, K. S. (1996a, August). *Internet addiction: The emergence of a new clinical disorder.* Paper presented to the American Psychological Association, Toronto, Canada.

Young, K. S. (1996b). Psychology of computer use: xl. Addictive use of the Internet: A case that breaks the stereotype. *Psychological Reports, 79,* 899–902.

Young, K. S.. (1998). *Caught in the Net: How to recognize and recover from Internet addiction.* New York: Wiley.

PART II

Privatization and
the Body Proper-ty

4

Pink Ribbons Inc.

The Emergence of Cause-Related Marketing and the Corporatization of the Breast Cancer Movement

SAMANTHA KING

Queen's University

It was very important for me, after my mastectomy, to develop and encourage my own internal sense of power. I needed to rally my energies in such a way as to image myself as a fighter resisting rather than as a passive victim suffering. At all times, it felt crucial to me that I make a conscious commitment to survival. It is physically important for me to be loving my life rather than to be mourning my breast. I believe that this love of my life and my self, and the careful tending of that love by women who love and support me, which has been largely responsible for my strong and healthy recovery from the effects of mastectomy. A clear distinction must be made, however, between this affirmation of self and the superficial farce of "looking on the bright side of things."

Like superficial spirituality, looking on the bright side of things is a euphemism used for obscuring certain realities of life, the open consideration of which might prove threatening or dangerous to the status quo.

—Lorde, 1980, p. 74

If I had to do it over, would I want breast cancer? Absolutely. I'm not the same person I was, and I'm glad I'm not. Money doesn't matter anymore. I've met the most phenomenal people in my life through this. Your friends and family are what matter now,

—Cherry, cited in Ehrenreich, 2001

IN THE CONTEXT OF A HISTORICAL MOMENT in which breast cancer is widely understood as an enriching experience of the sort Cindy Cherry described, Audre Lorde's words, penned on the March 30, 1979, and subsequently published in the *Cancer Journals* (1980), seem startlingly prophetic. Of course Lorde was not writing in a social vacuum, but out of her experiences as a postmastectomy woman and in response to several issues that emerged as she integrated the breast cancer crisis into her life: the invisibility and silence of women with the disease, prosthesis, amputation, the cancer-industrial complex, the relation between cancer activism and antiracism, heteronormativity, and her confrontation with mortality. Her purpose was to encourage women to interrogate and speak out about the meaning of cancer in their lives—"for silence," she wrote, "has never brought us anything of worth" (p. 10)—and to use their experiences to work for change. In the above-quoted passage, Lorde's specific concern was with the blame-the-victim mentality of the breast cancer establishment, exemplified by a doctor who had written a letter to a medical journal declaring that no truly happy person ever gets cancer.

So how did we get from a national mind-set in which breast cancer was viewed as a self-induced stigmatized disease and individual tragedy best dealt with privately and in isolation, to one in which breast cancer is viewed as an enriching and affirming experience during which women with breast cancer are never "patients," but always survivors? What were the historical conditions that once allowed a doctor to declare that the truly happy never get cancer, and what are the conditions that now enable us to think of breast cancer as a route to true happiness? And what have the effects of this shift been in terms of the ways in which breast cancer is understood and responded to?

These questions have been answered in part by a recent proliferation of academic and popular writing on the emergence of breast cancer activism in the United States. Taken as a whole, this writing recognizes that a conjuncture of factors enabled the materialization of breast cancer activism and the transformation of the U.S. public's attitude toward the disease: The women's health movement (Brenner, 2000; Ehrenreich, 2001; Leopold, 1999a, which formed in the late 1960s, created an environment in which women were encouraged to question their doctors and the patriarchal practices and structures of the medical-industrial complex, and to practice self-help and mutual support. During the same period, the decision of several famous women—most notably Shirley Temple Black (in 1972), Betty Ford (1974), and Happy Rockefeller (1974)—to speak publicly about their breast cancer diagnoses was crucial to the process of destigmatization (Altman, 1996; Ehrenreich, 2001; Leopold, 1999a Lerner 2001).[1] The 1975 publication of Rose Kushner's *Breast Cancer: A Personal History and Investigative Report*, in which she criticized the practice of performing one-step mastectomies without the consent of the patient, is also widely acknowledged as a turning point in the history of the disease (Brenner, 2000; Ehrenreich, 2001; Klawiter, 2000; Lerner 2001). Kushner's exposé prompted a decade of nationwide campaigning for informed consent legislation at the state level, and as activist and advocacy groups sprung up around the country, a national movement began to emerge.

Through a variety of research techniques (journalistic and academic) and disciplinary foci, authors such as Roberta Altman (1996), Sharon Batt (1994), Barbara Brenner (2000), Maren Klawiter (2000), Ellen Leopold (1999a, Barron Lerner (2001), Alisa Solomon (1992), and Carole Stabiner (1997) trace the consolidation of this movement into an effective political force. These authors view the founding of the National Alliance of Breast Cancer Organizations (NABCO) in 1986 and the creation of the National Breast Cancer Coalition (NBCC) five years later as central to this process.[2] As a result of NBCC campaigning, in particular, federal government funding for breast cancer has increased dramatically (from $40 million in 1981, to $407 million in 1993, to $605 million in 2005), and breast cancer activists now enjoy a more active role in research funding decision processes and in research agenda setting.

Maren Klawiter (2000) offers one of the most compelling accounts of this history, making visible the connections between changes in the medical management of breast cancer, the destigmatization of the disease, and the growth of activism. She shows how a multiplication of treatment regimens, a proliferation of support groups, and the expansion of screening into asymptomatic populations during the 1980s and 1990s helped produce new social spaces, solidarities, and sensibilities among breast cancer survivors and activists. In other words, changes in the treatment of women by the medical profession—changes preceded by fledgling activism—opened up numerous spaces in which women could talk openly about their experiences of the disease with one another, thus enabling the emergence of a multifaceted breast cancer movement.

This chapter builds on these analyses by tracing the materialization of the "breast cancer survivor" as a category of identification by focusing in particular on a hitherto neglected but absolutely central force in the emergence of the breast cancer movement: the role of corporate philanthropy.[3] More specifically, it explores how breast cancer-directed corporate philanthropy has shaped the emergence of the breast cancer survivor as a category of identification and the effects of this configuration on the ways that the "problem of breast cancer" is understood and responded to.

The absence of analyses of the role of philanthropy in literature on the breast cancer movement can be explained in part by an understandable commitment on the part of breast cancer scholars to focus on the resistive strategies of grassroots activism and to chart substantive changes in the funding and regulation of breast cancer research, screening, and treatment. So while most researchers have included fund-raising organizations such as the Susan G. Komen Breast Cancer Foundation in their accounts of breast cancer activism and have often been critical of the mainstream and corporate-friendly politics of such organizations (Batt, 1994; Brenner, 2000), they have not tended to explore how the discourses and practices of individual and corporate philanthropy per se have functioned in terms of the movement's public profile and persuasive power.

A complete picture would thus acknowledge that breast cancer foundations, nonprofit organizations, and fund-raising events have proliferated in the last two decades; that breast cancer research is a—if not the—favorite charitable cause for corporations seeking to attract female consumers through cause-related marketing campaigns; and that philanthropic approaches to the disease have even become part of federal and state health policy (through the introduction of the breast cancer fund-raising stamp and breast cancer research tax check offs, for example). It would also recognize that organizations such as the Susan G. Komen Breast Cancer Foundation (the world's largest nonprofit funder of breast cancer research) have played a central role in breast cancer policy making; raised millions of dollars for research; and offered what are among the most visible and accessible modes of breast cancer activism—in the case of the Komen Foundation, the Race for the Cure and numerous cause-related marketing campaigns[4]—currently in circulation. Indeed, although the conceptualization of breast cancer as a political issue has not dropped out of public circulation in the same way that residual discourses of stigmatization have not been entirely displaced, in popular discourse the fight against the disease is now constituted predominantly as a fight that does—and should—take place on the terrain of science and medicine funded through corporate philanthropy. An analysis of breast cancer-directed corporate philanthropy—and of the Race for the Cure and breast cancer–related marketing in particular—is thus crucial to a fuller understanding of the cultural appeal of breast cancer as an issue for public concern in the present moment and to identifying those "realities of life" or threats to the status quo that are obscured by the widespread determination to look only on the bright side of the disease (Lorde, 1980, p. 75).

Foucault, Philanthropy, and Governmentality

The pages that follow explore the popular appeal of breast cancer-directed corporate philanthropy by examining not so much why it has gained such appeal, but how this appeal is constituted, deployed, and understood by those who create and participate in it. Although my analysis is concerned with the popularity of events such as the Race for the Cure and practices such as cause-related marketing, it does not proceed from the assumption that these phenomena simply attract the participation of fully formed subjects and citizens. Rather, in their capacity as fund-raising ventures; marketing enterprises, practices and sites of consumption; physical activities; collective experiences; mass movements; and pedagogical tools, they are technologies of power, or a set of practices and discourses, that have constitutive effects (Foucault, 1979, 1980). Drawing on the work of Michel Foucault (1991), and contemporary theorists of governmentality such as Nikolas Rose (1999), I conceptualize these technologies as mechanisms of governance that help shape identities (e.g., "the breast cancer survivor"), cultivate political subjects (e.g., "the volunteer citizen"), and produce knowledges and truths about breast cancer and how best it might be responded to. Thus, through the course of my investigations, I explore the productive functions and effects of breast cancer philanthropy and examine its articulation to broader questions about the character of contemporary U.S. culture and citizenship.

By analyzing these technologies of power in a broader context, my aim is to highlight the ways in which government, or the conduct of conduct, has in the past two decades become centrally concerned with the production of civically active, self-responsible citizens. While citizenship responsibilities in this configuration are most frequently enacted through consumption, the ideal citizen is not, to quote Nikolas Rose (1999), "the isolated and selfish atom of the free market" (p. 166). Instead, in the contemporary organization of political responsibility, subjects are addressed and understood as individuals who are responsible for themselves and for others in their "community." Ideally, responsibility is not to be demonstrated by paying taxes to support social welfare programs or by expressing dissent and making political demands on behalf of one's fellow citizens. Instead, in the words of former President Bill Clinton, Americans must be taught that "to be a good citizen, in addition to going to work and going to school and paying your taxes and obeying the law, you have to be involved in community service" (Hall & Nichols, 1997, p. A12).

Thus, from former President Ronald Reagan's 1981 Task Force on Private Sector Initiatives, established to develop, support, and promote private sector leadership in community development and social service, to former President George H. W. Bush's Points of Light initiative, to Bill Clinton's 1997 Summit on America's Future held to solicit individual and corporate generosity as a "complement" to welfare reform legislation, to former President George W. Bush's faith-based initiatives, four successive federal administrations have sought to establish the organizational and subjective conditions through which to reshape relations between the state and the individual. They have done this not simply by rolling back the public welfare system with the hope that the charitable impulses of citizens and corporations will flourish, but by helping to create techniques, strategies, and programs—frequently in partnership with nonprofit or business entities—aimed at producing volunteer and philanthropist citizens.

Despite the association between volunteerism and freedom in U.S. culture and the pervasive view that the social state has stifled the innate generosity of the American people, the turn toward volunteerism and philanthropy does not mark a radical turn away either from government or from the role of the state in governing as the rhetoric of those who celebrate the "end of big government" suggests. Rather, it marks a shift toward a different form of governing and the emergence of an alternatively constituted state. In this context, this chapter highlights how government, or the "conduct of conduct" to use Foucault's formulation, is dispersed throughout the social body, rather than resting solely or even primarily with the state. This is not to trivialize the role of the state in governing, particularly in a conjuncture that has seen an "intensification, acceleration, and integration of governing strategies under a state of emergency, or permanent war" (Bratich, Packer, & McCarthy, 2003, p. 17), but rather to show how functions that we might traditionally associate with the state, or connections between the governor and the governed, occur at innumerable decentered, dispersed, and often private or commercial sites within the social body. The turn to volunteerism and philanthropy can thus be read as an effect of the desire to "govern at a distance" that theorists such as Nikolas Rose (1996) have identified as a central characteristic of neoliberal thought. Institutions, programs, and techniques designed to encourage volunteerism and philanthropy, for example, are mechanisms of governance that have varying degrees of autonomization from the state. Nonetheless, these networks and techniques are frequently established through alliances with the state, and, even when operating in deeply privatized settings (a National Football League advertising campaign, for example) often work to "elaborate core state interests" (Bratich et al., 2003).

Although my chapter is indebted to Foucauldian explanations of the neoliberal transformation of society (Burchell, Gordon, & Miller, 1991; Cruikshank, 1999; Rose, 1999), it also seeks to go beyond the rather totalizing accounts of this transformation that, in Larry Grossberg's words, constitute neoliberalism as "too much of an intentionalist project, and too much of a singular model" (Packer, 2003, p. 33). By focusing on the explosion of breast cancer-directed philanthropic activity as an articulation of a quite disparate and messy set of forces, this chapter shows how neoliberal thought is concretized in specific practices, and how practices that are engaged in without particular political intention can end up reinforcing or, sometimes, threatening the neoliberal formation. Building on the argument Bratich, Packer, and McCarthy (2003) made in their introduction to *Foucault, Governmentality, and Cultural Studies*, then, the chapter shows how breast cancer culture finds itself caught up in the processes of regulating conduct without a necessary reliance on the "codified, institutionalized" forms of governance. Moreover, by highlighting the ways in which neoliberal governmentality is implicitly racialized and gendered, such that participation in consumer-oriented philanthropic activity represents a yardstick against which the capacities of individuals to become "proper" Americans is measured, it brings into question what are rather universalizing accounts of neoliberal arts and rationalities of governing and the processes of subjectification that they enable.

The Emergence of Survivor Culture

Like all identity formations, the "breast cancer survivor" did not emerge from an easily traceable, singular point of origin. Rather, it arose out of a conjuncture of relatively autonomous, yet mutually implicated, social forces that gained strength in the last two decades of the twentieth century. Among the most significant of these forces was a concerted challenge to the traditionally hierarchical relations that defined interactions between medical researchers, doctors, and patients.

In the 1950s, writes Paul Starr (1982), "medical science epitomized the post-war vision of progress without conflict" (p. 336). But in the decades that followed, a variety of groups and interests emerged to challenge this model. Alongside the efforts of the women's health movement, leftists mounted a critique of the profit-driven medical-industrial complex, which they argued worked to benefit large corporations and shareholders rather than patients; liberals and conservatives began to question burgeoning health-care costs; and revelations of ethical abuses in clinical trials and other forms of medical experimentation led to campaigns for informed consent legislation (Epstein, 1998). From these forces emerged a greater skepticism of medical experts and a shift away from established notions of the "proper" medical patient as passive, unquestioning, and deferential.

The AIDS movement that took shape in the 1980s, however, really revolutionized the possibilities for disease activism in the United States. Rather than acting as what Steven Epstein (1998) calls a "disease constituency," which primarily functions to pressure the government for more funding, the AIDS movement became an alternative basis for expertise. In contrast to other models by which they could have positioned themselves in relation to medical science, AIDS activists did not reject science or seek to show that science and truth were on their side, but rather staked "out some ground on the scientists' own terrain" (p. 13). In other words, they fought AIDS both from outside and within medical science, as they questioned the uses, controls, content, and processes of scientific practice, they also claimed "to speak credibly as experts in their own right" (p. 13). As such, according to Epstein, it became the first social movement to actually undertake the transformation of "disease victims" into "activist-experts."

The efforts of activists to be involved participants in AIDS research and policy were inextricably intertwined with their struggle to eschew the widely held understanding of people with AIDS as "victims" of disease. Activists rejected this label arguing that it elicited fear and pity, suggested inevitable death, allowed "spectators" to distance themselves from those with the disease and thus remain passive, and connoted some character flaw or bad "lifestyle choice" that had invited the tragedy to befall them (Navarre, 1988; Zita Grover, 1987). Moreover, Max Navarre described how the fear and hopelessness that stem from constant reminders that "you are helpless, there is no hope for you" easily lead to despair (p. 143). Navarre and others aimed to enable people with AIDS to understand themselves—and for others to in turn understand them—not as the condition but as people with a condition. Self-empowerment, he and others believed, breeds hope, and "hope is one of the greatest healers" (p. 144). On the basis of such beliefs, in 1983 the National Association for People With AIDS adopted the Denver principles that declared that people with AIDS had the right and responsibility actively to determine their own experience with the syndrome. The opening declaration of the principles reads as follows, "We condemn attempts to label us as victims, which implies defeat, and we are only occasionally 'patients,' which implies passivity, helplessness,

and dependence on the care of others. We are 'people with AIDS'"
(Navarre, 1988, p. 148).

The recognition that identity categories—the means through which
people with disease are labeled and categorized—could significantly
shape the course of a disease and society's response to it has had
profound implications for the formation and strategies of health activist
movements in the wake of the AIDS epidemic. Through processes of
what social movement scholars call "social movement spillover"—when
new movements grow from the foundations of existing movements and
borrow from their strengths and strategies—the health activist groups
that emerged in the 1980s and 1990s, while diverse in their agendas and
strategies, shared a sense of the importance of disease identity categories
that suggested live, active, and empowered individuals. Among cancer
activists, this recognition was evidenced by the gradual disappearance of
the label "cancer victim" (and to a slightly less extent, "cancer patient")
from public discourse and its replacement with the "cancer survivor."

This shift was given institutional legitimacy and form in 1986
with the formation of the National Coalition for Cancer Survivorship
(NCCS). Their organization was the first, the NCCS claims, to define
an individual diagnosed with cancer as a survivor from "the moment
of diagnosis and for the balance of life." Since that time, NCCS has
been a leading force in advocating for "survivor's rights" by lobbying
for increased funding for cancer research and access to quality cancer
care and sponsoring educational publications and programming. The
founding of the NCCS was followed by the formation of other cancer
survivorship organizations (the American Cancer Society's Cancer
Survivors Network, for example) and a move on the part of existing
organizations to place survivorship at the center of their missions and
at the heart of their public relations activities. While in some cases a
professed interest in "survivorship" was just another term for commitment to research on prevention, treatment, and cure, in other cases
"survivorship" came to represent a new realm of scientific concern, a
hitherto neglected phase of the experience of cancer. An April 6, 1998,
Dallas Morning News article explained the development as follows, "As
many as 10 million Americans call themselves cancer survivors. Yet
until recently, their well-being has been largely unexplored by most
doctors and medical researchers" (Beil, 1998, p. 7D). As a result, the
cancer survivor became—or rather was constituted as—a subject of
scientific investigation and several leading cancer organizations insti-
tuted programs to encourage the study of the physical and mental
well being of people who had lived through the disease. In 1996, the
National Cancer Institute created the Office of Cancer Survivorship

to encourage the study of the "growing number of cancer veterans."
In 1998, the American Cancer Society and the Komen Foundation
followed their lead with the launch of similar efforts.

This short history offers an indication of the extent to which the
empowered patient—the activist-expert, the survivor—has become
institutionalized and incorporated into the fabric of the cancer establishment. This is nowhere more clear than in the case of breast cancer.
The movement remains extraordinarily diverse, with support groups,
grassroots collectives, charities, national lobbying organizations, corporations, and federal agencies working both in alliance and independently
to shape the course of the disease. But breast cancer groups that embrace
patient-empowerment as a way to mobilize critical engagement with
biomedical research, anger at governmental inaction, and resistance
to social discrimination—Breast Cancer Action in San Francisco, for
instance, or the Women's Community Cancer Project in Cambridge,
Massachusetts—are marginalized in mainstream discourse on the
disease. Instead, and as the two case studies that follow show, the version
of the breast cancer survivor that prevails in the national imaginary
is used to mobilize fund-raising for high-stakes, cure-driven scientific
research on the disease; to validate—usually without questioning—scientific authority and expertise; and to market an ever-increasing number
of goods to consumers eager to play their part in the fight against the
disease. The Susan G. Komen Breast Cancer Foundation's Race for the
Cure has been a central actor in the development of this particular
configuration of the breast cancer survivor—a configuration that relies
on and in turn reproduces an unbridled optimism about life with and
beyond the disease and, concurrently, an obstinate refusal to question
the status quo.

The Race for the Cure

Seven hundred women took part in the first Susan G. Komen Breast
Cancer Foundation Race for the Cure in Dallas, Texas, in October 1983.[5]
By 1999 the race was the nation's largest 5K series with events in 99
cities across the United States. Between 1988 and 1999, participation
in the series increased tenfold to nearly 600,000, grew by 44% between
1997 and 1998 alone, and reached 1.4 million in 2005. The National
Race for the Cure, held in Washington, DC, each June, is now the biggest
5K run in the world. In addition to the numbers who participate, the
appeal of the Race for the Cure is apparent in its capacity to attract
high-profile corporate sponsors, as well as the support and attendance
of politicians and celebrities at events across the United States.[6]

The stated purpose of the race is to raise money for breast cancer research, screening, and education (the series raised in excess of $72 million in 2004) and to promote breast cancer awareness, particularly early detection. In the Komen Foundation's publicity materials and in mass media discourse, the race is also configured as a mass-participation, authentically grassroots social movement that has succeeded in revolutionizing attitudes toward breast cancer and catapulting breast cancer to the top of the national medical science research agenda.

On June 6, 1999, I traveled to Washington, DC, to attend the 10th Anniversary National Race for the Cure. Already the world's largest 5K event, the 1999 race registered 65,000 runners and broke its own record for participation (52,000) set the previous year. Women with breast cancer and their colleagues, friends, and families traveled from all over the United States to take part, along with thousands of local residents from Maryland, Virginia, and Washington, DC, itself. As with other Races for the Cure across the United States, many participants entered as members of sororities and fraternities or as employees running on corporate, government, diplomatic community, and volunteer teams.[7]

While the race itself took runners through the streets of the nation's capital, the rally site was on the grounds of the Washington Monument, around which a huge area of grass and footpaths had been cordoned off. Immediately alongside the monument stood a 150 foot-tall, bright pink, looped ribbon—the now-ubiquitous representation of breast cancer charity and awareness in the United States. The rally stage was situated immediately in front of the Washington Monument; its backdrop consisted of three enormous black and white panels adorned with the names of the race's numerous corporate sponsors.[8]

The day's events began at 6:30 A.M. with the Sunrise Survivor Celebration. The recognition of breast cancer survivors is a central theme in Races for the Cure across the country. At each event a time is set aside in the program for a breast cancer survivors' ceremony and for many women it is the highlight of their day. The response of Nancy Statchen, a two-and-a-half-year survivor, is typical:

The whole experience was so inspiring to me, the survivors, their strength and vitality. . . . A year and a half after diagnosis, this event was the first time that I openly proclaimed my membership in this club. And how proud I am—women, all these incredible women. After being confronted with this demon, carrying on, stronger than ever, committed to helping join the cause. (Stachen, 1998)

At the National Race for the Cure, thousands of participants lined up and filed slowly into the survivors' tent—its entrance marked by a metal archway festooned with bright pink balloons—to enjoy a "survivors' breakfast" from the various corporate sponsors. The breakfast was followed, at 7:30 A.M., by the 10-Star Salute to Survivors' Parade (a feature that is common to all Race for the Cure events) and the prerace rally.

Led by Komen Foundation founder Nancy Brinker, thousands of breast cancer survivors (all sporting bright pink visors and t-shirts to distinguish themselves from other participants) marched down from the tent toward the main stage. Clapping and dancing to the words and music of Gloria Gaynor's "I Will Survive," they moved along a pathway lined on either side by a cheering crowd of thousands, and the National Mall was transformed into an immense sea of pink and white. As the music grew louder and the clapping more vigorous, this group of predominantly middle-aged White women took their place on the stage, their arms outstretched in the air, waving in time with the music.

Following a mass recital of the Pledge of Allegiance, Priscilla Mack, co-chair of the race, introduced the survivors to the crowd, "I am very proud to be surrounded by a sea of faith. Each survivor has to dig down deep and fight for her life. We applaud you and we stand behind you." Mack then proceeded to ask women who had survived breast cancer for 30 years or more to wave their hands and "be recognized." A handful of women raised their hands. As she counted down through the years until she reached one, the hands increased in number.

Standing close to the stage, I could not help but recall Audre Lorde's (1980) well-known entry in the *Cancer Journals* when she points to "socially sanctioned prosthesis" as "another way of keeping women with breast cancer silent and separate from each other" (p. 16). Lorde then asks, "What would happen if an army of one-breasted women descended upon Congress and demanded that the use of carcinogenic, fat-stored hormones in beef-feed be outlawed?" (p. 16). Here was an army of postmastectomy/lumpectomy women, assembled in the nation's capital, but surely not in a way that Lorde imagined.

This was an intensely moving moment, both for the survivors on the stage and the crowds on the mall, many of whom wore signs on their backs with the names of loved ones who had survived or died from breast cancer. For some women on the stage it was the first time that they had publicly declared their identity as breast cancer survivors (one of my interviewees told me that it had taken her two years to pluck up the courage to attend the race as a survivor). For others, the race marked the first time that they went without a wig in public. Moreover, these women were far from silent and stood as a powerful symbol of the sheer number of people affected by the disease, as well as the possibility of triumph over illness. Proud, vibrant, hopeful, and passionate, clad in brightly colored athletic apparel, and participating in vigorous physical activity to raise money for a worthy cause, these survivors seemed far removed from the alienated women with cancer of whom Lorde wrote so eloquently. Their self-presentation also contrasted starkly with the weak, pale, bed-ridden, cancer "victim" that had in prior decades stood as the dominant embodiment of the disease.

But, as commentators on the AIDS epidemic have argued, the deployment of positive images of disease raises complex political questions. While, as we have noted, AIDS activists recognized early on the importance of challenging the hegemony of pessimistic, often hateful, images of people with AIDS and the pervasive rhetoric of the "AIDS victim," it was also the case that overly bright and hopeful configurations of the disease and of survivorship had the capacity to both undermine demands that the syndrome be taken seriously and dissipate the rage of activists that was so crucial to sustaining the AIDS movement. The highly orchestrated survivor celebrations that are so central to the mission and appeal of the Race for the Cure highlight the individual strength, courage, and perseverance of women with breast cancer and offer an important source of hope and (albeit temporary) community, but they leave little room for the politically targeted anger that Lorde envisioned. The resulting rhetoric is so upbeat and so optimistic that one could deduce from these events that breast cancer is a fully curable disease from which people no longer die.

Indeed, anger or dissent of any kind were stark in their absence at the national Race for the Cure. During the pre- and postrace rallies the crowd heard various speeches from local celebrities, corporate executives (pharmaceutical companies that sell cancer products were particularly prominent), Komen Foundation members, and Al and Tipper Gore. We were also introduced to Secretary of State Madeleine Albright and numerous members of Congress, both Republicans and Democrats. The content of these speeches was overwhelmingly optimistic and focused predominantly on celebrating survivors and reiterating the importance of cure-oriented science underwritten by corporate support and generous individuals. Nancy Brinker's hope-filled words were typical:

> Today is a defining moment in the breast cancer movement, because we are making progress. Twenty years ago, when my sister Susan Komen asked me to do something to cure this disease, we couldn't

even imagine a day like today. Sixty-five thousand people turning out in our nation's capital to once again race, run, walk, and pray for the cure. It is coming! It is coming!

A representative from Bristol Myers Squibb Oncology emphasized the corporation's commitment to the cause and its faith in cure-oriented science, "We have come together to form a team to Race for the Cure. Bristol Myers Squibb continues to believe that by working as a team to raise awareness and fund research, a cure for this disease can and will be found." To a cheering crowd, the volunteer coordinator for the Komen Foundation declared, "When you think volunteerism, you think reach out and touch someone, and I just love that model. That model is the corporate logo of AT&T and they're a national leader in volunteerism." And executive co-chair of the race, Priscilla Mack, made this explicit when she declared, "With sponsors like these, we will find a cure!"

Not surprisingly, no questions were asked about—nor even any mention of—persistently high rates of breast cancer in the United States or elsewhere. Although the participation of thousands of survivors should be indicative of these rates, their presence was celebrated as evidence of the promise of individual struggle against the disease rather than of a social or medical crisis that kills 40,000 women each year in the United States alone. Survivors, in other words, stood as symbols of hope for the future, rather than of urgency in the present. Differences of age, race, and class in mortality rates—for example, the fact that although breast cancer mortality rates dropped slightly among all women in the 1990s, rates among Black women continue to rise—were also ignored or subsumed under the banner of the "survivor." Moreover, no demands for action—beyond calls for continued participation in the Race for the Cure—were made of the various representatives of the cancer industries or the state, nor indeed of participants in the race.

One could argue, of course, that the Race for the Cure is designed to raise money (more than $2 million in this instance) and celebrate survivorship, not to provide a platform for the expression of dissent as Audre Lorde had envisioned. One could also argue that the United States needs such celebratory and harmonious public gatherings. But doing so would be to ignore the implication of the race in a broader war of position over what constitutes "the problem of breast cancer" in the present moment and over what kinds of actions and identities are legitimate or effective in bringing about social change.

Placing the Race for the Cure in the context of the history of cancer in the United States is helpful here. Faith in the power of positive thinking, the promotion of research into finding a cure for cancer (instead of research focused on prevention), and the belief that large infusions of money into research can conquer anything have been remarkably durable features of the various manifestations of the alliance against cancer in the twentieth century (Patterson, 1987). The Komen Foundation's emphasis on finding a cure certainly articulates the race to the national prestige bound up with the fight against cancer in a way that a focus on prevention—and all that it connotes—does not. That is, the search for a "magic bullet" (a specific treatment that will root out and destroy cancerous cells for good) channels research questions and public attention toward individual pathology or deviation from a biological norm and away from social conditions, environmental factors, and other "external" variables that might serve to threaten the nation's image of itself.[9]

The focus on finding a cure for breast cancer, rather than on prevention, has been subject to critique from numerous scientists and breast cancer activists (see Batt, 1994; Brady, 1991; Solomon, 1992). Many of these critics also express doubt about the usefulness of mammograms—encouraging early detection via mammogram is the central focus of the Komen Foundation's "awareness" efforts—in the fight against cancer and point out, among other things, that even under optimal conditions, mammograms can miss up to 15% of tumors. They also argue that mammograms are not preventative but detective technologies and that the widespread promotion of mammograms as preventative is deceptive and even dangerous (some scientists-activists argue that too many mammograms can actually cause cancer). Furthermore, although early detection is touted by the breast cancer-industrial complex as increasing survival rates, many scientists and activists have argued that although mammograms might detect tumors earlier, they do not necessarily improve the survival of patients, but rather extend the amount of time in which women bear knowledge of their condition. In other words, they have very little impact on overall breast cancer mortality.

Because of its focus on early detection and cure-oriented science, the Komen Foundation has won generous sponsorship from pharmaceutical companies such as Zeneca and Bristol Myers Squibb, and mammography equipment and film manufacturers DuPont and Kodak. But the foundation also relies on the work of pharmaceutical and screening researchers to keep donations coming in, just as these corporation depend on the Komen Foundation to do public relations work for them—without constant promises that a cure is in sight the public would probably not maintain faith in these strains of research or keep giving to the Komen Foundation.

The optimism of the survivor celebrations, the focus on cure-oriented science, and the fund-raising goals of the Race for the Cure are thus mutually reinforcing. One 51-year-old Army officer and breast cancer survivor made this link explicit when she said of the race:

> It gives people a way to actively show their support to find a cure. When a person just donates money through the mail, they [sic] are unable to "touch" the results of their [sic] contribution. With the race, the supporters can be right there with the survivors who represent the positive aspects of their support through contributions. They can see the result of the research and new drugs—mothers, grandmothers and daughters who are still alive to share memories with their families. (Personal correspondence)

Barbara Ehrenreich (2001) offers a more critical perspective on the same set of links and warns against the dangers of this approach:

> In the overwhelmingly Darwinian culture that has grown up around breast cancer, martyrs count for little; it is the "survivors" who merit constant honor and acclaim. They, after all, offer living proof that expensive and painful treatments may in some cases actually work. (p. 48)

And of course in some cases they do work. But the voices of the chorus with faith in cure-oriented science—underwritten by the logic that "tidal waves" of money allocated to such research will simply overwhelm the disease (Leopold, 1999b, p. A19)—are growing ever louder. And in this context, recognizing that all might not be so well in the world of cancer becomes much harder as does asking questions that might reshape and redirect dominant approaches to fighting the disease.

Breast Cancer-Related Marketing

While the figure of the healthy, vibrant, honorable breast cancer survivor functions to maintain interest in and philanthropic support for cure-oriented science, it has also been widely deployed in the past decade as a marketing tool through which to sell (mostly) women concerned about the disease an enormous range of consumer items. An increasingly competitive domestic marketplace in the past two decades has seen U.S. corporations focus their attention on retaining, rather than creating, consumer loyalty for established brands. The emergence and widespread use of cause-related marketing exemplifies this concern and few causes have been taken up so widely, or with so much success, as breast cancer.

Over the past 10 years, upbeat and optimistic breast cancer campaigns have become a central and integral part of the marketing strategy of numerous corporations: American Airlines, Avon, Bally's Total Fitness, BMW, Bristol Myers Squibb, Charles Swab, Chili's, Estée Lauder, Ford Motor Company, General Electric, General Motors, Hallmark, J. C. Penney, Kellogg's, Lee Jeans, National Football League, Pier One, Saks Fifth Avenue, Titleist, and Yoplait, among others, have turned to breast cancer philanthropy as a new and profitable strategy through which to market their products. Moreover, the nonprofit and advocacy groups with which they have most frequently aligned themselves—the now-defunct National Alliance of Breast Cancer Organizations and the Susan G. Komen Breast Cancer Foundation—are two of the largest, most high-profile arms of the U.S. breast cancer movement.

In fact, the Komen Foundation is recognized as something of a pioneer of cause-related marketing. In an oft-recited story, Nancy Brinker, founder of the Susan G. Komen Breast Cancer Foundation, tells how she approached an executive of a lingerie manufacturer to suggest that they include a tag in their bras reminding customers to get regular mammograms. In response, the executive told Brinker, "We sell glamour. We don't sell fear. Breast cancer has nothing to do with our customers" (Davidson, 1997, p. 36). The success of the Komen Foundation in persuading businesses that breast cancer does have something to do with their customers and that an affiliation with the disease might actually encourage customers to buy their products is illustrated by subsequent events.

Nancy Brinker is now recognized as the leading expert in cause-related marketing and the Komen Foundation has more than a dozen national sponsors, a Million Dollar Council comprised of businesses that donate at least $1 million per year, and a slew of other corporate partnerships at both the local and national levels (Davidson, 1997). They even have a contract with a lingerie company—Walcoal—to manufacture an "awareness bra."[10]

In April 1999 the National Football League (NFL) became the latest corporation to sign on as a national sponsor of the Komen Foundation's Race for the Cure.[11] This arrangement—which partners a professional sports league that is the epitome of American hypermasculinity with a nonprofit group that is the epitome of pink-ribbon hyperfemininity—brought with it an immediate guarantee of differentiation and recognition. The announcement of the new partnership coincided with

an ongoing effort on the part of the NFL to show, in the words of
Detroit News writer Becky Yerak (2000), "That it's in touch with its feminine side" (p. B1). Yerak continues, "New advertising and marketing
campaigns by the National Football League . . . have begun muting
the usual machismo and shaping pitches more to women, children and
even men who aren't necessarily hardcore fans of the weekend showcase
or alpha males" (p. B1). This new approach to marketing was created,
in part, in response to a survey that found 40% of the NFL's weekly
television viewers are women and, of those 45 million, "20 million call
themselves avid fans" (p. B1). Hoping to maintain this market and to
capture the interest of new fans, the NFL turned to breast cancer and
the cultivation of a compassionate, yet strong, masculinity.

In a news release announcing the deal, Nancy Brinker and Sara
Levinson of the NFL described their new partnership as an opportunity
to spread the message of early detection to the NFL's huge fan base,
which includes more than 68 million women ("NFL sponsors," 1999,
p. 21). Situating the promotion of mammography at the center of the
campaign and pointing to the promise of this new alliance against
cancer, Brinker said of the deal:

> We are thrilled to have an organization like the NFL as a national
> sponsor of Race for the Cure. This partnership will allow us to spread
> the life saving message of early detection to millions of professional
> football fans, both women and men. With the support of NFL teams,
> players and fans, we can win the race against breast cancer. (p. 21)

The deal included a promise by the NFL to enhance marketing and
"grassroots" support of the Komen Race for the Cure events. Grassroots
activities were to include appearances by players and their families at
race events, national television advertising, breast cancer detection
information affixed to all "NFL for Her" merchandise, and race sign-ups
at NFL Workshops for Women (p. 21).

DeAnn Forbes, owner of a women-owned advertising agency that has
a contract with the Detroit Lions, explained the NFL's new approach
as follows:

> People are tired of seeing a guy in a uniform and another guy in a
> uniform. Human interest is what'll bring a broader audience. . . .
> Whether it's the average fan or novice, they want to know what drives
> these players. The only way you can really feel connected is to see
> them, hear them, know them. (Yerak, 2000, p. B3)

Thus, the NFL's campaign is designed to stimulate what is understood as the peculiarly female desire for human interest and personal interaction. Of course, as this discourse constitutes women—in contrast to men—as more emotional and more in need of such interaction, it also helps solidify historically embedded links between women, nurturing, and benevolence.

Beginning in October 1999, and to coincide with Breast Cancer Awareness Month, the NFL aired 6 television spots featuring NFL players to "help raise awareness and encourage fans to join in the fight against breast cancer" ("Real Men," 1999).[12] The spots, introduced in a news release headed, "Real Mean Wear Pink," aired during NFL games and primetime and daytime programming on ABC, CBS, ESPN, and FOX. Each spot is tagged with a logo bearing the NFL shield wrapped around a pink ribbon and a phone number that provides information about Race for the Cure events. The footage for the spots was filmed in July 1999 at the Race for the Cure in Aspen, Colorado.

Like much breast cancer-related marketing, the NFL's commercials place breast cancer survivors at the center of their narratives. Each of the commercials is visually similar: hundreds of middle-aged White women (along with smaller numbers of White men and children), wearing pink-and-white athletic apparel, walking and jogging along the tree-lined streets of Aspen. Interspersed with these images is footage of the featured players (four of whom are the only people of color visible in the commercials), erecting banners and signs, handing out water to participants as they run by, shaking hands with the men, holding hands with the children, and hugging the women.

In each commercial, the players describe their appreciation and admiration for the courage and pride of the survivors. These voiceovers are accompanied by long, lingering close-up shots of the faces of individual survivors. Jamal Anderson says, "There's nothing like the look of the survivor. And you look into their eyes and you can't help but be overwhelmed." "Man, these people are the true warriors," Tony Gonzales declares, "Man, they're out their struggling with life and death. It's just . . . it's an inspiration for me." While Hardy Nickerson explains:

> Once I got to the race and started talking to people and started hearing their stories, I think that was the most uplifting part about the whole Race for the Cure. Once you get around the survivors, man they tell you, "I've been a survivor for thirty years." "I've been a survivor for forty years." I found myself caught up and just wanting to talk to everybody and wanting to hear all the stories.

As the players express their admiration for breast cancer survivors, they also describe how their experiences at the race have inspired them to "do more" for the cause. Gonzalez says it is something he might "wanna do in the future," while Anderson suggests that their participation "might help make next year's race bigger" and that it "hopefully raised the awareness of what the Komen Foundation was trying to do." Hardy Nickerson points to the uplifting stories of survivorship as a motivation to bring more people into the fight against breast cancer: "Cuz the more you hear the stories, the more encouraged you get, and the more encouraged you get, the more you're able to encourage someone else. That's what life is all about." Kordell Stewart, who describes his mother's battle with breast cancer and her living 10 years after diagnosis instead of the one year predicted by her doctors, says, "It's about these people out here who are struggling with cancer and not knowing if they're gonna make it or not. But yet, if we come out here and just give a helping hand they might get an extra year or so. You just don't know how strong the mind is."

In tone and style—the sentimental, personal narratives, the soft focus shots, the pink-and-white color scheme, the centrality of familial relations, the uplifting music—the Real Men Wear Pink Campaign is in many ways a typical breast cancer-related marketing effort. What makes it a particularly interesting site for analysis, however, is that it condenses a range of issues relating to gender and racial politics, survivorship, corporate philanthropy, and the bright side of breast cancer.

The players who appear in these commercials, and whose participation in philanthropic activity is represented by an endless stream of news releases, on the one hand, their business—the NFL—and its social values. But, as public figures whose profession has been inextricably linked with inner-city criminality and violence through an unrelenting racialized media discourse of the past decade, they also serve another purpose (King, 2001). As exemplars of the "right side" of the NFL, they represent a willingness to embrace bourgeois, humanistic values such as the need to perform organized, charitable works and to transcend the imagined space of dependence, sloth, and violence from which they are said to have come. Indeed, the NFL responded to the negative public attention it received as a result of the arrests of Ray Lewis and Rae Carruth on separate charges of murder in the early months of 2000—attention that frequently cited welfare motherhood as a factor in NFL players' allegedly troubled lives—by focusing more heavily on its philanthropic activities in public relations communications (King, 2001). These commercials, therefore, have discursive effects that go beyond the realm of breast cancer to help produce and reproduce a racialized discourse of generosity that characterizes U.S. culture at this time. While these commercials offer a model for the ideal practitioner of American generosity, they also give shape to an idealized recipient of such generosity. The breast cancer survivors who appear in the NFL commercials are ordained with an inherent morality and wisdom—indeed, the awestruck voiceovers of the players in conjunction with the soft focus frames of the survivors faces suggest beatification—and are thus configured as higher-order citizens. But, perhaps paradoxically, the discourse of survivorship deployed through these commercials is also infantilizing. In her attempt to understand the popularity of stuffed bears and other commodities more commonly associated with childhood as gifts with a breast cancer theme, Barbara Ehrenreich (2001) wonders if in some versions of the prevailing gender ideology, "femininity is by its nature incompatible with full adulthood—a state of arrested development." "Certainly," she writes, "men diagnosed with prostate cancer do not receive gifts of Matchbox cars" (p. 46). Here Ehrenreich identifies (although she doesn't elaborate on) what I think is a key tension in mainstream breast cancer survivor culture: On the one hand breast cancer survivors are celebrated for their courage and strength and urged to feel empowered as actors within the medical system, but on the other they are asked to submit to mainstream scientific knowledge and depend on doctors and scientists to protect them from death. They—and the public at large—are told to obtain regular screenings, to demand insurance coverage for mammograms, and to explore a range of treatment options, but they are discouraged from questioning the underlying structures and guiding assumptions of the cancer-industrial complex.

While some feminist voices do raise such questions—What does cause breast cancer if only 30% of women diagnosed have known risk factors? If mammography, chemotherapy, and radiation have not succeeded in bringing down morality rates, what might? Why are more efforts not made to fund research into cause and prevention and particularly environmental factors in breast cancer incidence?—these voices, as I have indicated, are largely excluded from the mainstream of breast cancer culture. And while research on women's experiences with breast cancer suggests a wide range of psychological responses to the disease (in other words, the dominant image of breast cancer as the route to true happiness is not borne out by the research) the heterogeneity of these experiences does not easily penetrate dominant discourse on the disease and the approach of the cancer establishment to it.

Conclusion

Given how breast cancer survivors and the "problem of breast cancer" have been constituted in public discourse, the effectiveness of breast cancer activism is, perhaps not surprisingly, frequently explained not only by reference to well-executed political organizing, but also by allusion to the types of people who are thought to be most affected by the disease, in other words, to those identity categories—"wife," "mother," "future mother"—that are made visible through discourse on the disease. In a discussion of the success of the NBCC in raising the amount of federal dollars allocated to research in the *New York Times Magazine*, for instance, Susan Ferraro (1993) wrote:

> As the coalition's clout has grown, the powerful scientific and legislative communities that perhaps inevitably resist change have begun to hedge their objections to the advocates' assertions and demands. It's hard if not impossible to criticize mothers and sisters who are fighting cancer. (p. 61)

On the basis of this same logic, breast cancer has come to be known as "blissfully without controversy" (Goldman, 1997, p. 70).

The image of breast cancer as uncontroversial has been particularly influential in making the disease a priority for federal policy makers. In a coauthored essay, U.S. Representative Patricia Schroeder and U.S. Senator Olympia Snowe (1994) describe how the Congressional Women's Caucus selected breast cancer as an issue that would unite the group and enable it to build a strong middle ground as debates about reproductive freedom escalated within and outside the U.S. Congress in the 1980s. Indeed, the disease is often portrayed as one of the few issues capable of uniting an increasingly partisan Congress and has been used by antiabortion and pro-choice members and potential members of Congress to attract support from women constituents (King, 2004; Weissman, 1998). Carol Weisman cites the case of U.S. Senator Arlen Specter, a mostly pro-choice, fiscally conservative, Republican who had (famously) aggressively interrogated Anita Hill during the Clarence Thomas confirmation hearings and found himself in trouble with female voters. In the face of his Democrat opponent Lynn Yeakel's renowned television campaign drawing attention to his behavior at the hearings, and in an attempt to win back female voters, Specter became a key advocate of breast cancer initiatives. In the 1996 elections, conservatives such as U.S. Senators Rick Santorum of Pennsylvania, Jon Kyl of Arizona, Ted Stevens of Alaska, and John Warner of Virginia followed his lead by engaging in what the *New York Times* called the "battle of the breast" as they vied for the "breast vote" (Kolata, 1996, p. IV5). More recently, breast cancer became a key issue in the race for the 2000 Republican presidential nomination. When George W. Bush made television commercials featuring Republican Party activist and breast cancer survivor Geri Ravish criticizing McCain's record on financing breast cancer "issues," McCain responded with publicity countering Ravish's claims and highlighting Bush's own failures to support spending on certain breast cancer programs (Purnick, 2000, p. B1).

Of course, it is not inevitable that a disease that is seen as a threat to the strength of the nuclear family to reproduce itself be viewed as safe and uncontroversial. We have only to think about discourse on AIDS for a vivid counterexample. Whereas AIDS was from the beginning associated with—and made visible through—the "abnormal" identities and "deviant" lifestyles of gay men, Haitians, sex workers, and injecting drug users, however, breast cancer has been made visible through straight, White, married, young to middle-aged women. Thus, since its emergence in the 1980s as a key political issue it has been regarded as "safer" than AIDS and thus more attractive both to politicians seeking to attract women voters and corporations seeking to attract women consumers. In Amy Langer's words, "because AIDS was so public and so on the margin, breast cancer was by comparison relatively easy to square with corporate values" (Davidson, 1997, p. 36). John Davidson makes the distinction between AIDS and breast cancer more explicit. Drawing on the narrative of blame that is so common in discourse on AIDS, Davidson suggests that AIDS, unlike breast cancer, can be attributed to "amoral" acts:

> Unlike AIDS, breast cancer can't be attributed to questionable behavior. Breasts may be a sexual part of the anatomy, but they are also symbolic of motherhood and nurturing. Moreover, the 180,000 women stricken by breast cancer each year and the women who surround them—mothers, daughters, sisters, friends—represent a large and important group of consumers. (p. 36)

While there *is* a discourse in circulation that locates risk factors for breast cancer in individual behaviors that are associated with unhealthy or improper lifestyles—poor diet, lack of exercise, late or no child-bearing, and failure to get regular mammograms—this discourse operates more to detract attention away from external variables that might be implicated in high incidence rates (industrial pollution, for instance), rather than to demonize women with breast cancer. And, again, this is in large part because the "type" of woman that breast cancer is imagined to strike is not always already an object of suspicion and hatred.

What becomes apparent through this analysis of survivorship, breast cancer culture, and corporate philanthropy, then, is that nothing is inherently uncontroversial about breast cancer. Instead, the disease has been manufactured as such over two decades of organizing that has gradually been incorporated into conservative political agendas, the programs of large nonprofits in partnerships with the cancer industries, and corporate marketing strategies. The challenge thus becomes to disrupt the tyranny of cheerfulness that presides over breast cancer culture at this time so that those struggles and controversies that are at present pushed to the margins of discourse on the disease might find center stage and thus enable a more rigorous assessment of the status quo.

Notes

1. Extensive media coverage of the biology of breast cancer, methods of detection, available treatment options, and the psychological impact of losing a breast, followed their announcements.

2. NABCO, which closed its doors in 2004, was formed to provide "information, assistance, and referral to anyone with questions about breast cancer" and act "as a voice for the interests and concerns of breast cancer survivors and women at risk" (www.nabco.org). The NBCC was created from an initial meeting of 75 groups, including Breast Cancer Action of San Francisco, the Women's Community Cancer Project of Cambridge, and the Washington, DC-based Mary Helen Mautner Project for Lesbians with Breast Cancer.

3. I use the term *corporate philanthropy* to refer both to the activities of fund-raising organizations that rely on partnerships with businesses to support their work and to the philanthropic activities of businesses, which are increasingly tied to corporate strategy (i.e., growth and profit-making).

4. Cause-related marketing is a strategy by which corporations or brands associate themselves with a social cause such as breast cancer, child literacy, or homelessness. Most often, the association takes the form of donating a percentage of the profits on a particular product to a cause, but it can also take the form of free advertising (the National Football League pays for commercials promoting the Race for the Cure, for instance), or sponsorship of fund-raising events (Lee Jean's Denim Day, for instance, on which employees in participating companies pay $5 to the Komen Foundation in return for being permitted to wear jeans to work).

5. This section of the chapter is based on research conducted over the past 4 years. During this time, I attended Race for the Cure events in Illinois; Washington, DC; and Arizona, at which I took field notes and photographs, made tape recordings of speeches and ceremonies, and talked with participants and volunteers. I have also followed and occasionally taken part in discussions on the Komen Foundation's Talk Back online message boards and collected their publicity materials, newsletters, and annual reports. In addition to these sources, I have collected print media coverage of the Race for the Cure from 1983 to the present.

6. The 1999 Komen Race for the Cure series was "presented nationally" by J. C. Penney and "sponsored nationally" by American Airlines, Ford Motor Company, Johnson & Johnson, the National Football League, New Balance Athletic Shoes, Pier 1 Imports, and Tropicana Pure Premium Orange Juice.

7. The Race for the Cure is a carefully orchestrated and centrally managed affair. Although organizers of individual races are permitted to inject a hint of local flavor into their events, the foundation, headquarters in Dallas, determines the general format so that one gathering is remarkably similar to the next: each event has a pre- and postrace rally, a survivor recognition ceremony, a "wellness" area, and a spot where corporate sponsors promote their wares. Race T-shirts, signage, and other publicity materials are all embossed with the foundation's logo, and there is a template for the signs—imprinted with the names of loved ones who have survived or died from breast cancer—that participants pin to their backs. Much of the music that blasts from the loudspeakers during the events is the same across the nation and certain of the spoken passages from the pre- and postrace rallies are identical. So although the main focus of this chapter is on field research conducted at one race and while the analysis is concerned in part with the specificities of this particular event, my research at Races for the Cure in other locations suggests that any Race for the Cure in any town or city across the United States will look very much the same.

8. For evidence of the silence of the Komen Foundation on the relation between environmental factors and breast cancer incidence, see its Web site (www.komen.org); Nancy Brinker's book (1995), *The Race Is One Step at a Time*; and the foundation's three times a year newsletter, *Frontline* (recent issues are available on the Web site). The Komen Foundation's primary agenda is to encourage women to undertake early detection (via mammography, self-exam, and regular checkups) and, more recently, risk evaluation.

9. Throughout the year the foundation's corporate partners stage an array of special fund-raising events: American Airlines holds an annual Celebrity Golf Weekend; BMW organizes a series of sponsored test-drives; Bally's Total Fitness offers self-defense classes; Chili's restaurant chain stages an annual 10K run; Danskin holds a women-only triathlon series; *Golf for Women* magazine sponsors Rally for the Cure in which women pay to play in golf tournaments at country clubs across the United States; Jazzercize, in conjunction with the Atlanta Falcons, organizes Dance for the Cure; Johnson & Johnson coordinates the Virtual Runner Program, which allows supporters across the United States who cannot actively participate in the Race for the Cure to take part in a "virtual run" via the Internet; and *Self* magazine organizes a series of events called Workout in the Park in which participants give a donation in exchange for the opportunity to try out various fitness classes. Other corporations—including J. C. Penney, Titleist, Pinnacle, and Tomichi Studio—hold promotions in which they donate a percentage of the sale price of "breast cancer awareness products" to the Komen Foundation. Perhaps the most high-profile of this category of events is the Fashion Targets Breast Cancer campaign, in which Saks Fifth Avenue stores across the country hold "shopping events" to raise money for Komen and other national and local breast cancer charities.

10. The Susan G. Komen Foundation, one of the largest private funders of breast cancer research in the United States, was founded by Nancy Brinker in 1982 in memory of her sister who died of the disease. The foundation is most well-known for its national network of 5K runs, the Race for the Cure.

11. The NFL is perhaps more accurately described as a cartel rather than a corporation; it is an organization of independent firms (the teams) that restricts influence on the production and sale of its commodity and controls

wages. The Real Men Wear Pink Campaign was created and produced by the
NFL (which is funded by the pooling of profits from individual teams, NFL-
specific advertising revenues, NFL-specific television rights, and the sale of
NFL merchandise), as a league-wide rather than team-specific campaign.
However, individual franchises can and do invent their own breast-cancer
fund-raising events within the broad terms of the NFL's contract with the
Komen Foundation.

12. Five of the 6 television spots feature a different, high-profile player—Jamal
Anderson, running back with the Atlanta Falcons; Tony Gonzalez, tight end
with the Kansas City Chiefs; Hardy Nickerson, linebacker for the Tampa Bay
Buccaneers; Kordell Stewart, quarterback for the Pittsburgh Steelers; and
Jason Sehorn, defensive back for the New York Giants—describing their
experiences as volunteers at the race. The sixth spot is a compilation with
music but no voiceovers.

References

Altman, R. (1996). *Waking up/fighting back: The politics of breast cancer.* Boston: Little,
Brown.

Batt, S. (1994). Patient no more: *The politics of breast cancer.* Charlottetown, Canada:
Gynergy.

Beil, M. (1998, April 6). Life after cancer. *Dallas Morning News,* p. 7D.

Brady, J. (Ed.). (1991). *1 in 3: Women with cancer confront and epidemic.* San Francisco:
Cleis.

Bratich, J., Packer, J., & McCarthy, C. (Eds.). (2003). *Foucault, cultural studies, and
governmentality.* Albany: State University of New York Press.

Brenner, B. (2000). Sister support: Women create a breast cancer movement. In
G. Gordon, C. Burchell, & P. Miller (Eds.). (1991). *The Foucault effect: Studies in
governmentality.* Chicago: University of Chicago Press.

Brinker, N. (1995). *Race is run one step at a time: Every woman's guide to taking charge
of breast cancer.* Arlington, VA: Summit Publishers.

Cruikshank, B. (1999). *The will to empower: Democratic citizens and other subjects.*
Ithaca, NY: Cornell University Press.

Davidson, J. (1997, May). Cancer sells. *Working Woman,* pp. 36–39.

Ehrenreich, B. (2001, November). Welcome to cancerland. *Harper's,* pp. 43–53.

Epstein, S. (1998). *Impure science: AIDS activism and the politics of knowledge.* Berkeley:
University of California Press.

Ferraro, S. (1993, August 15). You can't look away anymore: the anguished politics
of breast cancer. *New York Times Magazine,* pp. 25–27, 58–60.

Foucault, M. (1979). *Discipline and punish: The birth of the prison.* New York:
Vintage.

Foucault, M. (1980). *The history of sexuality. Vol. 1: An introduction.* New York:
Vintage.

Foucault, M. (1991). Governmentality. In G. Burchell, C. Gordon, & P. Miller
(Eds.), *The Foucault effect. Studies in governmentality* (pp. 87–104). Chicago:
University of Chicago Press.

Goldman, D. (1997, November 3). Illness as metaphor. *Adweek,* p. 70.

Hall, M., & Nichols, B. (1997, April 25). Clinton: Citizenship means giving. *USA
Today,* p. A12.

King, S. (2001, Winter). An all-consuming cause: Breast cancer, corporate
philanthropy, and the market for generosity. *Social Text, 69,* 115–143.

King, S. (2004). Breast cancer activism and the politics of philanthropy. *International Journal of Qualitative Studies in Education, 17*(4), 473–492.

Klawiter, M. (2000). From private stigma to global assembly: Transforming the terrain of breast cancer. In M. Burawoy, J. A. Blum, S. George, Z. Gille, M. Thayer, T. Gowan, L. Haney, et al. (Eds.), *Global ethnography* (pp. 420–473). Berkeley: University of California Press.

Kolata, G. (1996, November 3). Vying for the Breast Vote. *New York Times,* p. 5.

Kushner, R. (1975). *Breast cancer: A personal history and investigative report.* New York: Harcourt Brace Jovanovich.

Leopold, E. (1999a). *A darker ribbon: Breast cancer, women, and their doctors in the twentieth century.* New York: Beacon.

Leopold, E. (1999b). Switching priorities in the breast cancer fight. *Boston Globe,* p. A19. Retrieved June 5, 2003, from Lexis Nexis Executive Database

Lerner, B. (2001). *The breast cancer wars: Hope, fear, and the pursuit of a cure in twentieth century America.* New York: Oxford University Press.

Lorde, A. (1980). *The cancer journals.* San Francisco: Spinster's Ink.

Navarre, M. (1988). Fighting the victim label. In D. Crimp (Ed.), *AIDS: Cultural analysis/cultural activism* (pp. 143–1678). Cambridge, MA: MIT Press.

NFL sponsors race for the cure. (1999, April 19). *New York Times,* p. 21.

Nixon plans to enlist citizens. (1969). *New York Times,* p. 21.

Packer, J. (2003). Mapping the intersections of Foucault and cultural studies: An interview with Lawrence Grossberg and Toby Miller, October 2000. In J. Bratich, J. Packer, & C. McCarthy (Eds.), *Foucault, Cultural Studies, and Governmentality* (pp. 23–46). Albany: State University of New York Press.

Patterson, J. (1987). *The dread disease: Cancer and modern American culture.* Cambridge, MA: Harvard University Press.

Purnick, J. (2000, March 6). Exploiting breast cancer for politics, New York Times, p. B1.

Rose, N. (1996). Governing "advanced" liberal democracies. In A. Barry, T. Osbourne, & N. Rose (Eds.), *Foucault and political reason: Liberalism, neo-liberalism and rationalities of government* (pp. 37–64). Chicago: University of Chicago Press.

Rose, N. (1999). *Powers of freedom: Reframing political thought.* Cambridge, UK: Cambridge University Press.

Schroeder, P., & Snowe, O. (1994). The politics of women's health. In C. Costello & A. Stone (Eds.), *The American Woman, 1994-95* (pp. 45–53). New York: Norton.

Sedgwick, E. K. (1992). Epidemics of the will. In J. Crary & S. Kwinter (Eds.), *Incorporations* (pp. 582–595). New York: Urzone.

Solomon, A. (1992). The politics of breast cancer. *Camera Obscura, 29,* 157–177.

Stabiner, K. (1997). *To dance with the devil: The new war on breast cancer.* New York: Delacorte.

Stachen, N. (1998, July 9). Posting to message board. Retrieved from www.komen.org, July 9, 1999.

Starr, P. (1982). *The social transformation of American medicine.* New York: Basic.

Weisman, C. (1998). Women's health: Activist traditions and institutional change. Baltimore, MD: John Hopkins University Press.

Yerak, B. (2000, January 7). Lions share market with women: Alpha males move over. *Detroit News,* p. B1.

Zita Grover, J. (1987). AIDS: Keywords. In D. Crimp (Ed.), *AIDS: Cultural analysis/cultural activism* (pp. 17–30). Cambridge, MA: MIT Press.

5

Regulation through Postfeminist Pharmacy

Promotional Discourse and Menstruation

JOSHUA GUNN & MARY DOUGLAS VAVRUS

University of Texas, Austin, and University of Minnesota

"I'M A REMIFEMIN-IST!" exclaimed the happy and healthy looking African American woman speaking to us from the television screen. We couldn't believe what we were seeing: a woman unapologetically using the word feminist in mainstream television. However, our hopes diminished as quickly as they appeared. This was an advertisement—for a menopause remedy. In it several healthy looking, smiling women engaged in various activities demonstrating their active lifestyles (e.g., without any signs of windedness, one woman proclaims her allegiance to Remifemin-ism while working out in a gym). Indeed, each woman spoke enthusiastically about Remifemin—a new (as of 2001) estrogen-free menopause treatment, which was allegedly making all of their lives better. Clearly, this ad feminism was being invoked to sell a product, not to praise either the movement or what it had done to improve women's lives.

But Remifemin was not the only treatment trumpeted as one that would help women immeasurably by tending to some aspect of their menstrual cycles. Beginning in early 2000, three menstruation-related campaigns emerged in U. S. mainstream media, each promoting a product claiming to treat a different phase of the menstrual cycle: Sarafem for premenstruation ("premenstrual dysphoric disorder"), Seasonale for menstruation (cessation of menstruation and its "excessive ovulation"), and Remifemin for menopause (reduction of hot flashes, etc., by becoming a "Remifemin-ist"). Each of these campaigns promoted a pharmaceutical cure for the ills alleged to derive from these aspects of menstruation. Articulating menstruation's phases to a pathological condition is not a novel technique for pharmaceutical promotions. What is new is the way these products are promoted through a second articulation—to "feminism." We place feminism in quotation marks here because we want to mark the contested nature of the term in this context, a crucial part of our argument. We argue that the Sarafem, Seasonale, and Remifemin campaigns, conducted in print media, on the radio, and on television, are part of a *post*feminist discursive formation that reshapes typical promotions of menstruation-related remedies into kinder and gentler strategies of medicalized self-surveillance. Drawing on Foucauldian ideas about governance and biopower, we argue that postfeminist discourses that subtly challenge feminism and circulate culturally in entertainment and news media, as well as in advertising, serve to make the pharmaceutical regulation of the menstrual cycle at once desirable and even literally palatable. Considered together (these emerged within a very short time and in quick succession), these three products make this medical surveillance of menstruation into what is virtually a lifelong project—from menarche through and beyond menopause. Ultimately, they mark menstruation as a disorder whose numerous symptoms must be stopped for the good of everyone: the sufferers and all those with whom they have relationships; to do otherwise, these promotions suggest, would be personally and socially irresponsible. To do otherwise risks a social-symbolic death.

This chapter reviews the promotional campaigns of Sarafem, Seasonale, and Remifemin for what they suggest about how postfeminism can be articulated to these discourses on the menstrual cycle, resulting in the potential incorporation of an almost lifelong technology of medicalized self-surveillance for women. To do this, we introduce the term *gyniatric apparatus* to point to the regulatory function of this discourse and to recognize that this use of postfeminism is aimed exclusively at women, through the manipulation of their hormones.

This chapter concerns governance by a subset of the health industries—the pharmaceutical industry—and, in particular, the creation and regulation of a particular population of postmenarche women consumers within what we will term the *gyniatric apparatus.*

The gyniatric apparatus comprises multiple elements: practices that involve everything from birth control, self breast exams, and dieting; policies as diverse as affirmative action programs to advocating on the behalf of women; habits concerning personal hygiene; and, of course, the discourse that renders the diversity and complexity of the apparatus as something coherent. The central, discursive logic that sets the gyniatric apparatus in motion is that of a pathology specific to the female body. The gyniatric apparatus defines the female body as a fundamentally abject body and regulates a population of these bodies

in various ways: most recently in ways specifically tied to menstruation, deploying postfeminism and its rhetoric of self-empowerment to
accomplish this task.

Biopolitical Regulation

> We need to see things not in terms of the replacement of a society of
> sovereignty by a disciplinary society and the subsequent replacement
> of a disciplinary society by a society of government; in reality one has
> a triangle, sovereignty-discipline-government, which has as its primary
> target the population and as its essential mechanism the apparatuses
> of security.
>
> —Michel Foucault (1991, p. 102)

In her elegant explication of Foucault's concept of biopolitics and
its relation to governmental rationality, Laurel Graham (1997) unfolds
Foucault's triangulation of sovereignty-discipline-government into a
continuum: At one end is the sovereign's right to *"take* life or *let* live"
as manifest in slavery and torture (Foucault, 1990, p. 138); moving
toward more abstract (and more internalized or invasive) tactics is
the abode of what Foucault terms "semio-critiques," rhetorics of
threat or virtual punishment that eclipse punishment itself; further,
"as we approach panopticism," suggests Graham, "the subject becomes
more active in working out the reasons to conform" to the will of
the state (para. 54). Moving further along the continuum, processes
of surveillance become internalized (and the necessity of the police
recedes; Gordon, 1991, p. 20), and self-discipline becomes the principal
means by which an agency "governs at a distance." The fundamental
difference among different points on this social continuum concerns
the ends of governance. A sovereign and disciplinary society administers
death in obvious, concrete ways. Contemporary logics of governance
seem increasingly immaterial, however, and seek to promote life by
defining and regulating populations. Whereas older tactics of discipline focused on the individual body as such, governmental rationality
aims toward the regulation of the abstraction of a group of people,
a "population" as a collection of types of bodies, to secure their
well-being or welfare. Foucault suggested these ends are pursued, as
opposed to achieved, by numerous dispositifs, apparatuses of security,
or what Ronald Walter Greene (1999) has helpfully dubbed "governmental apparatuses" (also see Deleuze, 1992; Hardt & Negri, 2000,
pp. 329–330).

Although one can identify a variety of disciplinary techniques and strategies in the contemporary West, Foucault's later observations about the art of government seem prescient as ours has increasingly become a society of control and self-surveillance, comprising multiple governing apparatuses that are not necessarily working in concert with a nation-state. This is not to say that disciplinarity has disappeared; institutions that house obvious disciplinary apparatuses—schools, prisons, churches—certainly remain. Rather, the move toward a society of control and self-discipline represents a contemporary horizontaliza-tion of disciplinarity, as the recognizable significance of institutions and traditional ensembles of sovereignty (e.g., the nation-state) erode.

The move toward the immanence of self-surveillance and discipline is intimately caught up in globalization. "The establishment of a global society of control that smoothes over the striate of national boundaries," argue Hardt and Negri (2000, p. 332), "goes hand in hand with the realization of the world market and the real subsumption of global society under capital." In light of the achievement of a nontranscendent, transnational capitalism, Foucault's understanding of governmental rationality asks us to consider several types of governance or regulation that are not necessarily articulated to traditional political institutions. In other words, government does not concern itself with overt political entities as much as it concerns itself with the conduct of human behavior, or the "conduct of conduct," in more general terms. Greene (1999) has suggested that in contemporary society the art of government is best described as an "abstract form of power materialized in the production of rules, procedures, and norms that judge and regulate the behaviors of a population," which, in turn, "transforms the possibilities for conduct" through the supplication of spaces for performance and the demarcation of limits (p. 3). Governmentality refers to a productive and regulating form of power that has become "less limited and bounded spatially in the social field" even though governing apparatuses operate by marking abstract or mental spaces of possibility—of potential conduct (Hardt & Negri, 2000, p. 330).

The nation-state can be said to comprise a governing apparatus that is no longer as powerful or prominent as the multiplicity of governing apparatuses that regulate consumerist populations (vis-à-vis a citizenry). The new articulations of the gyniatric apparatus govern particular female consumers as well. Before we describe the newer articulations of the gyniatric apparatus, however, it is helpful to describe the elements and function of a governing apparatus in general, how the governing apparatus operates as a constantly changing and evolving mechanism of deployment, or a dispositif, working to secure the welfare of a population, and the way in which discursive strategies work to articulate the specificity of an apparatus, or in other words, how discourse works to coordinate the elements of an apparatus into a functional, productive, and identifiable whole.

The Governing Apparatus

A *governing apparatus* is a material structure akin to a machine but not reducible to one insofar as the population regulated comprises humans who feel, act, and make choices in ways that are never guaranteed. It is at once both an abstraction and a concrete composition of elements that work together toward two ends simultaneously: it "identifies a population in need of calibration at the same time as it mobilizes that population to perform its own transformation" (Greene, 1999, p. 5). In other words, an apparatus fabricates or constructs a problem in relation to a particular group of individuals and encourages that group to self-manage the problem via any number of practices, techniques, and habits that catalyze modes of self-discipline. The logic of the apparatus is performative, however, meaning that regulation is a dynamic process that continuously redefines the problem and the population in discourse; there may be a historical origin of the specificity of a given apparatus and the discursive strategies associated with it, but this origin should be understood as a reconfiguration of older apparatuses and/or their disarticulated constitutive elements (again, practices, policies, institutions, techniques, etc.). In other words, apparatuses are not caused by this or that human being or group; they govern them, and they have done so since the emergence of the global society of control.

Greene (1999) has identified one example of a contemporary governing apparatus as the "population apparatus," a mode of governance that regulates human reproduction abstractly and transnationally through a complex assembly of discourses, institutions, practices, and procedures.[1] The population apparatus began to coalesce, argues Greene, in the theories of Thomas Robert Malthus, which were responsible for giving shape to a modern problematic—a looming population explosion—and for defining the "couple" as an object of regulation or governance to help address the problem. In his book-length analysis and critique of the population apparatus, Greene argues that since Malthusian rationality was set into motion, the population apparatus has expanded to include a host of practices (contraception), policies (domestic planning), political institutions (family planning agencies), and discursive strategies (rhetorics of crisis) that continuously reinscribe a kind of reproductive apocalypse, shifting to regulate new problem populations (e.g., the urban poor, the American woman, and the racialized Other in less-developed countries).

Insofar as Malthusian logics concern a looming or imminent problem that threatens the lives of a population, Greene (1999) identifies the central logic of the population apparatus as that of promoting and sustaining life (pp. 17–20). Foucault (1990) outlined this "modern" promotional and administrative character of contemporary governance at the end of the first volume of The History of Sexuality. There, Foucault detailed the transformation of political power from that of wielding or preventing death to that of promoting and "administering life," a historical unfolding of the productive nature of power as such (p. 138). In general, says Foucault, "power over life" came in two forms. The first form is that of discipline from without, "an anatomo-politics of the human body" or a microphysics of power that specifically addresses the body. In Discipline and Punish, for example, Foucault (1995) described discipline and the assemblage of techniques it organizes in terms of a gradual recession of conspicuous modes of domination (such as torture, the prison system, etc.) and the emergence of various machineries of power that subjected a "docile" body to regimented modes of conduct (e.g., "exercise," and later, self-surveillance; pp. 160–162; 195–228). In this earlier work discipline is not wielded by institutions, but is both a "type of power" and a "modality for its exercise" that focuses on the individual (p. 217).

The second kind of power over life concerns kinds or "species" of bodies and the characteristically sociological categories of demography and surveillance in relation to their being living things: "propagation, births and mortality, the level of health, life expectancy and longevity" are the (characteristically sexual) processes that this second kind of power over life seeks to manage (Foucault, 1990, p. 139). The practices that aim to manage the behavior and thoughts (collectively, the "conduct") of a given individual as a member of a particular population is termed biopower. Combined with the subjection-effect of so many disciplinary techniques, for Foucault the exercise of biopower marks the "threshold of modernity" in the sense that it heralds a moment when "the life of [a] species is wagered on its own political strategies" (p. 143).[2]

Biopower can be said to work through or within a governing apparatus in a peculiar way: Because of its attention to populations over that of the individual citizen, governing apparatuses function in terms of norms, not laws. Hence one consequence of the development of biopower, says Foucault (1990), was a decline in juridical forms of power and a transformation of the juridical subject into the self-disciplining subject

(p. 144). Instead of operating on a juridical model of the permitted and forbidden, security and biopower make discipline lateral and in terms of "a tolerable bandwidth of variation" (Gordon, 1991, p. 20), in particular because the management of life must abandon the punishment of death and its attendant, dichotomous logics. A government rationality of security gives "rise as well to comprehensive measures, statistical assessments, and interventions aimed at the entire social body" or population (Foucault, 1978, p. 146).

In terms of the rationality that structures the discourses associated with it, a governing apparatus, then, is not so much an apparatus of adjudication as it is of simple judgment and self-judgment concerning the normal and abnormal in relation to an identified norm. In the case of the population apparatus, for example, if the problem was an impending population explosion and the consequent crises of sustainability, then abnormal or deviant populations are identified as those unable or unwilling to regulate their reproductive behaviors; the discursive strategies that result often articulate the suspect population to other problematic discourses, such as those of gender, race, and so on (e.g., the racialized other, the AIDS crisis in Africa), to promote newer policies, practices, habits, or behaviors that work to encourage a population to normalize itself. Because the function of judgment in discourse is to articulate populations and various governing elements into an identifiable (i.e., coherent despite its complexity) governing apparatus, discursive strategies play an important role.

Discourses of the Interior: Health Care and Postfeminism

We suggest that the continuum of sovereignty-discipline-government mentioned previously should be conceived as a loop. Many reasons exist for doing so, such as the continued existence of sovereign agencies, disciplinary institutions, and so forth. The reason we highlight this, however, directly implicates the social field of health care: the progressive administration of life most typical of governmental rationality is never completely disarticulated from the threat of death; or rather, death remains a psychic limit or perceived point of recalcitrance. Punishment as a form of discipline is merely replaced with masochism as a means by which the individual self-surveils in relation to this or that norm. As a psychic negativity, then, death is no longer the consequence of transgression, but the consequence of an internalized failure to normalize; death in this sense is thus fundamentally an abstract symbolic or social death, in distinction from the threat—real or virtual—of the punishing death of transgression.

Normalizing discourses that operate in the shadow of (social) death can be characterized as "discourses of the interior." In the context of the emergence of notions of social and political deviance and abnormality, Gordon (1991) describes the conduct of conduct as the "postulation of an interior domain of mental norms [that] parallels and presupposes [the] promotion of an alert public sensorium of civil vigilance" (p. 37).[3] The "conduct of conduct," in other words, operates at the level of an interior—a subject, a psyche, an unconscious. Furthermore, the decentralization of state power through the interiorization of self-discipline by means of an ensemble of agencies, practices, and discourses (inclusive of vocabularies) is, in this sense, why Foucault characterized governmentality as a type of rationality.[4] (Although Foucault [1991b] did prefer "an analysis of . . . discourses in the dimension of their exteriority," he never argued that interiors—subjects, psyches, contents—did not exist; indeed, they must exist or governmental rationality would have never emerged [see Foucault, 1991b; and on the subject as a "fold," Deleuze, 1988, pp. 94-123]). Furthermore, although government rationality, and by extension any governing apparatus, is autonomous, it is an autonomy that must nevertheless become "internalized," or enfolded, to use Deleuze's metaphor, in order to regulate. Analogously, governmental apparatuses articulate populations to discursively emergent problems that are internalized in the process of self-discipline.

In this "folded-in" sense we turn to the discursive strategies of the pharmaceutical industry, which at the most abstract level is part of a diffuse transnational apparatus of medicalization that constructs and identifies diseases and provides for their remedy. The discursive strategy of this apparatus, then, calls diseased populations into being and supplies a means of self-surveillance and self-regulation principally by means of pharmaceutical products. Although, to be sure, the health-care apparatus works to sustain the life of a population (that is, works to prevent death), one discourse of that interior seems to be increasingly prominent: psychological health. Increasingly, discourses regarding mood have articulated everything from allergy suffering to diabetic symptoms to a diseased psychic existence; returning to the norm, averting (social) death, not only requires physical but also psychical standardization.

Like all governmental apparatuses, the health industry exists to administer and promote life and to maximize profit while doing so; however, in this age of health maintenance organizations (HMOs) and the rising cost of prescription drugs, undeniably the practical logic animating its policies, practices, tactics, techniques, and rhetorics is fundamentally economic. Indeed, precisely this strange articulation of the promotion of the security and welfare of multiple populations and the increasing impossibility of achieving or maintaining the norms of "good (mental) health" deployed in its discourse makes the apparatus viable as an economic or profit producing one—and a visibly coherent one as well.

This chapter focuses specifically on one part of the health-care apparatus—that which is concerned with the bourgeois female body—to demonstrate how a health-care apparatus in general works to fabricate and regulate a population for economic ends. This implies that what the health-care apparatus shares in common with governing apparatuses in general is the problem of the contemporary immanence of capital.

In traditional Marxian political economy, crisis theory held that capital was an imperial force that continuously expanded to avert the looming crisis of overaccumulation. More contemporary understandings of capital, however, characterize its movement as immanent—that global capital must move inside, to its interior, continually rearranging the forces and relations of production. Put more concretely: When capital has nowhere to expand and therefore can no longer exploit the labor of a given population, then it must do other things to remain dynamic. One thing capital has done, argue Hardt and Negri (2000), is shift to a post-Fordist economic structure that uses immaterial labor—the labor of exchanging knowledge and information (p. 290). Another thing that has happened is the manufacturing of commodities for which there is no human need. We suggest the latter strategy is one of the principal means by which the pharmaceutical component of the health-care apparatus maintains economic viability in immanent terms; it foregrounds obscure diseases (whose very diagnoses are often quite contested), especially mental diseases/illnesses or virtual social deaths, to continuously administer life.

The production of commodities that have no apparent use is, of course, nothing new; it simply requires a discourse of demand. What seems different in our neoliberal age are the ways in which economic interests articulate production to governing apparatuses that are always already at work. In other words, to create a successful circuit of production and consumption, pharmaceutical corporations must deploy promotional discourses that are articulated to established modes of governance, which have already been successful in regulating a given population; this necessity is not only born of the post-Fordist manner in which capital currently operates, but also, again, because capital is an immanent force: it must work on the interior. We suggest that the regulation and governance of the female body, through the gyniatric apparatus, is one of many apparatuses that have been articulated to the larger machinations of the health industry.

Postfeminism and the Gyniatric Apparatus

In the promotional literature pharmaceutical companies produce concerning menstruation, postfeminism is deployed in a gender-specific fashion to encourage self-surveillance through the menstrual cycle. Postfeminism derives from feminist discourse, yet dispenses with much of it as unnecessary for contemporary circumstances. The gyniatric apparatus constitutes a population and then deploys postfeminist discursive strategies that regulate that population by moving it away from feminism and encouraging commodification, interiorization, and a bourgeois existence instead. Substituting interiorized concerns for feminism's collective politics of activism, postfeminism nevertheless works in the effort to regulate a population of bourgeois women through its relentless focus on the subject as consumer (Vavrus, 2002). Rayna Rapp (1987) notes that postfeminism works by depoliticizing feminism and reducing "feminist social goals to individual 'lifestyle'" (p. 32, emphasis in original). This aspect of postfeminism makes it ideal for the gyniatric apparatus's exercise of biopower: in this case, the use of pharmaceutical drugs intended to manage menstrual symptoms, and, by extension, the women who would consume them. The norms the gyniatric apparatus generates are those that concern the physical and social health of a population of bourgeois women whose participation in postfeminism's discursive practices helps to ensure their distance from the abject quality of their bodies—as the untreated abjectness of female bodies has been promoted as the abnormal, even grotesque, alternative to the cleansed, medicated body.[5] That is, the pharmaceutical industry relies on the female body being coded as abject to do much of its work; left untreated, abject bodies constitute an abnormal population. Only those bodies willing to submit to pharmaceutical treatment can be regulated properly by the governance of the gyniatric apparatus.

Feminist analyses of medical discourses on premenstrual syndrome (PMS), menstruation, and menopause have problematized them for the way they pathologize a necessary bodily process as they signify sexual difference: the feminine is marked as pathological Other to the masculine norm. Yet, to ensure the success of these campaigns (and perhaps to mitigate effects of any errant feminist critiques that make their way into popular media) the manufacturers of Sarafem, Seasonale, and Remifemin must promote these remedies as woman-friendly. Although appropriating feminism for this purpose would be one means of accomplishing such a gyniatric end, such a strategy would be risky for many advertised products: feminism critiques many of the constructed identities on which advertising of all kinds relies. *Post*feminism, on the other hand, is ideal for articulating a range of products to a putatively woman-friendly discourse: the postfeminist subject is encouraged to think in terms of commodification and consumption, and numerous other consumer products have begun to market to this identity.

We begin with Sarafem and its target: PMDD. According to Figert's (1996) book on the politics of PMS in the psychiatric and psychology communities, the discussion of whether to even consider PMS a legitimate medical problem was a hotly contested one. Many psychologists and psychiatrists believed that moving premenstrual symptoms into the realm of the medical would serve only to play into preexisting dangerous notions about women being at the mercy of their hormones once a month and neglecting their homes and families. In 1983, when a working group was formed to study the question of whether the American Psychiatric Association (APA) should include PMS in the *Diagnostic and Statistical Manual of Mental Disorders* (DSM-III)'s appendix (called the DSM-III-R), several groups, including the APA Committee on Women, protested vigorously. This group's chair, Hortensia Amaro, wrote to the APA that including PMS as a mental illness "has ominous implications for perpetuating damaging stereotypes of women and for fostering an unnecessarily pathological view of women's experience" (quoted in Figert, 1996, p. 41).[6] To make PMS sound like its "psychological symptoms . . . are unpleasant mood states or dysphoria" (p. 40), the APA Working Group renamed it "Premenstrual Dysphoric Disorder" or PMDD. After much struggle and the rejection of the protesters' concerns, PMDD became a part of the DSM-III-R in 1987, after finally having been renamed Late Luteal Phase Dysphoric Disorder (LLPDD). However, because of the protesters' concerns, LLPDD was placed in a category titled, "proposed diagnostic categories needing further study" (p. 48). Today, and after more controversy about the medical status of PMS, it is listed in the DSM-IV's regular text (as opposed to its appendix) and known once more as Premenstrual Dysphoric Disorder (PMDD; pp. 149–150). However, some psychiatrists and psychologists still do not accept PMDD's status as a mental disorder (Figert, 1996; Vedantam, 2001).

Figert's (1996) study, which includes interviews with many of the principal actors in the struggle over PMS's diagnostic status, reveals the political machinations that lay behind what might seem to be a straightforward inclusion of a medical diagnosis in the most important manual that exists for psychiatric and psychological diagnoses. However, as Figert describes it, the inclusion process was far from smooth. The timing of the deliberations that preceded LLPDD's inclusion in the DSM-III-R coincided with a commercial shift, as well. That is, by the early 1980s, products that claimed specifically to treat PMS symptoms began to appear on grocery and drug store shelves, and numerous PMS-related greeting cards, buttons, bumper stickers, self-help books, and clothing appeared at the same time. Figert refers to the appearance of such items as the constitution of the "PMS industry" and notes that it was a cash cow, composed of the "3 Ps (products, pills, and prescriptions)" (p. 18). In a section entitled, "What's at Stake in the Construction of PMS?" Figert argues that:

> for some women, the publicity and legitimization of PMS and its symptoms as real, a natural part of their body and its processes, have led to a positive sense of control over this phenomenon. However, a more negative image of PMS as something that controls women once a month, that makes them "crazy" and subject to their hormones, is much more pervasive in our contemporary Western culture. This image has allowed women to use PMS as an excuse to express their emotions or to account for their otherwise "strange" behaviors. Other people (husbands, children, doctors, lawyers, judges, juries, co-workers) have also used PMS to explain women's behaviors—often within a scientific or medical framework that then gives physicians and scientists "expert" legitimacy over women's bodies and minds. (p. 21)

Following Figert (1996), we suggest that Sarafem's emergence is one P in the 3 Ps Figert points to earlier, and one that was marketed both to attend to Eli Lilly's exigencies and to recognize (however unknowingly) the regulatory potential of postfeminist discourse along with its importance as a commercial vehicle. Sarafem was marketed to the public using both television and print advertisements. One of the two television advertisements (Eli Lilly had produced three, but the first was deemed by the Food and Drug Administration to be too aggressive) included two brief but dramatic and silent vignettes, each of which conveyed the frustration of experiencing PMDD. In the first, a woman storms around her house, finally violently throwing a pillow against a couch. As her male lover or husband follows her into this room, she looks at him and then appears to yell; his face shows his bewilderment and his stance—arms crossed in front of his chest—signifies his hostility toward her. The second vignette occurs in the dressing room of a clothing store where a woman is trying on clothes and finding everything too tight, apparently because of premenstrual bloating. Her expression reveals her exasperation about the experience, and she thrusts the clothing into the arms of the friendly-looking salesperson (also a woman). The voiceover suggests that these instances of irritability and mood swings could be even more severe than a simple case of PMS: "Think again. It

could be PMDD." The female actors in the television ad each appears
to betray what is expected of her, according to stereotypic notions that
still abound about women: one of the women is so affected by PMDD
that she is prevented from partaking in that quintessentially female
activity of shopping. The other apparently causes harm to her romantic
relationship. The print advertisements are less dramatic and, instead
of depicting unpleasant scenarios, they show women who appear to
have treated their PMDD—apparently with Sarafem. One, found in *TV
Guide*, features the upper half of a grinning woman bending into the
advertisement's copy, her torso cut off by the frame of the ad. "Mood
swing" is at the top of the page in large block letters; however, "mood"
is crossed out with green ink strokes, followed by smaller block letters
below it: "Think it's PMS? Think again." An inch or so below that is the
following: "It could be PMDD," followed by Eli Lilly's pitch:[7]

> Irritability, sadness, sudden mood changes, tension, bloating. If you
> suffer from many of these symptoms month after month and they
> clearly interfere with your daily activities and relationships, you could
> have PMDD. PMDD—Premenstrual Dysphoric Disorder—is a distinct
> medical condition that is characterized by intense mood and physical
> symptoms right before a period.

At the bottom of this ad is a picture of the half pink–half purple Sarafem
pill, perched above these words: "More like the woman you are." The
other print ad that circulated for Sarafem was very similar to the first,
but featured a facial shot of a serenely smiling woman under the word
"irritability" in block letters, this time with the "irrit" crossed out with
strokes of green ink. The remainder of the ad's text was identical to
the first.

Not only do these Sarafem ads rest on hide-bound expectations
about women, they promote a product that purports to restore women
to their authentic, presumably balanced selves—far from the ravages
of menstrual hormones—through the ingestion of a pill composed of
synthetic substances created in pharmaceutical laboratories. They also
present symptoms that many women *and* men might feel, either cyclically
or more often,[8] as a result of conditions that may have little to do with
individual chemical imbalances and much to do with structural factors,
such as workplace or economic conditions. In glossing over any other
possibilities for the generalized symptoms, Eli Lilly makes its product
part of the gyniatric apparatus's deployment of postfeminism. In other
words, the marketing of Sarafem focuses on PMS as a marker of an
abject, out-of-control body and thus uses postfeminism's consumerist

heteronormativity. The female actors who display symptoms of PMDD are being prevented from shopping and from being nice, even submissive, to a male spouse or lover; they are not engaged in riotous behavior or doing anything else especially disturbing. This is characteristic of the postfeminist character of mainstream media, and it suggests to viewers and readers that to avoid treatment is to risk the appearance of mental illness—a (social) death that is exemplified by relatively mundane behaviors. To treat one's PMDD is to enter the world of "swing" and "ability." These ads normalize both PMDD as a universally accepted diagnosis and Sarafem as a treatment; taken together, they also normalize the attributes of the clearly preferred population as being those of happy, smiling women.

Like Sarafem, Seasonale has been promoted as a treatment for menstrual symptoms. However, rather than simply treat the symptoms, Seasonale eliminates them altogether except for four very short periods a year (allegedly to make women feel better about taking the drug). Unlike Sarafem, Seasonale had not been advertised on television or in print media at this time because it did not receive FDA approval until September, 2003; however, the concept of menstruation cessation—achieved through Seasonale or something like it—has been floated as a news item in a variety of media: television, radio, newspapers, medical journals (including the *Journal of the American Medical Association* [*JAMA*]), news magazines, and various Internet sites (Warren, 2002, p. 6, .n. 5). The principal actors behind the development and promotion of the concept of menstruation cessation are Doctors Elsimar Coutinho and Sheldon Segal. Coutinho is the author of the book *Is Menstruation Obsolete?*, translated from Coutinho's native Portuguese by Segal (with a literal translation, the title is *Menstruation, A Useless Bleeding*; Warren, 2002, p. 13). Coutinho and Segal's rationale for promoting the cessation of menstruation is that Western women (who experience menarche earlier now than ever before, have fewer children than ever before, and experience menopause later than ever before) are experiencing hormonal poisoning as a result of an "excessive" number of menstrual cycles they endure throughout their lifetimes (Warren, 2002, p. 6). In an interview with Warren, Coutinho is quoted as saying that his work is helping women because the "estrogen surge" that occurs during menstruation is toxic and "'so embarrassing' that women have to 'use a lot of soap and all kinds of perfume to get rid of it'" (p. 13).

Coutinho and Segal's work on this project has been accepted by prestigious medical journals such as *JAMA* and *The Lancet*. In one issue of *The Lancet*, two physicians argue that the elimination of menstruation would help "women individually and society as a whole" (in Warren,

2001, p. 3). Yet not all experts are as sanguine about menstruation cessation. As Warren (2001, 2002) and Stein (2003) point out, several hormone experts, physicians, and researchers react to the prospect of menstruation cessation with uncertainty and even negativity. However, mainstream media treatments have been positive overall. In other words, although skepticism and concern exist in the medical and scientific communities about the elimination of menstruation, no such skepticism emerges in the glowing stories that have appeared in media texts. For example, Warren (2002) includes a quote from *Cosmopolitan* magazine, whose author suggests that without those pesky menstrual periods, you "have three to five extra days in the month you can wear white pants or go skinny dipping" (p. 18). Another author, this one writing in the London *Independent*, points to another great feature of the lack of a period, "your stomach stays flat so you can show off your midriff all year round" (in Warren, 2002, pp. 18–19). It's dubious, at best, to think that either of these authors is revealing advantages that "help women individually and society as a whole," as *The Lancet*'s physician-authors believe menstruation cessation will. But even so, the promotion of menstruation cessation and Seasonale, as Warren points out, is risky because it (ironically enough) encourages women to flood their bodies with hormones to stop the "overdose" of hormones (Coutinho's theory) that results from menstruation. Women can trade one set of problems—those that accompany menstruation—with another: those incurred through the ingestion, implantation, or injection of synthetic hormones.

The medical rationale for using Seasonale, expressed by Coutinho and in *The Lancet*, is also the site at which the gyniatric apparatus operates. By couching the promotion of Seasonale in the language of self-help that benefits individual women and "society as a whole," Coutinho and his supporters can regulate the constituted population of menstruating women by casting Seasonale use as both a remedy for individual suffering and as a public service. Suggesting that "good" women will take Seasonale simultaneously brings into existence a deviant population: all those women who will opt not to take Seasonale, who will thus continue to "poison" themselves, make their fashion choices more difficult and experience what Coutinho believes is an "obsolete" process. The Seasonale-taking subject, on the other hand, has consented to surveiling her own and her sisters' cycles and managing them as a part of the gyniatric apparatus's governance. In other words, taking Seasonale to eradicate the menstrual cycle demonstrates tacit approval for the regulating conditions set out by Seasonale's backers. Moreover, it requires these individuals' interpellation into the postfeminist discourse that insists that as much distance as possible be placed between women and anything suggesting the female grotesque (in this case, symptoms that accompany the menstrual cycle as well as menstruation itself).

Worth mentioning, however, is that Sarafem and Seasonale represent the potential financial gain of their manufacturers and, in the case of Seasonale, their discoverers, too. Sarafem not only represents an appropriation of postfeminism by a pharmaceutical company, but also another trend as well. That is, like several other successful drugs whose patents were running out, Sarafem is a renamed and repackaged version of a soon-to-be-generic drug—Eli Lilly's wildly successful antidepressant Prozac. And although the disease it was targeted to cure—PMDD—can be found in the DSM-IV, medical experts are far from unanimous about whether it can be considered a legitimate disease or should ever have been included in any edition of the DSM at all (Figert, 1996). Seasonale, on the other hand, is just one of several possible repackaged birth control hormones—pills, implants (Norplant), and injectables (Depo-Provera). The latter, Norplant and Depo-Provera, were developed by Sheldon Segal and Elsimar Coutinho, respectively, the two doctors whose work has been most publicly associated with the argument that menstruation suppression is a good thing (Warren, 2002). If Sarafem or the cessation of menstruation (the latter would obviously negate a need for the former) were to become an acceptable means of dealing with the inconveniences of menstruation, then Eli Lilly, Coutinho, and Segal stand to make a great deal of money.

The last remedy we examine, Remifemin, arguably poses no threat of overdosing on synthetic hormones: Its active ingredient is black cohosh root, an herb that has been used to treat menopause (and other problems) since the nineteenth century (NIH, 2003, p. 2).[10] And although the National Institute of Health's office of dietary supplements does not endorse its use (on the basis of too few studies documenting its efficacy or long-term effects), its Web site provides a fairly detailed explanation of what *is* known about black cohosh.[11]

Remifemin treats symptoms, and, unlike hormone replacement therapy (HRT), does not go further to eliminate osteoporosis or cardio-vascular disease, for example. But, like HRT, Remifemin is marketed in such a way as to become one more treatment in what Bunton (1997) calls "health-related consumer culture." Bunton elaborates on such a culture by adding that it is based on a "more general privileging of bodily appearance, youthfulness, vitality, health and beauty and the 'aestheticization' of everyday life associated with consumer culture" (p. 232). The Remifemin television ad described in the introduction to this chapter features physically fit women who, through their gym workouts, appear to be aiming at least to sustain their fitness, if not to build on it. The Remifemin print ads found in various magazines feature a blue-eyed, blond haired woman smiling broadly as she announces, "my menopause symptoms faded 1, 2, 3. . . . You bet I'm a Remifemin-ist!" On the GlaxoSmithKline Web site, the same woman tells readers, "I'm a Remifemin-ist because I saw a dramatic reduction in my menopause symptoms in just 12 weeks!"

These "Remifemin-ists" lay claim to a postfeminist ideology, the particulars of which are these: postfeminism takes feminist gains for granted, yet, while doing so, replaces feminist ideology with individualistic, consumer-oriented practices intended only for very specific women, specifically, those who have sufficient income to support the consumption habits of at least a middle-class life. Remifemin's focus on individual self care for the purpose of personal independence is revealed in its ads' repeated invocation of the term "feminist," appended to the rest of its trade name. By using "feminist" in its ads for Remifemin, GlaxoSmithKline suggests that it desires some of the connotations of feminism, but without implicating itself any further in the *politics* of feminism. The term *feminist* most likely resonates with women beginning to experience symptoms of menopause, as they are from the early baby boomer generation and could well have been involved or simply interested in second-wave feminist activism (undoubtedly, they have reaped the rewards of feminist activism, whether or not they acknowledge this). Also, Remifemin's herbal active ingredient marks it as a treatment that feminists might be more inclined to embrace as feminist critiques of medicine have generated a large literature on, among other topics, synthetic treatments for menopause. GlaxoSmithKline's tactic here could prove to be a successful hailing gesture to the second-wave feminist as she wends her way through the labyrinth of menopause treatments, their benefits, and side effects.[12]

The advertising industry is no stranger to the use of feminism in the texts it produces. From Virginia Slims cigarette ads featuring the "You've come a long way, baby" slogan to Enjoli perfume ads that belt out, "I can bring home the bacon, fry it up in a pan," while reminding women to "never let him forget he's a man," slivers of feminism are sliced and doled out to media audiences. Some media critics argue that the ease with which feminist politics can be packaged and commodified suggests that the movement has sold out and become "commodity feminism" (Goldman, Heath, & Smith, 1991). Our argument suggests that something more is at work than simply a trend to commodifying some of the beliefs of feminism. We argue that postfeminist discourse indeed relies on the commodification of feminism, but goes beyond it to construct a population of bourgeois women who can be regulated by an apparatus that marks them as deficient—and therefore deviant—unless they accept postfeminism's ideology. In the case of the pharmaceutical industry's attempt to alter women's experiences with menstruation, this occurs in promotions that suggest good women are those who, for instance, can continue to shop for clothing even while they are premenstrual. Good women are those who rid themselves of their menstrual cycles so that they can buy and wear midriff-revealing tops.

But such postfeminist discourse is not limited to its insistence on articulating good women to consumption; it also articulates good women to the emotional labor of relationship maintenance, whether it occurs within or outside of their families. Although feminism paved the way for women to have more power in their workplaces and made acceptable the idea that women could—and should—work in occupations other than those in the so-called helping and services professions, postfeminism jerks women back from this utopic vision to insist that women who participate in the wage labor system should also be primarily responsible for the nurturing and filial concerns of home. Relying on an essentialist view that marks women as biologically tethered to nurturance and domesticity, postfeminism asks women to do both the wage labor and the unremunerated labor of the private sphere (Vavrus, 2002). Postfeminist discourse, then, marks as good women those who tend to their menstrual cycles. Good women do not throw pillows out of exasperation with their male partners, nor will they angrily thrust piles of too-small clothes at female salespeople. Good women smile through their menopause symptoms. Good women do not "embarrass" themselves by smelling bad through their estrogen surges (in this discourse, good women have put estrogen surges behind them). Good women thus demonstrate that they are committed to being among the population of happy women whose cycles—and by extension, everyday lives—can be regulated through the gyniatric apparatus.

Conclusion

Warren (2002) points out that what is at stake with Seasonale can be understood in Foucauldian terms. We suggest that her point is a valid one in considering Sarafem's and Remifemin's postfeminist governance as well. Just as plastic surgery, Botox, or other "surface" interventions work to "sculpt" a more perfect female, synthetic hormones work on both the surface and in depth to create a female made sexier through a kind of androgyny. The move to erase menstruation from women's biology can lay claim to creating both these surface and inner changes in women—from improving their looks (flatter stomachs and flawless complexions), their dispositions (no more premenstrual snarling or depression), their health (no more endometriosis or ovarian cancer), and their generally unruly bodies (no more smells, "accidents," or strange cravings for chocolate or sex). The net effect is what, following and expanding on Foucault, numerous feminists have framed as the "female, docile body" (p. 9).

Sarafem, Seasonale, and Remifemin encourage internalizing docility for women through a gyniatric apparatus. Postfeminist discursive practices constitute an important part of this apparatus and aid significantly in the pharmaceutical industry's governance of a population of post-menarche, bourgeois female bodies. By articulating menstruation and menopause treatment to individualized self-care, materialized through commodification and consumerism, postfeminism operates in the service of biopower.

However totalizing this discourse may seem, particularly where it is articulated to an apparatus of governance, biopower leaves us an out. That is, in its blindness to the particular disciplining of the individual on the basis of dichotomies, a governmental rationality of security, in its exercise of biopower, also helps to generate:

> a new kind of counterpolitics. As governmental practices have addressed themselves in an increasingly immediate way to "life". . . individuals have begun to formulate the needs and imperatives of that same life as the basis for political counter-demands. Gordon, 1991, p. 5)

To wit, just as discipline produces deviancy, so too does the emergence of biopower produce counterconducts that are able to thrive precisely because the norm has replaced the rule.

One important reason that the emergence of biopower is significant is that the "life" it concerns is always capable of outwitting any biopolitics of regulation, for example, rallies for reproductive rights (see Gordon, 1991, p. 5) and even resistance to the pharmaceutical pathologization of the process of menstruation (see Stein, 2003). The potential "reversibility" of biopolitics means that the arena of possible action is *always open*. Biopower is the apotheosis of a managerial abstraction that closes down some possibilities as it opens others. In this case, the advertisements and media reports that promote Sarafem and Seasonale have been met with skepticism by feminists, some journalists, and medical researchers. That their criticisms, although not commensurate with the products' promotions, reach mainstream media at all exemplifies what biopower may permit.

Notes

1. Another example is "rhetorical pedagogy," which works to produce public citizens and circulate them within a public (Greene, 2002, pp. 434–443).

2. That something as horrific as genocide can occur at all, argues Foucault (1990), means that power has been exercised at the level of "the large-scale phenomenon of population" (p. 137). As we understand it, the significance of this formulation is precisely that a governing rationality is operating at a very high level of abstraction that has finally dispensed of a juridical mode in favor of what Habermas (1984) has termed "universal humanity." Presumably the direct, political consequences of this are, on the one hand, the ability to contend with subjects as biological/living subjects (as opposed to the abstraction of "citizen" or some other notion), yet, on the other hand, a simultaneous ability to bury the sentiment of face-to-face encounter with the faceless horde. In other words, the abstract citizen has been replaced by the faceless mob.

3. This interiorizing movement is not to be understood, however, in terms of consciousness per se, but rather, as an "enfolding," a rendering of the "inside as an operation of the outside . . . as if the ship were a folding of the sea" (see Deleuze, 1986). From our reading, this is not to say that Foucault (1990) denies the existence of an interior (for certainly an enfolding or envagination is the creation of an interior however much its operations depend on the outside), but rather, that one can best explain the workings of the modern subject in terms of exteriors.

4. Among Foucault's (1991a) many definitions of the term is that *governmentality* is the "ensemble formed by the institutions, procedures, analyses and reflections, the calculations and tactics that allow the exercise of this very specific albeit complex form of power, which has as its target population, as its principle form of knowledge political economy, and as its essential technical means apparatuses of security" (p. 102).

5. Mary Russo's *The Female Grotesque* (1994) points to the place of abjection in the historical, virtual prohibition of female bodies from the public sphere and in the marginalization of nonelite women (p. 12). Her project is to elevate the grotesque in feminism to make it "heterogeneous, strange, polychromatic, ragged, conflictual, incomplete, in motion, and at risk" (p. 1). This move is one that Russo believes poses a direct challenge to the normalization of the bourgeois within feminism. Russo defines the grotesque body as "open, protruding, irregular, secreting, multiple, and changing; it is identified with non-official 'low' culture or the carnivalesque, and with social transformation" (p. 8). Historical representations of women's social movements articulate them to groups of grotesques (see Douglas, 1994, e.g., about the use of grotesque imagery in descriptions of second-wave feminists), and, Russo adds, "we may begin a long list which would add to these curiosities and freaks whose conditions and attributes which link these types with contemporary social and sexual deviances, and more seemingly ordinary female trouble with processes and body parts: illness, aging, reproduction, nonreproduction, secretions, lumps, bloating, wigs, scars, make-up and prostheses" (p. 14).

However, she argues that precisely because of contemporary feminism's failure to truly incorporate the grotesque—to be at peace with it—feminism has become what she believes is a politically exclusive movement that may be in danger of narrowing itself into irrelevance for vast numbers of women. To extend Russo's argument, we suggest that recoding the grotesque and its abject qualities as positive moves feminism away from the postfeminist dimension of the gyniatric apparatus.

6. Figert (1996) notes that the damaging stereotypes of women associated with PMS can be found in discussions of women and their menstrual cycles since ancient Greek times. She points out that more recent discussions of PMS have focused on remedying PMS symptoms so that women can return to their rightful place as stabilizers of their homes and families, and can get back to doing any wage labor that might be expected of them. In other words, PMS— and its female sufferers—are viewed as disruptors of the social, familial, and even economic order (pp. 8–10).

7. Like so many pharmaceutical ads in print media, Eli Lilly's name is nowhere to be found in the text of the ad; it appears only at the bottom of the following page, along with the pagelong list of possible side effects and cautions.

8. See Rivers (1996, chap. 3) for a discussion about men reporting PMS-like symptoms in themselves—as long as they are not referred to as PMS symptoms.

9. As of 2004, Seasonale advertisements began to appear regularly on both network and cable television.

10. However, its use may cause breast cancer to spread, according to a recent study (Center for Science in the Public Interest, 2003).

11. Interestingly, this same Web site includes information about Remifemin, stating that it is one of the commercialized preparations for black cohosh root. The numerous other commercial preparations of it listed from a Google search are not displayed on this page of the National Institute of Health's (NIH) Web site.

12. This labyrinth has become even more difficult to navigate with the news that HRT trials have revealed that replacing lost estrogen with synthetic estrogen and other hormone blends can have serious side effects, such as conditions leading to stroke and heart disease. Thus, Remifemin's play for second-wave feminists may not be necessary as more women—feminism-sympathetic and otherwise—look to non-HRT treatments for their menopause symptoms.

References

Bunton, R. (1997). Popular health, advanced liberalism, and *Good Housekeeping* magazine. In A. Petersen & R. Bunton (Eds.), *Foucault: Health and medicine* (pp. 223–248). New York: Routledge.

Center for Science in the Public Interest. (2003, October). Black cohosh warning. *Nutrition Action Healthletter*, p. 7.

Deleuze, G. (1988). *Foucault* (S. Hand, Trans.). Minneapolis: University of Minnesota Press.

Deleuze, G. (1988). Foldings, or the inside of thought (subjectivation). In G. Deleuze (Ed.), *Foucault* (pp. 94–123). Minneapolis: University of Minnesota Press.

Deleuze, G. (1992). What is a dispositif? In T. J. Armstrong (Trans.), *Michel Foucault: Philosopher* (pp. 159–168). New York: Routledge.

Douglas, S. J. (1994). *Where the girls are: Growing up female with the mass media.* New York: Times Books.

Figert, A. E. (1996). *Women and the ownership of PMS.* New York: de Gruyter.

Foucault, M. (1995). *Discipline and punish: The birth of the prison* (2nd ed.) (A. Sheridan, Trans.). New York: Vintage.

Foucault, M. (1991a). Governmentality. (R. Braidotti, Trans.). In G. Burchell, C. Gordon, & P. Miller (Eds.), *The Foucault effect: Studies in governmentality* (pp. 87–104). Chicago: University of Chicago Press.

Foucault, M. (1991b). Politics and the study of discourse. (C. Gordon, Trans.). In G. Burchell, C. Gordon, & P. Miller (Eds.), *The Foucault effect: Studies in governmentality* (pp. 53–72). Chicago: University of Chicago Press.

Foucault, M. (1990). *The history of sexuality. Vol. 1: An introduction* (R. Hurley, Trans.). New York: Vintage.

Goldman, R., Heath, D., & Smith, S. (1991). Commodity feminism. *Critical Studies in Mass Communication, 8*(3), 333–351.

Gordon, C. (1991). Governmental rationality: An introduction. In G. Burchell, C. Gordon, & P. Miller (Eds.), *The Foucault effect: Studies in governmentality* (pp. 1–51). Chicago: University of Chicago Press.

Graham, L. (1997). Beyond manipulation: Lillian Gilbreth's industrial psychology and the governmentality of women consumers. *Sociological Quarterly, 38,* pp. 539–566. Retrieved April 22, 2003, from Expanded Academic Index database.

Greene, R. W. (2002). Rhetorical pedagogy as a postal system: Circulating subjects through Michael Warner's "publics and counterpublics." *Quarterly Journal of Speech, 88,* 434–443.

Greene, R. W. (1999). *Malthusian worlds: U.S. leadership and the governing of the population crisis.* Boulder: Westview.

Habermas, J. (1984) *The Theory of Communicative Action, Vol 1: Reason and the Rationalisation of Society.* London: Heinemann

Hardt, M., & Negri, A. (2001). *Empire.* Cambridge, MA: Harvard University Press.

National Institute of Health (2003). Questions and answers about black cohosh and the symptoms of menopause Retrieved June 25, 2005, from http://___.nih.gov/factsheets/blackcohosh.html.

Rapp, R. (1987). Is the legacy of second-wave feminism postfeminism? *Socialist Review, 18*(1), 31–37.

Rivers, C. (1996). *Slick spins and fractured facts: How cultural myths distort the news.* New York: Columbia University Press.

Russo, M. (1994). *The female grotesque: Risk, excess, and modernity.* New York: Routledge.

Stein, R. (2003, March 10–16). Liberation or manipulation? A controversial drug that suppresses menstruation is close to FDA approval. *Washington Post* (National Weekly Edition), p. 31.

Vavrus, M. D. (2002). *Postfeminist news: Political women in media culture.* Albany: State University of New York Press.

Vedantam, S. (2001, May 7–13). What's in a name? A controversy rages over the marketing of Prozac as a new drug for a women's disorder. *Washington Post* (National Weekly Edition), p. 31.

Warren, C. A. (2001). *Poison blood.* Unpublished manuscript.

Warren, C. A. (2002). *The toxic (and inconvenient) female body: The new medical campaign against menstruation.* Unpublished manuscript.

6

Productive Bodies

Women, Work, and Depression

KRISTIN A. SWENSON

Butler University

You took my joy; I want it back.

—Lucinda Williams

DEPRESSION AS A MODERN PHENOMENON is culturally constructed primarily as a feminine malady. According to the Prozac Web site, the prime risk factors for depression include having low self-esteem, anxiety, and feeling that life is out of control, all qualities commonly associated with women.[1] Another risk factor is the biological workings of the female body itself, including menstruation, pregnancy, childbirth, and menopause. Not only is the female body a cause and a site for depression, but the multiple roles of parent, spouse, employee, and homemaker contribute to women being twice as likely as men to experience clinical depression.[2]

Antidepressants such as Prozac claim to regulate the chemical makeup of the brain to alter the depressed person's affective being.[3] Reversing the symptoms of lethargy, Prozac is described often as a "productivity" drug that transforms the medicated depressed person into an energetic, enthusiastic, and productive subject (see Metzl, 2003). Prozac and other antidepressants are prescribed for the production of an individual who is able to keep pace with the multiple roles required of contemporary women today. The traditional roles of married women have always included housework and primary child-rearing responsibilities, as well as lesser-acknowledged affective roles, such as the maintenance of interpersonal and social relationships. In the last 50 years, married women's roles have expanded to include not only an active social and family life, but also the demands of balancing wage and home labor. The predominance of depression in women and their use of antidepressants link the female body, work, and affective personal and social relations to the requirements of productivity in a postindustrial economy. The confluence of these factors presents us with a privileged site from which to seek an understanding of cultural, social, and economic production today.

The mass movement of women into wage labor coincides with the onslaught of modern psychotropic medication. In the early 1950s, antidepressants were discovered when serotonin was linked to emotional function and in 1952 the American Psychiatric Association published the first *Diagnostic and Statistical Manual* (DSM). In 1955, Miltown, the first mass-marketed tranquilizer, became widely available and prescribed (see Solomon, 2001; Metzl, 2003). Simultaneously, in the 1950s a significant increase of married and older women entered the paid labor force as part-time workers.[4] This confluence of events altered the entire terrain of work: who was working, where they worked, the length of the workday, and the forms of socialization occurring in the workplace.

The first generation of psychotropic medication treated symptoms of anxiety in women whose primary role was that of a housewife. As more women moved into paid labor, both the symptoms and treatment of depression changed to reflect the shifting affective and daily experiences of women. Depression, previously dominated by symptoms of anxiety and restlessness, was later redefined by symptoms of listlessness, sadness, and melancholy. In early advertisements of psychotropic medications, women appeared angry, aggressive, and agitated. A 1965 advertisement for Valium presented a large image of an aggressive woman with her jaw clammed shut, her teeth exposed, her eyes squinting with hostility, and her brow furrowed in obvious agitation. Under the heading, "Reduce psychic tension" the text proclaims, "Symptoms of psychic tension, anxiety or depression are often intermingled and rarely appear as separate, distinct elements" (*American Journal of Psychiatry*, 1965, pp. xii–xiii, reprinted in Metzl, 2003, p. 16). This historic moment categorized women's symptoms of depression as comprising both anxiety and melancholy. In the first DSM (1952) under the heading "depressive reaction," anxiety is the first symptom mentioned prior to connecting it with other symptoms of depression (pp. 33–34). In contrast, a recent ad for the duel antianxiety and antidepressant drug, Zoloft, portrays a crying egglike figure with a rain cloud overhead. Affirming one's feelings of depression, the text reads, "You know when you feel the weight of sadness. You may feel exhausted, hopeless, and anxious. Whatever you do, you feel lonely and don't enjoy the things you once loved." This ad demonstrates that the symptoms of anxiety are subordinated to those of depression. This inversion suggests an alteration not only in a shift of affective symptoms but also a historical transformation in the experience of the depressed. With tranquilizers such as Miltown and later Valium, the agitated, threatening, and discontented woman was sedated to keep her in the proper role of mother, homemaker, and wife. With antidepressants, the depressed is uplifted and energized to maintain her productivity in all her roles from wage earner to caretaker.

The medical treatment of depression was transformed by the social changes in the labor force, essentially targeting female workers as the main market for antidepressants. As the workplace incorporated women, and the responsibilities of work was not just to perform job tasks, but also to fulfill requirements that previously existed only in the social sphere, the workplace had also to incorporate a particular form of subjectivity embodied in the medicated depressed woman. As a result, depression can be understood as productive for capital in two ways at once: first, through the pharmaceutical industry, in the production and consumption of chemical treatments; and second, through the production of new forms of subjectivity. I contend that the depressive, by caring for the self through medication, has become the ideal productive worker in the now feminized sphere of paid work.

This chapter argues that the relation between women, work, and depression reveals the changing status of work; the process by which women have been incorporated into wage labor; how labor has altered to reflect feminine characteristics; and the form of self-governance required to participate in today's labor force. To this end, I briefly discuss Michel Foucault's (1990) concept of a "discipline society" and Gilles Deleuze's (1995) notion of a "control society" to understand the historical shift in work from the production of goods to the production of services. Next, the Marxist political theorist Antonio Negri (1992) is deployed for his argument that explains how collective social moments are subsumed by capital over time. The history of predominantly White married women's entrance into the labor force in the 1950s demonstrates the process by which women and their qualities—including depression—were subsumed into wage labor. These qualities are then "put to work" and are now considered the primary requirements for today's employee as illustrated through a reading of the highly rated reality television show *The Apprentice*. In today's labor force, depression encourages a form of self-governance that is the kernel of the subjective experience of both men and women in contemporary professional work.

Governmentality and the Affect of Contemporary Work

The process by which women in the United States entered the paid labor force in post-World War II America exemplifies Foucault's (1990) notion of biopower. The control of life through intensified form of power and politics is defined in two ways: first, through the formation of "the body as a machine" (p. 139) that is disciplined accordingly to produce certain results; and second, the body is formed and understood as a biological entity that can be organized through the control of life, death, health, and "all the conditions that can cause these to vary" (p. 139). The first of these deals with the body at the level of capital (biopower) and the second with the body at the level of the state (biopolitics).[5] Foucault's disciplinary society locates sites of discipline in various institutions including the family, the school, the factory, the hospital, and the prison, each with its own set of rules and organization of time, space, and movement. Foucault recognizes that capitalism "would not have been possible without the controlled insertion of bodies into the machinery of production and the adjustment of the phenomena of populations to economic processes" (p. 141). This is evident in the feminization of the labor force in which the movement of the female population into wage labor both produces, and is the result of, new forms of discipline that correspond to this historical transformation.

Deleuze (1995) argues that with the increase of rapid technological advances beginning after World War II, the world saw a shift in emphasis from a society of discipline to a society of control. Deleuze articulates the difference between discipline and control with the difference between *molds* and *modulations*. In a disciplinary society the factory disciplines the individual; in a control society, there is no mass mold, but rather a process of continual "remolding" without a set or static pattern. The difference is a change in *quantity* to *quality* and from *effect* to *affect*. Discipline works on the body to effectuate a particular model of being, while control works *through* the body by modulating affectations. As Deleuze explains, "Disciplinary man produced energy in discrete amounts, while control man undulates, moving among a continuous range of different orbits" (p. 180). This alteration in the primary formulation of work leads to a shift in the forms of self-governance. The primary requirement of flexibility in the contemporary workforce reflects how a system of control relies on affective relations rather than explicit commands to organize behavior in both the social and economic realm.

In Antonio Negri's (1992) essay, "Twenty Theses on Marx: Interpretation of the Class Situation Today," he argues that transformations in the mode of production occur in response to large-scale collective movements. Each transformation is a result of a process whereby social relations and cooperation create new forms of experience and existence that capital responds to by creating new processes of valuation. Negri's argument is this: Capital never changes on its own. History is always a relation between labor and capital where capital reflects new movements in the labor force. In response to the events of May 1968, he argues that "capital has followed this revolutionary force, it has repressed it, it has sought to close it off in new technical dimensions of production and command" (p. 157). Negri is arguing that the events of May 1968 in France, as well as corresponding movements throughout Europe and the United States, reflect a qualitative change in the relation between labor and capital. As a result of the social movements of the late 1960s, the form of value, or the formal way in which capital is capable of producing surplus-value, has changed to include functions that previously existed primarily in social relations. This form of response to a social movement, as opposed to a workers' movement, represents Negri's account of the rise of biopower as the subsumption of social relations and specifically the affective experiences of individuals, into capitalist production and exploitation.

The formulation that Negri (1992) explains, that is, that capital subsumed the revolutionary social movements of 1968 with the creation of a new form of production, helps to explain how a social and personal experience such as the change in the quality of depression in women can be made productive for capital during this time. Negri's account overemphasizes the importance of collectively organized social movements and neglects the "subtle revolution"[6] in daily life. In either case, the workings of capital have arguably changed to incorporate these mundane social relations into the new and quickly advancing forms of technological production. This is the process that Negri, following Marx, refers to as real subsumption. Even with his inclusion of the social revolutions in the 1960s, Negri's Marxism privileges the proletariat as the prime movers of history. This type of Marxism, while privileging the relations of human labor, systematically neglects the mundane aspects of everyday life, especially the feminine sphere of social labor.[7] For example, capital subsumed social relations in the 1950s as employers opened their doors to women as part-time laborers, not because of a revolutionary movement, but rather because of the banal existence of consumer demand. While Marxism is unable to recognize the importance of this sphere of social relations, capital, on the other hand, readily acknowledges it.

The Feminization of Labor

Jessica Weiss (2000) explains that the decrease in the labor force preceding World War II is the condition that permitted older and married women to enter into wage labor. The low birthrates during the Great Depression resulted in a decreased labor supply in the 1950s. The labor force was further affected as women began to marry earlier and left paid labor for unpaid labor. In response, employers, in need of workers, relaxed their policy of hiring single women only and began to employ married women. Employers were willing to make part-time work available, accommodating married women with school-aged children. As women entered the paid labor force and as the need for laborers increased after World War II, hiring requirements altered to include the female worker and capital accommodated the lifestyles of married women to benefit the ends of production.

Capitalism accommodated life to meet the needs of production by subsuming human relations into its fold. In this sense, employers "cooperated" with the lives of married women in the form of part-time labor, allowing women to continue their social roles as mother and spouse. "In every moment of the development of the capitalist mode of production," argues Negri (1992), "capital has always proposed the form of cooperation" (p. 154). However to produce productive labor, Negri continues, "this form had to be functional with the form of exploitation" (p. 154). Hiring married women as part-time workers exploited their labor with substandard pay and an absence of benefits. Corporations cooperated with the existing social relations of women's primary roles as mothers and wives by offering the flexibility of part-time labor to accommodate labor needs while maintaining traditional forms of exploitation. Capital does not only respond to collective social movements; but more important, capital is *always* responding to the real social experiences of living labor.

Jane Jenson, Elisabeth Hagen, and Ceallaigh Reddy (1988) explain that as the services sector increased in economic importance along with the availability of part-time work, more employment opportunities were available for women and many middle-class married women became active participants in wage labor (pp. 5–6). Women's participation in the labor force and their relation to work was different from that of the traditional male worker. Women entered into and out of the paid labor force throughout their life cycle because most middle-class women quit work when they wed and reentered the workforce when their children were school-age or when the family desired additional income to purchase consumer items including the new technological household appliances (Weiss, 2000).

Howard Kaltenborn at the 1957 National Manpower Council meeting explained the rationale behind hiring married women:

> These older women, as a group, constitute the least effectively utilized sector of our working population. [We] will [have] to employ them in increasing numbers in business, industry, and government in order to meet the nation's manpower needs and to insure the continued prosperity and growth of our national economy. (cited in Blackwelder, 1997, p. 161)

Kaltenborn recognized that married women were an untapped paid labor force and could be subsumed readily into labor, exploited as part-time wage earners. The recognition that this previously untapped source for wage labor was ripe for exploitation was not lost on employers. As the National Manpower Council advocated the hiring of female laborers for part-time work, its members touted the benefits of hiring married part-time workers by explaining that they could easily be laid off during an economic downturn and rehired during growth periods. Part-time work and flexible work schedules exploited the previously untapped female labor force while saving employers a significant amount in wages and benefits (see Blackwelder, 1997, pp. 162–163).[8]

During the 1960s the number of wage earning women increased from "23 million to well over 31 million, and female labor force participation increased from 37.7% to 43.3%" (Blackwelder, 1997, p. 177). Women entered the wage-earning labor force in increasing numbers, but unlike the 1950s, middle-class and working-class mothers maintained a constant relationship to wage labor, and many, including mothers with infants and toddlers, accepted full-time employment (see Blackwelder, 1997; Jenson et al., 1988). During the 1960s and 1970s, the labor demand expanded and women continued to fill the needs of the growing economic and services industry. Regardless of class and family status, more women were seeking employment out of economic need as the cost of living continued to rise. By the 1970s, the services industry surpassed manufacturing and by the 1980s services-sector jobs accounted for 65% of the national income (Blackwelder, 1997, p. 6). The labor market was in continual need of services-sector employees and because services positions were traditionally segregated as women's work, and as women's financial status required the necessity to earn a wage to support themselves and to contribute to their families, women were further ingrained into the labor force.

In the 1980s the economic downturn affected the labor force in its entirety. As Jenson et al. (1988) explain, the expanse of global capital on the world market shifted the economic structures of advanced industrialized countries. "The link between mass production and stable demand collapsed in the face of a process of increasing internalization of capitalism and interpenetration of domestic economies by one another" (p. 9). The effects of the ebbs and flows within global capital resulted in a significantly altered labor force. In the face of recession, businesses responded by downsizing, cutting costs by turning full-time labor into part-time labor, stagnating wages, and replacing human bodies with new technologies. Businesses drastically altered their structure by shortening product production time and increasing flexibility in response to an unpredictable global market (see Blackwelder, 1997, p 206; Jenson et al., 1988, pp. 9–10).

Peter S. Albin and Eileen Appelbaum (1988) explain that in the unstable 1980s economy, temporary work began to replace both full-time and part-time work. Although the proportion of female part-time laborers had remained constant since the late 1970s, "the part-time employment of women [became] increasingly involuntary" (p. 148) as women who had previously had full-time positions were now redirected to part-time work. Moreover, "involuntary part-time employment of women, which accounted for 12% of part-time workers in 1970, counted for 22% by 1986" (p. 148). Although part-time employment paralleled "the expansion of traditional service industries, the growth of temporary employment . . . outpaced the American economy as a whole" by the late 1980s (p. 148). In addition, with the intensification of computers and newly developing rapid communication systems, the labor force altered as large companies that at one time employed a significant amount of full-time employees, began maintaining a "core" of full-time employees, supplemented with temporary laborers (p. 149). These temporary laborers were disposed of at the whim of the economy, not unlike the part-time female laborers of the 1950s.

In this precarious and volatile economy, the laborers who possessed traditional female characteristics were the most likely to survive. In this new economy, an employable employee needed to be flexible, open to change, able to keep up with rapidly altering communication systems, while navigating the rocky terrain of global capital. Emily Martin (1994, 1995) articulates that the physical body of the worker, and the organizational system of the corporation, must both be "flexible." She (1995) writes, "The successful and ideal organization is no longer a monolithic, hierarchical bureaucracy but a fleeting, fluid network of alliances with great organizational flexibility" (p. 225). The worker must be "innovative, flexible, whole in mind and body, nimbly managing a multitude of relationships and circumstances to maintain a vigorous state of health" (p. 225). Women's traditional ebbing and flowing in and out of the labor force, their ability to multitask and manage wage labor while managing the "second shift" at home, along with their agility in riding the waves of employment opportunities by accepting part-time and temporary labor, positioned women as the most qualified employee. The labor force has further subsumed women, their qualities, characteristics, and social relations while deepening their relation to capital and intensifying their exploitation.

Donna Haraway (1991) explains the restructuring of work "as both literally female and feminized, whether performed by men or women" (p. 166). Harraway explains:

> To be feminized means to be made extremely vulnerable; able to be disassembled, reassembled, exploited as a reserve labor force; seen less as workers than servers; subjected to time arrangements on and off the paid job that make a mockery of a limited work day; leading an existence that always borders on being obscene, out of place, and reducible to sex. (p. 166)

This feminization required of the postindustrial professional worker is reminiscent of the traditionally feminine roles of mother, wife, homemaker, and caretaker, only now this intensification of feminization applies to work itself.

It is with much irony that the first season of Donald Trump's reality show, *The Apprentice* (Burnett & Trump, 2004), with its feared words "you're fired," was rated the number one show during our most recent economic downturn. *The Apprentice* presents a hyperbolic example of the demands of the contemporary workforce along with the flexibility required of today's professional worker. In each episode, two teams are given a task to complete and the team that completes the task most successfully wins for the week and is thereby temporarily relieved of the possibility of being "fired." Mirroring the structure of the professional workforce, with its use of organized teams rather than individual job positions, each team developed a name for their so-called corporation: Versacorp and Protégé. With each task, the team elected a project manager that both directed the team and was held responsible for its success or failure. The project manager of the losing team selected two team members to accompany him or her into the "boardroom" for possible termination. The team members then had to defend their performance and answer to Trump and his two associates' scathing comments. Trump would then fire one of the three team members present. The show proceeded accordingly for 13 weeks until a winner was selected. The "winner" was then awarded the opportunity to work for one year as president of one of Trump's companies.

These 13 weeks of work and competition are organized as entertainment in the form of reality television. Nonetheless, the "real life" outcome—the "opportunity to work"—differed from other reality competitions in which the winner leaves with a cash payment and ostensibly the possibility of *not* having to work.[9] This show exhibited both the active participation in work tasks as they exist in contemporary corporate America and, because of its competitive component, makes a statement as to the form and quality of contemporary professional work and the form and quality required of the worker who is to succeed in today's economy. Each week the contestants were required to perform divergent tasks that ran the gamut from selling lemonade on the streets of New York City, to negotiating with known celebrities for a fund-raising event, to renovating and renting a New York apartment. Notably, the tasks are not representative of the job position for which the candidates would be "applying"; rather the tasks themselves are immaterial. The team and candidates that succeeded were those that best demonstrated the qualities of the postindustrial worker. That is to say, it is not that a candidate can *do any particular thing,* but rather that the candidate is flexible enough to *do anything.* Particular skills were not required; instead, what was necessary was the ability to develop affective relationships both inside and outside of work. In the case of *The Apprentice,* the social adeptness or ineptness of the candidates was illustrated not only during the workday, but also in the required communal living arrangement. Work does not end.

The teams were initially divided by gender. Choosing a corporate name was the fist task of each team. The name Protégé Corporation recognized the objective and role of each candidate in her relationship to Donald Trump. The name Versacorp recognized the versatility and flexibility that both corporations and their employees must embody. The teams and their members were required to move easily from one set of tasks to the next, from one skill set to another, and were to adapt quickly to unpredictable changes and opportunities. This quick adaptation required the potential employees to use all of their resources including their material bodies. Although, presenting some ethical concerns to both the teams and the audience, the contestants readily sexualized and racialized their bodies to complete the job tasks. For example, whether taking the opportunity to use one's sexual qualities to sell alcohol at Planet Hollywood, as the women were accused of doing, or to capitalize on one's gender and race by presenting oneself as a famous athlete, as an

African American man was accused of, the strategy was similar in kind: the candidates employed the resources they had available, including their marked material bodies and the opportunities to exploit them. The candidates also had to shift language codes quickly. In one task, the teams had to sell their choice of goods at the flea market whereas the following task required the candidates to negotiate with celebrities. One candidate misread the codes of conduct in her celebrity meeting by insisting that the celebrity spend four days with the highest auction bidder, which mortified her team and led one member to accuse her of being "a loose cannon." When the candidates had been whittled down to the four, they were each formally interviewed by four of Trump's high-level employees and most trusted advisors. Their conclusions to each candidate are telling: Kwame's perceived low energy was a concern; Nick had charisma and could sell a product but no one believed that he had anything more to contribute to the corporation; Bill was well liked and successfully defended himself for not having an MBA; and Amy, the sole woman who had made it to the final four, was reported by one advisor as "boring to talk to" and resembling a "Stepford wife"; sexism is obviously not dead. Importantly, just because work requires feminine characteristics, this does not imply that "women win." In this new feminized sphere, a show such as *The Apprentice* demonstrates that although work is feminized, feminine characteristics, when exhibited by women, may still carry a negative connotation. This is exemplified by the numerous moments in which the socialization of women was portrayed as "cattiness," "bitchiness," and "competitiveness," whereas similar traits exhibited by men was characterized positively as an example of leadership qualities.

In the final week of competition, Bill and Kwame each constructed a team of former candidates to work under their supervision. Bill was given the task of successfully executing a national golf tournament. Kwame was challenged with the task of successfully managing and executing a pop concert event. While both candidates and their teams succeed in their projects, Bill was ultimately selected as "The Apprentice." Although both candidates were definitely qualified, their differences are significant. Kwame represented the traditional, Ivy League MBA candidate; he was the quintessential "corporate man" in the best sense.[10] In contrast, Bill had what he referred to as "entrepreneurial blood" and was openly enthused and flexible. Kwame, on the other hand, was perceived as not taking opportunities when they arose. This was demonstrated when Kwame did not break what he thought were the rules, and therefore he made the "mistake" of not taking the *opportunity* to terminate a team member who was sabotaging his performance and frustrating other team members. Kwame was perceived as too hands-off; whereas although Bill and his overt enthusiasm may have at times annoyed his team, he was reviewed positively and completed the tasks with fewer mishaps and fewer significant teammate problems.

The conclusion one can draw from *The Apprentice* is that the requirements that were originally demanded from women as part-time labor are now pervasive in contemporary work. This feminization of labor does not result in better working conditions for women, but rather new working conditions for everyone. The effects of a feminized labor force—a labor force that is unstable, flexible, amorphous, ungrounded, and based on service and social relationships—is a labor force in which new sentiments appear as workers strive to maintain some footing on a ground that is continually slipping away.

Feminine Qualities Put to Work

Paolo Virno (1996), in an essay titled, "The Ambivalence of Disenchantment," deftly identifies the affective qualities that today's worker must embody, and the process by which these qualities are both acquired prior to entering the labor force while being simultaneously subsumed into the labor force itself. This process demonstrates, once again, the "cooperation" of capital with social relations to appropriate and exploit life as it is lived: biopower's production of life.

The primary qualities of the wage laborer include the ability to be habitually multitasking; the capability to keep pace with rapid conversions (e.g., software updates); the skill of adaptability in every enterprise; the flexibility of shifting from one set of rules to another; the facility for a multiplicity of language games; a command of the rapid flow of information and communication; and, finally, the dexterity to successfully navigate within the realm of "limited possible alternatives" (Virno, 1996, p. 14). Importantly, Virno argues that "these qualifications are not products of industrial discipline as much as results of a socialization that has its center of gravity *outside of the workplace*" (p. 14, emphasis in original). As was illustrated in *The Apprentice*, the candidates were not selected because of expertise in the field in which they were going to work, but instead, because of general social skills that are acquired prior to specific professional training. Virno continues to argue that this is "a socialization punctuated by discontinuous and modular experiences, by fashion, by the interpretation of the media, and by the indecipherable *ars combinatoria* of the metropolis intertwining itself in sequences of fleeting opportunities" (p. 14). This is a double movement for Virno. On one hand, the process of socialization, the process of experiencing the self and the world "appears independent of production outside the initiatory rituals of the factory and the office" (p. 14–15). On the other hand, the "continuous change in the organization of labor *has subsumed* the complex of inclinations, dispositions, emotions, vices, and virtues that mature precisely in a socialization outside of the workplace" (p. 15, emphasis in original). In this shift from a disciplinary society to a control society, the site of the workplace no longer "molds" the body into performance; rather, the workplace itself has mutated to absorb the affectations of social relationships that mature prior to work.

The subjectivity of today's wage earner is constituted by the ambivalence generated through the blurred spheres of work and life, and thus by the deteriorating ability of work to ground the subject. Because work now occupies the entire field of social relations and because the subjectivities that are productive for capital are characteristically feminine, then the sicknesses associated with femininity are absorbed by capital as well. Stated simply, those aspects of life that have traditionally been experienced outside and prior to work are now a requirement for work itself. The relation between women, depression, antidepressant medications, and work reveal tensions between the dominant form of subjectivity—the flexible feminized worker—and the form of capitalist organization.

Jonathan Michel Metzl (2003) explores the proliferation of psychotropic medication and its relation to traditional gender roles in print advertisements and psychological journals from 1955 through 2002. He aptly notes, "The process whereby—unlike most other types of medications—psychotropic medications become connected with both curing disease and maintaining certain specific notions of gender roles is a mechanism of action that evolved over the latter half of the twentieth century" (p. 12). Significantly, as the number of women entering the labor force after World War II increased, psychotropic drugs entered common cultural parlance. Metzl argues that with the shift toward psychotropic drugs and away from psychoanalysis, "women were assumed to be the source of an epidemic of 'cultural anxiety,'" and in psychotropic drugs such as Miltown, "culture found its restorative cure" (p. 27). With psychotropics women were kept content and in their place as the traditional mother and spouse regardless of their new subject position as wage earner.

In the 1960s and 1970s, as women were gaining more power in the workforce and fought to alter the patriarchal social structure, psychotropic pharmaceuticals were advertised to calm down angry and irate feminists who would rock the social boat demanding equality in wages and opportunity. A 1965 ad in the *American Journal of Psychiatry* offered Valium as a panacea for women who were tense and frustrated, "With adjunctive support from Valium, . . . patients generally find life more bearable despite continued situational problems." The advertisement also claims that Valium was found "effective in controlling tension-associated symptoms such as insomnia restlessness and other psychic and somatic complaints" while also aiding the patient's ability to "withstand the stress and strain of environmental pressures" (ad reprinted in Metzl, 2003, p. 16). While social injustice may have been the cause of women's frustrations and anxieties, their condition was articulated as pathological, and psychotropic medication was the remedy prescribed to cure their restlessness and agitation.

Early psychotropic drugs such as Miltown and Valium were drugs of sedation and attempted to produce sedate women who did not complain about their social or work roles. Drugs such as Valium were advertised as calming tonics whose purpose was to sooth and quiet the unsettled, restless, and discontented woman. In a 1970 Valium advertisement, the single woman of 35 was diagnosed as "psychoneurotic." Jan, the "35, single and psychoneurotic" female in the advertisement, is described as one of the many "unmarrieds with low self-esteem." Valium was the prescribed cure for the subjective position of singleness and helped to relieve the "emotional 'storms' of psychoneurotic tension and the depressive symptoms that can go hand-in-hand with it" (ad reprinted in Metzl, 2003, p. 148).

This hypothetical Jan crossed the traditional expectations of femininity not only by not getting married, but also for not being "marryable" and would come to realize that her dissatisfaction is her fault and her fault alone. Jan would be drugged into submission to conform to the traditional standards of her day, not only the social relations of coupling, but we can also imagine that Jan, without a husband and as a mature single woman, must support herself. Jan takes her depression into the workplace, and while depression like other sickness could be understood as a detriment to productivity, with psychotropic medication, Jan is able to go to work and not just be present, but be productive and content with her constricted role. Even at this historic moment, Jan's diagnosis as being "sick" places the blame squarely onto herself rather than on external social and economic limitations. She is culturally constructed as pathological because of her deviance from the prescribed social roles of her time. Jan is given Valium to calm her discontent, to maintain the status quo, and most importantly, to produce her subjectivity as quietly productive. To be clear, even Jan is being calmed of her anxiety and the agitation her particular role in society produced; her status as a medicated depressive still produces her as an affective body that meets the needs of the workplace. As society and the economy shift and change over time so will both the symptoms and narrations of women's depression.

Depression, unlike other illnesses, turns the subject against herself. In Friedrich Nietzsche's (1996), *On the Genealogy of Morals*, he eloquently describes depression as "a feeling of physiological inhibition" (p. 109). This definition describes the inability of the body to move, to produce, to be of use. The depressed body is "listless" and experiences a "certain fatigue and inertia" (p. 108–109). Depression differs, notes Nietzsche, from other illnesses in that the depressed are directed toward self-blame and the burden of healing is placed on them. Whereas in other forms of sickness one may blame an external force, with depression "you alone are to blame," states Nietzsche; "you alone are to blame for yourself!" (p. 104). This self-blame leads to feelings of guilt and shame, which in turn directs the depressed toward an orientation of the self "an intro-spective turn to their *ressentiment.*"[1] This turn toward self-resentment and blame is employed, argues Nietzsche, in order to "*exploit* the bad instincts of all the suffering to the end of self-discipline, self-surveillance, self-overcoming" (p. 107, emphasis in original). Hence, the instinct toward self-resentment is fallacious in that it leads to disciplining one's own behavior and actions; it produces self-monitoring and self-assessment; and encourages that one "get over" one's self, that the depressed de-press their listless physiologically inhibited bodies. This is an important move: First, the depressed are responsible for both their illness and its cure, turning the depressed subject into its own object. Second, this move releases external forces from any agency or cause of depression. In sum, the depressed are the reason for their illness and the agent of its "cure." There is no external blame directed outward toward social conditions or forces; rather, the self is the originator of sickness and as such, the self must discipline and govern itself appropriately.

Traditionally, work in a disciplinary society was often the cure prescribed for depression. One form of self-discipline that the depressed were encouraged to perform is labor, and specifically, mechanical labor. "There is absolutely no doubt," states Nietzsche (1996), "that it brings considerable relief to a life of suffering: this state of affairs is nowadays called, somewhat dishonestly, the 'blessing of work'" (p. 112). Mechanical labor and all of its attendants provide:

> absolute regularity, absolute and unconscious obedience, a way of life which has been determined once and for all, time which is fully occupied, a permitted degree of 'impersonality,' even a disciplining with a view towards impersonality, towards the forgetting of the self. (p. 112)

Work is the prescribed remedy for the listless body. Mechanical labor disciplines the body through external forces and produces the body as a cog in the wheel of production. This is most reminiscent of a disciplinary society in an industrial economy; work is mechanical work and the remedy for depression is to "lose oneself" in work. Thus, depression itself *works* to discipline and govern the self in the production of work. Capital is served on two fronts at once: the production of a working subject produced through a disciplining of the self, and the production of a working subject that views work as a means of becoming healthy through the lose of the self.

While depression has increased since 1955 for both sexes, the forms of labor that developed during the same period no longer provided relief from depression in the manner that Nietzsche (1996) describes. This new form of labor replaced "absolute regulatory" with the management of fluid relations, and as such, depression altered to reflect the change in both the economy and social relations. In 1992 the *New York Times* reported on the first international study of major depression. The study found that the possibility of experiencing depression is three times higher for people born after 1955 than their grandparent's generation (Goleman, 1992). This depression is described as not just feelings of sadness, "but a paralyzing listlessness, dejection and self-deprecation, as well as an overwhelming sense of hopelessness" (p. C1). This increase in depression is consistent with the increase of work-related disability claims attributed to depression. According to an analysis of MetLife's database of disability claims, depression accounted for 55% of the psychiatric claims, as reported in *Mental Health Weekly* (2003). The report noted that white-collar employees were more than twice as likely as other working populations to submit a psychiatric claim. From studies such as this, we can determine that depression is on the rise for contemporary workers and especially high in white-collar employees. Regardless of the cause of depression, more people are reporting that they meet the symptoms of a depressed person and those that seek medical assistance are being prescribed antidepressants and reporting success.

The narratives of Prozac read as libratory text. Prozac is the productivity drug that inflates the once physically inhibited body. Peter Kramer (1994) describes those on Prozac as "optimistic, decisive, quick of thought, charismatic, energetic, and confident" (pp. 16–17), all qualities required of today's wage earner. As the qualities of work are now primarily feminine and as work occupies the entire field of social relations, Jacquelyne Zita's (1998) contention that "the higher prevalence rates of depression among women can be read as a gendered function of women's over socialization into relational and interpersonal

orientations" (p. 75) is congruent with the process whereby social relations are intergraded into the sphere of work.

As workplaces increasingly operate on a more feminized model of
flexibility, multitasking, and the necessity of productive social relationships, the increase of depression is likely and documented in studies
such as those discussed earlier. Depressed people still blame themselves
for their depression, but in the age of pharmacology and advanced
biology, the depressed person can also blame his or her biological
makeup and take antidepressants to "regulate" this chemical aberration.
As depression becomes more pervasive, advertisements for depression
become less obviously gendered, although still definitely gendered. In
the Zoloft advertisement described earlier, the image presented is not
a human image, but rather an egg shaped blob that has a tear escaping
from an eye. A rain cloud follows the depressed egg. The text informs
us that depression "affects over 20 million Americans" and that "while
the cause is not known, depression may be related to an imbalance of
natural chemicals between nerve cells in the brain." The ad presents
depression as sexless and locates the cause of depression in the physical
body. While the egg itself appears sexless, eggs connote femaleness
in their relation to reproduction. Perhaps this sexless egg is the apt
expression of depression today. First it demonstrates that depression
is biological and that it is primarily centered in the femaleness of the
body. Second, because female eggs are necessary for the reproduction
of the species, we can begin to see that depression is now necessary
for the "reproduction of the conditions of production," to appropriate
Althusser's (1971) phraseology (p. 127).[12] That is to say, as work has
appropriated feminine affectivity and its attendant depression, the egg
aptly expresses that the ability to reproduce symptoms of depression
are now necessary for the reproduction of the conditions of production:
the reproduction of the conditions of depression make us all productive
for capital because we are now encouraged to medicate ourselves for
the sake of productivity.

In the DSM-IV (2000) a work-related example of depression is
presented: "a Realtor may become preoccupied with self-blame for
failing to make sales even when the market has collapsed generally
and other Realtors are equally unable to makes sales" (p. 350). While
this example focuses on an objective condition, the inability to reach a
goal, the model presented can be extended to understand the affective
condition of the depressed worker today. That is to say, that while a
depressed person may blame oneself for the objective conditions such as
the lack of making sales, this essay argues that the process of self-blame

is often extended beyond objective conditions to include the inability to manipulate or control fully the amorphous condition in which the worker is required to survive. The depressed takes on as his or her own fault the mutable, unstable status of his or her own subjectivity. This subjectivity, as has been argued, is mirrored in the model of capitalist organization of postindustrial labor. Both the environment of work, and the essential condition of the subject within it, lack stability and are defined by their fluidity, mutability, and essential lack of ground. While this condition of subjectivity and work is dominant today, the depressed blames the self for his or her lack of ground or stability in all areas of life. Therefore, the example in the DSM-IV is already dated because it suggests a concrete objective relation as the site for self-blame. This would assume that if one did get the sales or attain the goal than one would not be depressed. Today, the pervasive form of depression can be understood as literally objectless. The only stability the depressed person has is the internalization of the unstable relations in which he or she lives.[13] This condition allows for a particularly intense form of self-governance; whereas the depressed is diagnosed as "sick" he is, nevertheless, because of the self-blame for his own instability, arguably, the most willing and able worker in this economy.

Conclusion

Antidepressants in the age of a feminized labor force produce a feminine subjectivity that is productive for capital. The depressed subject is still directed toward the self—today by mass-mediated institutions—but the remedy that the self is directed toward is that offered by psychotropic pharmaceuticals. The blame for depression still lies within the individual. There is no external object to blame and because this blame is directed toward the self, it becomes a form of self-resentment, requiring the individual to seek his own treatment and to "overcome" himself; literally, to become someone else at the level of one's affective being. The shift to biopower produces a different form of governance that works through the body to alter its biological functions to produce the affects that correspond to the qualifications necessary for work. Antidepressants assist in the production and performance of affective qualities that are necessary for today's model worker, suggesting that depression can be productive, and perhaps necessary, within contemporary models of work.

The relation between depression and work continues to intensify. In a disciplinary society, the depressed were encouraged to seek refuge in mechanical labor as a means to forget one's self and therefore, one's depression. In a control society, little difference exists between the relationships at work and those in the social sphere. The ability to escape one's depression becomes nearly impossible. No longer is refuge found in forgetting that one is depressed. Through the *management* of depression, one is never able to *forget* that one is depressed. In both social and work relations, the process of continually monitoring, managing, altering, and becoming that constitutes the medicated depressed person's relationship with the self, mirroring the process in which contemporary life is lived.[14]

Notes

The author is grateful to Brynnar Swenson for the enthusiastic and ongoing discussion of the ideas presented in this chapter. The author also wishes to thank Lori Reed and Kirt H. Wilson for their comments on earlier versions of this chapter.

1. The Prozac Web site, www.prozac.com, expresses these symptoms as a sign of depression. This chapter is in no way a critique of those of us who have experienced depression nor a critique of those who have used medication to ease our depression. This chapter seeks to understand *a* relationship between women, work, and depression.

2. According to the DSM-IV-TR (2000) "Major Depressive Disorder (Single or Recurrent) is twice as common in adolescent and adult females as in adolescent and adult males" (p. 372). "Women are two to three times" more likely to experience dysthymic disorder, the most common and pervasive form of depression, than men (p. 378).

3. Importantly, other female maladies including bulimia, panic disorders, and irritable bowl syndrome are also considered affective disorders and seem to suggest that the female body is dysfunctional at the level of its affect. Recognizing the other common female affective disorders is illustrative of the point that the affect I am speaking of is not reducible to emotion, but rather is "the transduction of asignifying velocities across bodies" (Griggers, 1997, p. 111). Brian Massumi (1997), in his article "The Autonomy of Affect," notes that affect differs from emotion and that "affect is intensity," and "follows different logics and pertain to different orders" (p. 221) than emotion.

4. Women have always been a part of the labor force. Black and poor women have always worked, in both paid and unpaid labor, and have long experienced the exploitation of capital. Middle-class women have been historically called on as a paid labor force during times of economic and national crisis such as during the Great Depression and World War II. The significance of the post-World War II labor force is that married and predominately White women were still needed to meet the demands of the economic recovery.

5. I thank Brynnar Swenson for pointing me to this distinction.

6. "Subtle revolution" is a term appropriated from Ralph Smith's (1979) book, *The Subtle Revolution: Women at Work.*

7. For an account of why economics and gender exist in "different economies," and why Marxism is structurally blind to the economy of gender relations, see Gail Rubin's (1975) work, "The Traffic in Women: Notes on the 'Political Economy' of Sex."

8. This progressive move is fascinating in that it *presupposes* the feminist movement of the 1960s and 1970s. Regardless of the success or failure of this particular equal rights agenda, the movement of women entering the labor force, and capital's response to this movement, demonstrates that as early as the 1950s, with regard to White middle-class married women, capital was already recognizing the productive aspects of progressive movements. Far from resisting what will become the feminist movement, capital, by responding to the "subtle revolutions" of the transformation in women's daily experiences, is able to exploit the newly skilled yet inexpensive female laborer.

9. Interestingly, the number of applicants for the first season of *The Apprentice* exceeded those of any previous reality show according to Trump. On *Larry King Live* (April 18, 2004), Trump reported that 215,00 people applied for the first season of *The Apprentice* and 500,000 applicants were received for the second season.

10. Kwame's status as a young African American male and Bill's status as a young White male makes difficult a simple correlation between the two performances.

11. *Ressentiment* is the term that Nietzsche (1996) used to describe how the weak construct themselves through negating the strong. What is significant about his turn toward depression is that the "direction of ressentiment" (p. 106) is changed from negating an external entity and redirected toward a self-negation.

12. For an understanding of the processes of "the reproduction of the conditions of production," see Althusser's (1971) essay, "Ideology and Ideological State Apparatuses (Notes Towards an Investigation). Althusser argues that production is always already dependent on the material practices of reproduction and, like Virno (1996), these practices occur prior to work through what he coined "the ideological state apparatus." In my dissertation, I take Althusser's formulation of the ideological state apparatus further by arguing that we now have an "affective state apparatus" that works not only through ideology but also through the control of our biological affective being through such things as the so-called lifestyle drugs.

13. While this form of depression has become dominant, its symptoms have always existed, often understood as melancholy (see Freud's [1963] essay, "Mourning and Melancholia," in *General Psychological Theory*). The loss of a stable subjectivity is both made into an object and internalized in the depressed person. Judith Butler (1997) reflects on the incorporation of a lost object when she states, "If the object can no longer exist in the external world, it will then exist internally, and that internalization will be a way to . . . postpone the recognition and suffering of loss" (p. 134). Julia Kristeva (1989) put it this way: "My depression points to my not knowing how to lose—I have perhaps been unable to find a valid compensation for the loss? It follows that any loss entails the loss of my being—and of Being itself" (p. 5).

14. The goal of this chapter is to understand our current sociocultural condition. This is what Foucault and others have done in their work. This is what I believe Fredric Jameson (2004) suggests when he states, "I think it is only in the light of the study of late capitalism as a system and a mode of production that we can understand the things going on around us today . . . and understanding cultural production today is not the worst way of trying to understand that system and the possibilities it may offer for radical or even moderate change" (presented at the "End of Theory" conference at the University of Chicago and reprinted in *Critical Inquiry*, 2004).

References

Albin, P., & Appelbaum, E. (1988). The computer-rationalization of work implications for women workers. In J. Jenson, E. Hagen, C. Reddy. (Eds.), *Feminization of the labor force: Paradoxes and promises* (pp. 137–152). New York: Oxford University Press.

Althusser, L. (1971). *Lenin and philosophy and other essays.* London: New Left Books.

American Psychiatric Association, Task Force on DSM-IV. (2000). *Diagnostic and statistical manual of mental disorders: DSM-IV-TR.* Washington, DC: American Psychiatric Association.

American Psychiatric Association, Committee on Nomenclature and Statistics. (1968). *Diagnostic and statistical manual of mental disorders.* Washington, DC: American Psychiatric Association.

American Psychiatric Association, Committee on Nomenclature and Statistics. and National Conference on Medical Nomenclature. (1952). *Diagnostic and statistical manual of mental disorders.* Washington, American Psychiatric Association Mental Hospital Service.

American Psychiatric Association, Task Force on Nomenclature and Statistics, & American Psychiatric Association. Committee on Nomenclature and Statistics. (1980). *Diagnostic and statistical manual of mental disorders.* Washington, DC, American Psychiatric Association.

Blackwelder, J. K. (1997). *Now hiring: The feminization of work in the United States, 1900–1995.* College Station, TX: A&M University Press.

Burnett, M., & Trump, D. (Producers). (2004). *The apprentice* [Television series]. New York: NBC.

Butler, J. (1997). *The psychic life of power: Theories in subjection.* Stanford, CA: Stanford University Press.

Deleuze, G. (1995). *Negotiations, 1972–1990.* New York: Columbia University Press.

Depression, stress, account for much psychiatric claims. (2003, December 8). *Mental Health Weekly, 13,* pp. 42–45.

Foucault, M. (1990). *The history of sexuality.* New York: Vintage Books.

Freud, S. (1963). *General psychological theory: Papers on metapsychology.* New York: Collier.

Goleman, D. (1992, December 8). A rising cost of modernity: Depression. *The New York Times,* p. C1.

Griggers, C. (1997). *Becoming-woman.* Minneapolis: University of Minnesota Press.

Haraway, D. J. (1991). *Simians, cyborgs, and women: The reinvention of nature.* New York: Routledge.

Jameson, F. (2004). Symptoms of theory or symptoms for theory? *Critical Inquiry, 30,* 403–409.

Jenson, J., Hagen, E., & Reddy, C. (1988). *Feminization of the labor force: Paradoxes and promises.* New York: Oxford University Press.

Kramer, P. D. (1993). *Listening to Prozac.* New York: Viking.

Kristeva, J. (1989). *Black sun: Depression and melancholia* (L. S. Roudiez, Trans.). New York: Columbia University Press. (Original work published 1987)

Martin, E. (1994). *Flexible bodies: Tracking immunity in American culture from the days of polio to the age of AIDS.* Boston: Beacon.

Martin, E. (1995). Flexible bodies: Health and work in an age of systems. *The Ecologist, 25,* 221–226.

Martin, L., Gutman, H., & Hutton, P. (Eds.). (1988). *Technologies of the self: A seminar with Michel Foucault*. Amherst: University of Massachusetts Press.

Massumi, B. (1996). The autonomy of affect. In P. Patton (Ed.), *Deleuze: A critical reader* (pp. 217–239). Oxford: Blackwell.

Metzl, J. (2003). *Prozac on the couch: Prescribing gender in the era of wonder drugs*. Durham, NC: Duke University Press.

National Manpower Council. (1957). *Womanpower: A statement, with chapters by the council staff*. New York: Columbia University Press.

Negri, A. (1992). Twenty theses on Marx: Interpretation of the class situation today. *Polygraph, no. 5*, 136–170.

Nietzsche, F. W. (1996). *On the genealogy of morals: A polemic: By way of clarification and supplement to my last book, Beyond good and evil* (D. Smith, Trans.). New York: Oxford University Press.

Rubin, G. (1975). The traffic in women: Notes on the "political economy" of sex. In R. R. Reiter (Ed.), *Toward an anthropology of women* (pp. 157–210). New York, Monthly Review.

Smith, R. E. (1979). *The subtle revolution: Women at work*. Washington, DC: Urban Institute.

Solomon, A. (2001). *The noonday demon: An atlas of depression*. New York: Scribner.

Virno, P. (1996). The ambivalence of disenchantment. In P. Virno & M. Hardt (Eds.), *Radical thought in Italy: A potential politics* (pp. 13–24). Minneapolis: University of Minnesota Press.

Weiss, J. (2000). *To have and to hold: Marriage, the baby boom, and social change*. Chicago: University of Chicago Press.

Zita, J. N. (1998). *Body talk: Philosophical reflections on sex and gender*. New York: Columbia University Press.

PART III

Transnational Body Politics

7

The Pill in Puerto Rico
and Mainland United States

Negotiating Discourses of Risk and Decolonization

LAURA BRIGGS

University of Arizona

IN 1962, STEROIDAL ORAL CONTRACEPTIVES—the various versions of the Pill—were at the center of a major controversy, one that was to have far-reaching effects. A growing number of reports cited blood-clot problems among women taking the Pill, including a number of fatalities. Some were calling for the Pill to be taken off the market. The pharmaceutical companies, with the support of the U.S. Food and Drug Administration (FDA), were hesitating and arguing that the evidence linking the Pill with thromboembolism was merely circumstantial. They undoubtedly had a strong financial incentive to wait for more evidence; in 1962 Searle pharmaceutical alone had sales of $56.6 million (Reed, 1983, p. 364). Physicians were split, with a minority suggesting that the well-known carcinogenic risks of estrogen alongside the emergent problems of an apparent correlation with thromboembolism argued at least for extreme conservatism in prescribing the Pill. This state of uncertainty persisted until 1975, when researchers agreed that a by then considerably modified pill was safe for healthy, nonsmoking women younger than age 35.

This was a foundational moment for the women's health movement in the United States. The controversy over the Pill proved in retrospect to be the beginning of the end of the unchallenged authority of physicians, researchers, and the FDA to pronounce about women's health. Journalists, physicians, and patients wrote a series of books about the unrecognized and unacknowledged dangers of the Pill, with titles such as *The Bitter Pill* (Grant, 1985), *Pregnancy as a Disease* (Merkin, 1976), and *First, Do No Harm: A Dying Woman's Battle Against the Physicians and Drug Companies Who Misled Her About the Hazards of the Pill* (Greenfield, 1976). Perhaps the best-known of these books was Barbara Seaman's

(1969) *The Doctors' Case Against the Pill.* Out of this controversy activists
founded the National Women's Health Network, which was and remains
an important source of unofficial information and an organizing center
for lobbying and activism around women's health issues (McLaughlin,
1982). This controversy was joined to others: the thalidomide tragedy
of 1962, in which a tranquilizer given to pregnant women caused severe
limb deformities in their offspring, and a subsequent disaster with
another hormonal drug, DES, which was administered to pregnant
women to prevent miscarriage and later discovered to cause significant
reproductive health problems for girls born of those pregnancies.
These events together marked the beginning of a kind of women's
health activism that is still visible, for example in the legal and medical
battle over silicone breast implants (and, as Samantha King argues in
this volume, that has been co-opted in the philanthropists' campaign
for funding for breast cancer research). Ironically, as Paula Treichler
(1992) has noted, it was in and through these battles over women's
health that the FDA established regulations that AIDS activists would
work hard to undo).

I want to revisit this foundational moment and the events that led
up to it because our essential paradigms for understanding what was at
stake then are in important ways misleading. Where we have basically
suggested that it was something to do with the dispensability of "women"
as such—a lack of concern about (all) women's bodies—that allowed
researchers and physicians to encourage healthy women to use an
untried and potentially dangerous medication, this was only part of
the story. It was a struggle constructed also by the belief that many risks
could be taken with contraceptives for working-class and Third World
women, a trajectory in which First World women were in some sense
bystanders. The research on the Pill belonged to a particular cold war
moment, in which technological and scientific interventions were quite
explicitly meant to solve economic and political problems, in this case,
Third World poverty and Communism. At a time when the health risks
of estrogenic contraceptives were unknown and the argument for giving
healthy women a potent steroidal medication was quite controversial,
researchers and funders grounded the rationale for the development
of the Pill in overpopulation, the belief that Third World poverty was
caused by excessive childbearing, and that this poverty, in turn, caused
nations to "go over" to Communism. Within a few years, U.S. forces
would be distributing birth control pills in South Vietnam, even as they
dropped napalm on civilian populations in the North (Sheehan, 1988).
The pill's use by middle-class, First World women was an unintended
and unforeseen consequence of that initial research, and was first

prescribed in nonexperimental settings as an "off label" use of a drug that was approved by the FDA only for "menstrual irregularities." This story got lost in the 1960s as researchers hastened to defend themselves against the charge that they had illegitimately used Puerto Rico as a laboratory of dispensable bodies for the benefit of First World women. Yet an exploration of the moment of the development of the Pill, the ways physicians and researchers described its benefits when it came under attack, and the history of birth control in Puerto Rico shows that the testing was done there because Third World women were the population for whom the Pill was intended. As we think these days about the ethics of AIDS drug testing by U.S. firms overseas, it bears remembering that the effects of the globalization of drug testing and medical research are never simply contained "over there," but influence the treatment of working-class people in the United States, and sometimes even middle-class and affluent people.

My intent is certainly not to suggest that "over there" one has questions of race, colonialism, development, and poverty, while in places such as the United States, one encounters "women" and issues of gender and feminism. At the same time, to reiterate an argument of two decades of feminist scholarship on race, it is important to note how "women" are differentially imbricated in webs of meaning about race and nation. For example, one of the architects of the Pill research in Puerto Rico, Clarence Gamble, promoted very different policies and practices for women based on race, class, and region. He vigorously promoted "simple" methods for "simple" people, backing contraceptive foam in Puerto Rico rather than the diaphragm because, he believed, it was easier to use (Williams & Williams, 1978, p. 4). At the same time, he was writing articles for medical journals on the problem of the "college birthrate"—that college-educated men and women were having too few children (1947). He wrote of a project to promote birth control in Puerto Rico that it was:

> designed to discover whether our present means of birth control, intensively applied, can control the dangerously expanding population of an unambitious and unintelligent group . . . it has been said that birth control has been injurious to the race since it has been used by the intelligent and foresighted. It seems to me that only by some . . . demonstration can this accusation be refuted and our nation protected from an undue expansion of the unintelligent groups. (C. Gamble to Youngs Rubber Corporation, personal communication, March 24, 1947)

He was flatly contemptuous of working-class people in Puerto Rico (and elsewhere) and their ability to help themselves. Of a contraceptive program carried out through home visits, he wrote that "the jibaroes [*sic*] may not have enough energy to use the method, but if this doesn't persuade them I feel that nothing will" (C. Gamble to W. Wing, personal communication, May 23, 1955). At the same time, he could urge the reproduction of the educated few as crucial to the well-being of the world. As Gamble (1947) wrote in the *Journal of Heredity*:

> In this intricate technological age, highly trained specialists in large numbers are required to man the great complex of delicate organizations, industrial, political, educational, etc. that constitute a modern nation. The greatest single reservoir of those possessing the requisite abilities, the ability to plan, to guide, to execute with intelligence, is the group of college-trained citizens. . . . By reason of these considerations, the fecundity of this group is a matter of great significance. Since children tend to inherit the intellectual capacity of their parents, the average of the children of graduates will be above that of the nation as a whole. (p. 11)

With this kind of eugenic logic producing a bifurcated account of contraception, in which working-class and non-White people should use it a lot and affluent and well-educated people should use it very little, it confounds matters to think of the testing of the Pill in Puerto Rico as simply an experiment on women *qua* women, albeit particularly vulnerable ones. Rather, we need a more subtle account of what we might call "race/gender," or more awkwardly but more accurately, race/nation/class/gender—the ways that in this case Puerto Rican women became a keystone in a narrative that held that people colonized for decades by the United States were impoverished, not because of international politics, tariffs, trade, and economy, but because of their reproduction.

Precursors to the Pill

Gamble and the Puerto Rican context were not unique. A tradition of thinking of certain birth control methods as more appropriate for some populations than for others, what Patricia Hill Collins (1999) describes as the eugenic rhetoric of birth control, stretches back to the second and third decades of the twentieth century. Currently in the United States, we find that contraceptives such as Norplant and Depo Provera are overwhelmingly used in clinics and hospitals that serve working-class people (Roberts, 1997). In the 1920s and 1930s, as Margaret Sanger, the American Birth Control League, and other organizations tried to popularize the diaphragm as the most effective method available, scientists and organizations such as the Rockefeller Foundation argued that for working-class and colonized people—who by definition were understood to be not very bright—spermicides and other similar methods would be simpler and easier to use. In the United States, a principle promoter of this position was Robert L. Dickinson and his National Committee on Maternal Health (NCMH). As Dickinson wrote, "The requests which our Committee receives from foreign lands like China, India, and the Near East and from some of the slum districts here stresses the need of protection much more simple than the vaginal cap [diaphragm], or even...jelly" (R. L. Dickinson to Hon. Mrs. M. Farrer, personal communication, July 19, 1927). As the Great Depression wore on in the 1930s, Clarence Gamble, also a member and supporter of the NCMH, took this orthodoxy to the working-class whites in the Southern Appalachians and Puerto Ricans on the island, arguing that spermicidal foam was the answer to their economic woes. In 1936, over the objections of members of the American Birth Control League, Gamble closed down diaphragm clinics in Puerto Rico and substituted house-to-house canvassing by field workers equipped with foam powder and jellies (Briggs 2002). Social workers who had previously worked in the program found the shift distasteful; Gladys Gaylord wrote him that "my experience in Puerto Rico leads me to believe that it would be unwise to use any but the most approved methods. When I was there, [we] were loathe to back anything that was not guaranteed a high percent of success . . . in the critical situations which come into the clinic." As Gaylord noted, Gamble knowingly substituted a fairly effective method for one known to be much less so (G. Gaylord to C. Gamble, personal communication, October 26, 1936). Nevertheless, Puerto Rican physicians and birth control activists, unable to raise sufficient funds for clinics without help from the mainland, ultimately acceded to Gamble's wishes.

In the 1940s and 1950s, researchers' ideologies of what kinds of birth control were best for working-class and colonized people changed, although the notion of a two-tiered system of contraception did not. As eugenic fear of the feeble-minded poor gave way to anxiety over the explosive danger of overpopulation, the dominant characteristic of the birth control method needed shifted from "simple" to "strong." During this period some physicians began to advocate sterilization, not merely for institutionalized women, but for working-class women generally (efforts in Indiana and California were made to vasectomize institutionalized men, but they were decidedly a minority of those sterilized (Kevles, 1985, p. 108). Puerto Rico, as the only place in the United States (and one of the few in the world) where sterilization was legal in cases other than of mental illness or "feeblemindedness," was an early experiment in this respect. First in the private hospitals and then in the public hospitals, physicians in Puerto Rico began to perform a large number of *la operación*. It was a movement fueled in equal parts by physician pressure, public education campaigns blaming the island's "underdevelopment" on the profligate reproduction of working-class people, the massive movement of women into factory work that made caring for young children difficult or even impossible, and the history of bad and ineffective birth control on the island (Ramírez de Arellano and Seipp, 1983).[1]

Besides sterilization, the other major initiative in the direction of "strong" contraception was the pill. During the cold war, addressing Third World poverty through economic development became a major priority for a U.S. government trying to stave off the threat of Communism. If poor people were not so poor, the logic went, they would not "go over" to Communism in a violent effort to alleviate their economic situation. As economist Elmer Pendell (1956) insisted, in language apparently designed to explain the dangers of overpopulation and Communism to third graders:

> Population causes frequently lead to political consequences. Sometimes people have bartered their freedom for the promise of food. Sometimes people have rebelled against government because their poverty was too bitter. But neither the promise of food nor the struggle for freedom has often give[n] any sound basis for hope—because both food and freedom depend largely on conditions of reproduction. (p. 21)

For Pendell, then, not only does overpopulation cause poverty, which causes Communism, but birth limitation is the only road to both "freedom" and an end to poverty. Minimizing the "population explosion" was a significant goal of "development." And, as a *New York Times* editorial put it, "if significant reductions in population growth are to be achieved there must be a technological breakthrough in contraception similar to that in food production" (quoted in Djerassi, 1992, pp.-118–119). Just like the "green revolution" in agriculture, technology could provide an answer to Third World overpopulation; the problem was simply to find it.

In this context, researchers began to look at contraceptive technologies that had been previously thought too dangerous to pursue: specifically, hormonal contraception. While physician-participants and journalists traditionally characterize the development of the Pill as the inevitable result of a series of scientific and technological discoveries, sociologist Adele Clarke (1998) has argued provocatively that one of the most interesting questions about the history of the science of contraceptive research is often why it happened so late (see also Diczfalusy, 1979; Goldzieher & Rudel, 1974; McLaughlin, 1982; Vaughan, 1970). The basic science of the estrogen-progestin contraceptive pill was well-known in 1940; why did clinical trials not begin for another 16 years? Indeed, the idea of hormonal, systemic contraception had been around since the turn of the twentieth century, and numerous studies in the 1920s and 1930s found that estrogen and progesterone were effective in inhibiting ovulation. German biologist Ludwig Haberlandt showed in the 1920s that material from the corpus luteum (the "yellow body" left on the ovary after ovulation has occurred) could induce sterility in rabbits, and proposed that this line of research could lead to a contraceptive for human women (Perone, 1994). In the early 1930s, Corner and Allen isolated an extract from the corpus luteum in crystalline form, which they termed "progestin" (Allen & Weintersteiner, 1934). A. W. Makepeace and his collaborators (Makepeace, Weinstein, & Friedman, 1937) conducted animal tests on the inhibition of ovulation with progestin in 1937 and found it worked.

Meanwhile, on the estrogen side of the equation, Raphael Kuzrock (1937) reported in 1937 that estrogen caused ova to remain in the fallopian tubes and not descend into the uterus for implantation. He, too, suggested that this held promise for "hormonal sterilization" in humans. In this period, admittedly, the only commercial source for steroidal hormones was the distilled urine of mares and pregnant women—as Nelly Oudshoorn's (1994) account of its collection and the neighbors' complaints of the smell at the Dutch pharmaceutical company Organon have made unforgettably clear. This made hormones costly to produce and certainly created a drag on development of hormones for contraceptive use (pp. 73–108). Yet even this problem was solved by 1940, when Russell Marker (Marker & Rohrman, 1939, 1940) announced that he had created a synthetic progestin from Mexican yams. By the mid-1940s, Fuller Albright (Sturgis and Albright, 1940), who had been working on estrogen therapy for painful and irregular menstruation, had even proposed a method for clinical application—in a textbook, no less—where he wrote:

Since preventing ovulation prevents pregnancy, one could employ the
same principles in birth control. . . . Thus, for example, if an individual
took 1 mg. diethylstilbestrol [DES, a synthetic estrogen] by mouth daily
from the first day of her period for the next six weeks, she would not
ovulate. (Albright quoted in Reed, 1983, p. 316)

Indeed, when Gregory Pincus presented the earliest results from the
line of research that became the first contraceptive "pill" at a conference
in 1955, the session's chair, Sir Solly Zuckerman, felt that he had shown
nothing that was not already well-known: that progestin inhibits ovulation (Marks, 1998; Vaughan, 1970, pp. 34–35). The scientific obstacles
to producing a birth control pill had been solved by 1940, and the point
seemed obvious by 1945, yet it was another decade before there were
clinical trials. Other forces than the purely scientific were at work both
in inhibiting and promoting birth control research.

Risks, the Pill, and Overpopulation

The principle reason why this line of research was halted in 1940 was that
it seemed too great a risk for too little gain. The "pill" would represent a
major break with previous conventional wisdom about pharmaceuticals;
it was the first such systemically active compound given to a population
that was healthy, that did not even have a disease that might counterbal-
ance the dangers of a steroidal drug of unknown effects. Researchers
had no way to know whether or not the Pill was safe. If many people
were aware in 1940 that making a contraceptive pill was possible yet
still did not, it was because it seemed impossible to predict the side
effects. Indeed, this was Zuckerman's warning to Pincus at the 1955
Tokyo conference where his initial results were presented; he said:

We need better evidence about the occurrence of side effects in human
beings. It is not enough though . . . that we take presumed negative
evidence about the lack of side-effects from animal experiments to
imply that no undesirable side-effects would occur in human beings.
There is an urgent need for prolonged observation before we draw
any firm conclusions. (Vaughan, 1970, p. 39)

In fact, three pharmaceutical companies—Searle, Parke-Davis, and
Pfizer—possessed patents and animal studies in 1955 that would have
enabled them to begin clinical trials with the hope of turning a considerable profit, but there was no competition. Those at Parke-Davis and
Pfizer believed that clinical trials would be dangerous and unethical;

Searle, in contrast, went to Puerto Rico. In the 1970s, a member of the World Health Organization's Contraceptive Task Force praised Searle in retrospect "for their sang-froid, vision, and courage in marketing the first oral contraceptive preparation in a hostile atmosphere. . . . This was a period in history when several other drug houses declared that it would be incompatible with their ethical principles to manufacture fertility regulating agents" (Diczfalusy cited in Gunn, 1987). While some of this opposition was simply anti-birth control, the hesitancy of the other players ought to alert us to real and palpable concern present in the 1950s about side effects of reproductive drugs. Common sense dictated that caution was appropriate in giving steroidal compounds with powerful, systemic effects—many of which were unknown—to a population of healthy women. Pharmaceutical companies had plenty of reason for concern about clinical trials in healthy, reproductive-age women.

The decision to pursue this research a decade later had everything to do with belief that the dangers of overpopulation presented a new "disease" that justified some degree of risk-taking. The best spokesmen for the "overpopulation" position were those researchers who developed the Pill, teams led by maverick reproductive biologist Gregory Pincus and the cautious, Catholic obstetrician John Rock. The two could not have been more different, but they arrived at identical reasons to explain their interest in Pill research. Pincus (1965) wrote that "a recognition of the population explosion" prompted him to consider hormonal contraceptive research (p. 6); one of his postdoctoral fellows, Min-Chueh Chang echoed this, saying that he and Pincus had often discussed contraception methods, "particularly after the 'population explosion' made the headlines after World War II" he said (Perone quoted in Goldzieher, 1194, p. 13). These concerns, too, informed the decision by Planned Parenthood Foundation of America (PPFA) to fund Pincus and Chang's research; addressing overpopulation was a major organizational priority; the group hired William Vogt as executive director after he wrote a book on overpopulation (1960). After the development of the Pill, overpopulation continued to be an issue in Pincus's writing. He began a 1959 piece in the *Washington Post* with the following words:

The control of the population explosion now upon us by the limitation of births is particularly demanding in countries where the birth-rate pressure curtails already limited economic development. Conventional contraceptive methods have been known and publicized widely in these countries, but the acceptance of them has been most unremarkable. . . .

Accordingly, there has been an increasing demand for a simple, easily practiced, generally acceptable, inexpensive means of contraception. Generally this demand has been for some easy medication. (p. E8)

Urging that in the wake of the atomic bomb, scientific research must take responsibility for its social effects, Pincus (1965) wrote elsewhere that biologist had a positive social responsibility to address "overpopulation." He called for biologists to form a Federation of Population Scientists and to undertake further research on limiting fertility (Pincus, 1965, pp. 6–9).

Perhaps the most dramatic example of the importance of the over-population argument to research on the Pill is John Rock. A devout Catholic, Rock was by all accounts a man for whom moral and ethical considerations were paramount. Unlike Pincus, he never became rich from the success of the Pill—he refused to invest in Searle stock because he disliked the idea that people would think he had become wealthy from risks taken with others' bodies—and equally unlike the former, he had no love of the role of maverick. Moreover, he was known as a physician who was elaborately kind to his patients, had a faithful following, and who as a researcher was particularly concerned about side effects (McLaughlin, 1982, pp. 124–127). Not only did Rock (1963) become involved in the Pill research, but in 1963, he published a crusader's book, *The Time Has Come: A Catholic Doctor's Proposal to End the Battle Over Birth Control*. Addressed to the Catholic hierarchy and laity, it argued that the population explosion had rendered the Church's opposition to birth control obsolete, and more, profoundly wrong. He wrote:

Though the population problem daily grows more destructive of the values to which all men aspire, action by some governments and by the dominant international agencies is paralyzed mainly because of the religious controversy over fertility control. As long as the Catholic Church proscribes the methods of birth control known to most effective, it is said, no public institution—of the United States or the United Nations—will forthrightly tackle the population problem. (p. 5)

In short, he provides an excellent study—not of the unethical handling of the Pill trials—but precisely the opposite, of how global political concerns made the Pill trials *ethical* for many North Americans and later, for the burgeoning Puerto Rican middle class.

The Science and Clinical Trials of the Pill

In Puerto Rico, the road to the clinical trials was inaugurated with the founding of the Population Association and its transformation into Pro Familia, groups composed mostly of women that operated within the tradition of feminism that believed strongly in modernization, technology, and science as a road to social progress. On the continent, the project was launched in a similar way: Margaret Sanger, champion since the Progressive Era of technology as the means of better contraception, guided heiress Katherine Dexter McCormick toward funding endocrinological research on hormonal contraception. In 1951, at Sanger's urging, Gregory Pincus, already known for unconventional, radical work in reproductive biology (he had lost his appointment at Harvard University following his well-publicized claim to have induced parthenogenesis in rabbits) began work on hormonal contraceptives under a small grant from PPFA. In 1953, McCormick took over the funding of his work, and even as PPFA lost interest, began to fund it as extensively as Pincus could find use for the money (Reed, 1978, pp. 340–341). After leaving Harvard, Pincus had struggled for funding for his Worcester Foundation for Experimental Biology; he worked for numerous funders, including Searle pharmaceutical, the Rockefeller Foundation, and PPFA—a biological entrepreneur par excellence (Reed, 1978, pp. 343–354; Vaughan, 1970, pp. 26–28). With McCormick's interest, however, hormonal contraceptive research became lucrative as well as an appealing line of work for addressing the social problems of the developing world.

For Rock, Pincus, and the teams they directed, conducting clinical trials of the Pill in Puerto Rico simply made sense. In the popular press and the development literature, Puerto Rico had become a kind of poster child for overpopulation, which is to say, a classic example of the precise problem their science was meant to solve.[2] Moreover, as Gamble had shown in years of research on spermicides, Puerto Rico had many well-trained physicians and researchers who were experienced in birth control clinical trials. Perhaps most importantly, Rock, Pincus, and their sponsors at Searle found on the island many like-minded people, very concerned about "overpopulation" who were prepared to go to considerable lengths to secure "strong" contraception. The physicians and organizations that conducted the research and compiled the results—Doctors Edris Rice-Wray and Adaline Pendleton Satterthwaite, the Asociación Puertorriqueña Pro Bienestar de la Familia, and Gamble himself—all articulated their support for the testing of the Pill in terms of strongly held beliefs in the importance of addressing overpopulation. Interestingly, however, both the original researchers dealing with actual patients in Puerto Rico—Rice-Wray and Satterthwaite—opposed its approval, arguing that its side effects were too severe for it ever to be an effective tool in the fight against the population explosion.

Rock and his group of graduate physicians (Doctors Angelika Tsacoma, Luigi Mastroianni, and John Kelley) were initially using steroids for the opposite ends of Pincus's lab: to try to induce pregnancy in women who were inexplicably infertile. These clinicians used synthetic estrogenic and natural progesterone treatments, hypothesizing that the problem might involve underdeveloped reproductive organs and that simulating pregnancy could help. After four months, they stopped the treatment, and 13 of their 80 previously infertile subjects became pregnant (Asbell, 1995; Rock, Garcia, & Pincus , 1957). Working with Pincus's group (Chang, Robert Slechta, Anne Merrill, and J. Choiniere), Rock's group of clinicians began in 1954 to use the researchers' more active synthetic steroids, and tried to measure whether infertile patients were ovulating during the administration of these compounds. They initiated a regime of urine testing and basal body temperature monitoring to look for secondary effects of ovulation (e.g., pregnandiol in urine, sharp rise in morning temperature) in patients they believed were normally regular ovulators. Tsacoma even did laparotomies on 10 patients who were already scheduled for hysterectomies, looking for corpus lutea (yellow bodies), evidence on the ovary of recent ovulation (see Asbell, 1995; Maisel, 1965; McLaughlin, 1982, Oudoshoorn, 1994, Pincus, 1956; Ramírez de Arellano & Seipp,1983; Reed, 1978, Vaughan, 1970).

This research suggested that ovulation was inhibited, particularly with two steroids, initially reported to be 19-nor-17-ethinyl testosterone and 17-ethinyl estaeneolone. These names, although laborious, are interesting; the first is related to testosterone, the second, to estrogen. Later, among both historians and scientific researchers, the story came to be told that Pincus and Rock were interested only in progesterone-related compounds. This narrative was important because it described a "natural" mode of contraception in which chemicals merely simulated pregnancy, inhibiting repeated ovulation in the same way many mammalian females do during pregnancy, through excreting progesterone.[3] (In Rock's (1963) words, "They provide a natural means of fertility control such as nature uses after ovulation and during pregnancy" (p. 167). This also had implications for the kinds of side effects that were considered (Pincus [1956] argued that few were to be expected, since the human female body was "naturally" adapted to large amounts of progesterone, and supported an ethical argument about the "morality" of this sort of contraception because it mimicked a natural process. Moreover, testosterone and estrogen had and have profound social identities beyond their chemical character as steroids (Fausto-Sterling, 1992, pp. 90–155; Fausto-Sterling, 2000, pp. 170–194; Oudshoorn, 1994, pp. 1–41). They have been reified as "sex hormones," and, indeed, have been frequently rendered in popular culture as the essence of maleness or femaleness.[4] That both are present in men and women, and both are systemically active—not just affecting secondary sex characteristics but multiple bodily systems—has historically been less important than other cultural meanings. Yet all hormones are closely related steroids, and once chemists began to tamper with them, to change them sufficiently to render them patentable, it was probably more appropriate to consider all of them simply as steroids, as Pincus's early publications did, then try to name them as related to a particular hormone. As every introductory organic chemistry student knows, there is more than one way to name a carbon ring. In fact, that is precisely what happened. The 19-nor-17-ethinyl testosterone mentioned earlier came to be referred to as norethynodrel—a progestin, no longer a testosterone—and became the basis for the first Pill. As time went on, the Pill's character as a progestin became increasingly a part of its identity, although throughout the 1960s, no one could say for sure *how* it worked, whether in fact it simulated pregnancy or did something else. By 1963, a reviewer for a medical journal article noted in the margin that norethynodrel could just as easily be named as a testosterone, an estrogen, or a progestin—but commented, "testosterone looks funny in print. . . . Nah, we'd never print it."[5] Whatever the nature of global concerns about excessive population, those targeted to receive steroidal contraceptives were still importantly *women*, and the compound simply could not be named testosterone.

The responses to the next set of small-scale trials suggest again how fundamentally the targets of this project to offer a technological "fix" for overpopulation were women. In the next group of female patients, no new information was gleaned, and Pincus and McCormick showed themselves willing to use less-than-consenting populations, a "cage of ovulating females," in McCormick's phrase (Marks, 1998). In these clinical trials, one targeted female students at the new medical school in Puerto Rico, and another used mental patients in Massachusetts—female and male—at a facility where McCormick had been a regular contributor. (There was also a short-lived effort by Pincus to use Puerto Rican female prisoners.) For the medical students, the demanding daily regimen of pill-taking, temperature-measuring, vaginal smears, monthly urine collection, and endometrial biopsy proved impossible to maintain, even though their grades were apparently based on their participation in the study. No meaningful data were collected. Although the mental patient group could be more successfully monitored daily, female contraceptive effect was difficult to gauge in a population that was presumed not to be heterosexually active. These studies, then, offered little except the general information that these steroidal compounds posed no immediately appreciable systemic danger to users. However, they once again raised the issue of side effects; as with Rock's infertile patients, several complained of dizziness, nausea, headache, and menstrual irregularities (McLaughlin, 1982; Marks, 1998; Oudshoorn, 1994; Ramírez de Arellano & Seipp,1983; Vaughan, 1970; Pincus, 1958).

Researchers also followed another lead in this series of cases: steroids had previously been documented to cause male infertility, too. Among the psychotic men in Massachusetts, urine samples and biopsied testicular tissue showed—albeit inconclusively—that the steroidal compound they tested stopped sperm production (Pincus, 1957). The implications of this were never pursued; no effort was made to develop or further test the Pill as a contraceptive for men. Something about giving steroidal compounds to men was less appealing than controlling women's fertility. This choice was probably overdetermined; several explanations come to mind: McCormick and Sanger, as funders, were interested specifically in a female-controlled method and the discourse of overpopulation targeted women. However, another issue was noted that probably also contributed: one of the male mental patients was described by a nurse as acting "effeminate" during treatment. Although no physiologic effects such as breast development were reported, the suggestion that these steroids could make men act like women, or like homosexuals, was apparently enough. What behavior a psychotic man who was unable to cooperate with researchers could have exhibited to make him seem "feminine" to the nursing staff is difficult to imagine. But such possible side effects dovetailed with the perception of hormones as powerfully the "essence" of maleness or femaleness and seem to have been sufficient to deter further such research.

The next round of testing in 1956 involved a much larger series of cases, and these, too, were organized in Puerto Rico. Two groups of women, one residents of a housing project in Río Piedras, and another, patients of Ryder Hospital (usually, women turned down for sterilization because they had fewer than the three children required (Satterthwaite & Gamble, 1962) were enrolled in an effort to understand whether the Pill prevented pregnancy, and whether it was acceptable and could be used effectively by those who "most needed" contraception, specifically working-class women living in "overpopulated" and "underdeveloped" countries. Each group consisted of 200 to 300 women by 1957. Many feminist scholars and activists, as well as popular writers, have argued that the Puerto Rico trials were shoddily conducted in that they took inappropriate risks with women's health (Gordon, 1995; Marks, 1998; Oudshoorn, 1994, pp. 122–132, Ramírez de Arellano & Seipp, 1983, pp. 105–123). It might also be said that they failed on their own terms; they neither lowered the birth rate among trial participants nor was the Pill acceptable to the women who took it. Half the trial participants in both groups dropped out, and a good percentage of these left the trials because they found the side effects—severe headache, nausea, vomiting, midcycle bleeding—too unpleasant and not worth the trouble.[6] Additionally, a significant number of pregnancies occurred in both groups. In the first year and a half, among the 295 participants from Río Piedras, 19 became pregnant—or a percentage of 14 per 100 woman-years of exposure.[7] Pincus (1958) misreported this in the text of his article announcing the success of the pill, as five pregnancies. He acknowledges another 14 in a footnote.) Moreover, the pregnancy rate among those who stopped using the Pill was 79% within 4 months, a very high rate caused by the "rebound effect" of heightened fertility post-Pill (Cook, Gamble, & Satterthwaite, 1961). All of this was close enough for Pincus—the pregnancies during the study were explicable in terms of pills missed, whether under orders from a physician to relieve side effects or because of forgetfulness—and most occurred after women were no longer enrolled in the study. Those who were truly miserable with side effects quickly left the study. However, its real effect on the community of women who took the Pill was a rate of side effects (including those so severe as to require hospitalization) high enough that new recruitment for the study became quite difficult (A. Satterthwaite to C. Gamble, personal communication, Aprile 21, 1957), and a net *increase* in the pregnancy rate.

The trials—and the Pill generally—have been criticized as an example of male and masculinist science being callous about women's bodies, as we have seen (Seaman, 1969). But it bears underscoring that the people most directly involved with running these trials were women—and feminists. Sanger and McCormick supported and shepherded the work of Pincus and his lab, even when PPFA dropped it. Although Pincus was subsequently embraced by the medical community and sharply criticized by feminists, where he sought sympathetic audiences in the late 1950s is interesting. The first public venue in which information about trials of a contraceptive pill was published was not a scientific journal, but *Ladies Home Journal* (Maisel, 1957), and the first conference at which they were presented was an annual PPFA conference. In Puerto Rico, two North American female doctors—who, one suspects, found a wider scope for professional respect and work on the island than on the mainland in the 1950s—conducted the trials. Dr. Edris Rice-Wray, medical director of the Asociación and director of the Health Department work in Río Piedras, and Penny Satterthwaite of Ryder Hospital were the primary physicians recording the effects of the Pill. Each had a Puerto Rican female counterpart still more intimately involved in the trials: in Río Piedras, nurses Mercedes Quiñones and Iris Rodríguez of Pro-Familia, and in Humacao, with Ryder, social worker Noemí Rodríguez. These were no mere lackeys in this process, but well-educated, professional women who came to birth control work because they believed in the cause. Both Rice-Wray and Satterthwaite continued contraceptive research elsewhere when they left Puerto Rico, the former with the Pill in Mexico, the latter, with the IUD in Thailand (Reed, 1974; Rice-Wray, 1962). Like their male colleagues in the study, both also cited concerns about "overpopulation" as the motivating force that brought them to this work. Satterthwaite (Reed, 1974), the missionary, told the following story:

> On my way to Puerto Rico . . . [I met] Dr. Ralph Allee. He said to me, "Here [*sic*] you're going to Puerto Rico, out to save lives and to deliver babies, and full of enthusiasm. Have you ever thought about what you may be doing to complicate the future of the [island]." Here was an agricultural man . . . worrying about food supply. And so he was perhaps the first one that really faced me up to a responsibility.

Rice-Wray (1957, p. 78), similarly, wrote, "Puerto Rico is one of the most densely populated countries in the world. We are all interested in finding some reliable contraceptive which is cheap, acceptable to the people, easy to take and something the people themselves would be interested in taking." She later also used similar language to characterize the situation of Mexico (Rice-Wray, Schultz-Contreras, Guerrero & Aranda-Roselli, 1962). Of the motivation of Iris and Noemí Rodríguez and Mercedes Quiñones it is more difficult to say anything definite because they wrote no letters or articles for the study, which makes guessing at their frame of mind difficult. Nevertheless, they acted in a way consistent with both the leadership and membership of Pro Familia and the other *asociaciones* during the previous 20 years. From one point of view, they practiced the art of the possible, seeking to promote birth control and hence jumping onto whatever project some North American group or company was willing to fund. From a more cynical perspective, they collaborated with North Americans in the project of making over the "backward" working-class into modern families, through coercive means if necessary.

To notice the cooperation between feminists and Searle Pharmaceutical is not to say they behaved in precisely the same way. Both Satterthwaite and Rice-Wray treated side effects with much greater seriousness than Pincus or Searle Pharmaceutical. They were very concerned, and both recommended that the Pill not be used further. In her initial report to the company, Rice-Wray wrote that Enovid "causes too many side effects to be generally acceptable" (Rice-Wray, 1957, p. 85). Satterthwaite wrote letters to Gamble in which she said that she was "a little alarmed about changes in the cervices of these women who have been taking the pills," particularly those who had begun the study with cervical erosions that subsequently seemed worsened (Satterthwaite, 1957). She continued to insist on regular endometrial biopsies to test for any signs of reproductive cancers—even though the biopsies had to be sent all the way to Boston to be read due to lack of laboratory facilities on the island. Her doubts about the Pill's safety made it increasingly difficult for her to continue working on the pill trials, especially when Pincus played fast and loose about the distinction between "his" cases—those directly under his supervision at Río Piedras—and Satterthwaite's, for example reporting her results together with his (as if it were a single group) at the 1959 Planned Parenthood conference, even though she felt the results were not yet ready for public scrutiny (Satterthwaite, 1959). But the final straw was when, after her considerable concern about reproductive cancer risk associated with the Pill, and three cases within her sample, Pincus announced at a news conference that he believed the Pill had a *protective* effect against cancer and had gotten a grant from the American Cancer Society to study it (Reed, 1974). Even under pressure from Pincus, Satterthwaite refused to back down from her belief that the side effects women reported were real and significant. By the mid-1960s, Satterthwaite had decided firmly that the IUD was more acceptable, safer, and easier to use, and advocated its use over the Pill (Satterthwaite, 1965). Pincus, meanwhile, ran a placebo trial and concluded that the suggestion of the possibility of side effects was what was causing them due to "the emotional super-activity of Puerto Rican women." Thereafter, potential participants simply were not warned (Ramírez de Arellano & Seipp, 1983).

In sum, an underlying logic of risk brought the clinical trials of the Pill to Puerto Rico. Researchers had been motivated initially to do research on the Pill because they were concerned about overpopulation, and Puerto Rico stood as one of the paradigmatic examples of overpopulation. When Thomas Parran, head of the U.S. Public Health

Service, thought of overpopulation, he mentioned "such countries as China or India (or Java or Puerto Rico)" (T. Parran to R. Fosdick, personal communication, October 28, 1946). Where most researchers had been deterred in developing a steroidal contraceptive by concerns over dangers associated with its systemic effects, the "threat" of over-population was a factor that overrode such concerns. Medical researchers were accustomed to cost-benefit thinking: the risks of a drug ought to be less significant than the danger posed by the disease it was used to treat. The cost-benefit ratio of contraceptives was harder to figure within this calculus; no side effects were worth the risk if the people taking the drug were healthy. However, "overpopulation" shifted this equation: the dangers of overpopulation were construed as life-threatening and hence worth a great deal of risk.

Another reason exists to think of Pill research as overdetermined by the colonial context. Very early trials of an oral contraceptive were actually proposed for Puerto Rico. In 1941, the pharmaceutical company Hoffman-Laroche, apparently in collaboration with Sanger and Gamble tried to test an oral contraceptive—designed in Africa[8]—in Puerto Rico. Sanger proposed it to José Belaval, a Puerto Rican ob/gyn active in Gamble's projects, on a trip to the island, and he readily accepted (J. Belaval to M. Sanger, personal communication, January 21, 1941; M. Sanger to J. Belaval, personal communication, February 8, 1941; C. Gamble to J. Belaval, personal communication, April 4, 1941; C. Gamble to C. Gould, personal communication, January 25, 1941). Belaval even arranged for facilities with Presbyterian Hospital (C. Gould to Presbyterian Hospital, San Juan, personal communication, July 17, 1941), but he found no takers for the drug, a problem Gamble attributed to his "working too high on the social scale" (C. Gamble to C. Gould, personal communication, August 12, 1941).

Mainland Use and Debates

Between 1957 and 1962, millions of mainland women began to use this miraculous new drug that was reported to be 100% effective in preventing pregnancy and, because it was an analog of the body's own hormones, completely safe. The FDA cleared Searle's Enovid as a contraceptive for general use in 1960 after many physicians had begun prescribing it as an "off-label" use of a drug approved for menstrual irregularities.[9] Its popularity was built informally—through word-of-mouth and articles in women's magazines[10]—and caught Searle by surprise. When Pincus and Searle had overlooked and obscured reports of side effects—in Rice-Wray's series was that 50% of the women had dropped out because of side-effects (1957), while Satterthwaite (1957, 1958) believed that there were significant, potentially precancerous changes in the cervices of patients using the Pill—they had had Third World overpopulation in mind. When the FDA presented reports of thromboembolis in British and North American women using the Pill to them, the Pill's defenders continued to cite "overpopulation" as the major reason to continue to support it.

In my research, I followed this debate through several organizations, but found one particularly revealing and candid source: the editor's files for Rockefeller University's *Medical Letter*. The *Medical Letter* was sent to physicians and described new drugs, questions about side effects, and controversies over older ones. In the first years of the 1960s, following FDA approval of the Pill as a contraceptive, the *Medical Letter*'s editor, Harold Aaron, sent a series of drafts of articles out about the Pill to all the major players in the field—policy makers, researchers, corporations, and physicians. The reviewers of these articles were and, unfortunately, must remain anonymous because of restrictions attached to the papers by their donor and enforced by the archive. These reviewers were not, however, obscure; they encompassed some of the most significant researchers and advocates in the field. Together, they produce a fascinating ensemble of voices and suggest a great deal about what questions and arguments seemed possible to those involved in making decisions about the Pill.

In 1960, the *Medical Letter* ran an article that was warmly positive about the Pill. Its tone was one of certainty; it assured readers that a considerable amount was known about the effect of estrogen-progestin oral contraceptives. The only hint of concern about the effects of these drugs was that one reviewer insisted that a line that described the Pill as being "as safe as the condom and the diaphragm" be changed to "as effective as," arguing that unknown side effects were still possible.

By 1962 and 1963, however, the *Medical Letter* was grappling with how to report 28 cases of thromboembolic disease, including one death, which had been reported to the FDA and linked with the use of the Pill. Articles in the newsletter tried to strike a balance between warning of potentially serious effects on the one hand, but on the other not overreacting to anecdotal reports when there was little agreement over what the rate of clotting disorders should be in the general population, and whether 28 out of approximately 1 million users was too high (or whether there were others who had not been recorded as having to do with the Pill). However, guarded language met with little approval by either side. One article reproduced a pharmaceutical company's advice to physicians that they "should be alert to the possible occurrence of thrombophlebitisis or phlebothrombosis . . . even though a causal relationship has not been proved or disproved." One reviewer shot back acerbically, "such alertness is without preventive value . . . but it should aid in the recognition of vascular accidents otherwise ascribed to other or obscure causes," adding with a note to the editor "e.g., coronary occlusion [heart attack], or shouldn't we be nasty?"[11] Another, however, felt that any warnings at all about oral contraceptives had to be counterbalanced by a reference to overpopulation. This reviewer argued:

> All the adverse information is offered without adequate comment on the possible value of the drug. . . . In the interests of accuracy, it should be pointed out that this method of contraception is far and away more reliable in the sense of effective *in general use* than any other method of contraception that has ever previously been available. . . . It has also been established for women of low intelligence who have achieved no success at all with older methods. . . . Is it not rather ungenerous to make no mention at all of the possibility that this may make a major contribution to the biggest problem facing the world to-day, namely the population explosion. It is now generally known that in the underdeveloped countries, conventional methods of contraception have made no impression. The oral contraceptive . . . may prove to be one of the most important developments of the century.[12]

Aaron complained that the question of how to write the Pill article excited more controversy than anything in his memory.[13]

Yet this controversy generated regular responses. Those who defended the drug consistently did so on the grounds that the threat of overpopulation on a global scale outweighed the potential risks associated with it. Where one reviewer asked, "Would it not be a major catastrophe if we discovered, too late, that prolonged usage of this therapeutic regimen was carcinogenic?" and added, "I believe it should not be prescribed at all except in formal controlled experiments."[14] Yet another wrote that the Pill was "excellent in [the] indigent with low motivation."[15] Still another railed against the soul-searching over whether a method should be tested for 10 years before being introduced into the market:

> In relation to introducing a completely effective contraceptive method with a five year safety record we would remind you of the belabored but none-the-less ominous "population problem," and point to the very high degree of consumer acceptance, and hence demographic effectivity, of the 'pill' approach to contraception.[16]

The international wing of Planned Parenthood took the most extreme position. At the same time physicians were worrying over whether their U.S. and British patients should be monitored monthly or more often if they were on the Pill, Mary Calderone of PPFA announced the organizational guidelines for their World Population Emergency Campaign. To render the Pill portable to "high population areas," she suggested an initial pelvic exam, a second visit shortly afterward to answer questions, and thereafter monitoring every six months or less. Thromboembolism was not a concern, she insisted, "In the opinion of PPFA's Medical Committee the only contraindication to prescription of orals is pre-existing fibromyoma" (M. S. Calderone, Med. Dir,. Planned Parenthood Federation of America to Executive Directors and Chairmen of Medical Advisory Committees, personal communication, May 23, 1962).

This correspondence about the controversy over thromboembolism—and, implicitly, the larger health risks of the pill—suggests a great deal about how researchers, pharmaceutical companies, physicians, and policy makers weighed the dangers to women's bodies at a time when neither direction provided clear evidence. There was reason to believe that the possibility was present of serious, even lethal health consequences. Equally, however, it was possible that the Pill was safe, and it was indisputably very effective. In mid-1962 the question fundamentally could not be decided with the information then available. These responses suggest that the choices these players made were profoundly influenced—or at least justified by—their imagination of the sorts of bodies the Pill was most likely to affect. Those who defended the continued widespread use of the Pill imagined and described Third World bodies. Those who did not describe such bodies did not urge the continued use of the Pill.

The irony of all this, of course, is that the Pill very quickly had profound and long-lasting effects on the bodies and lives of the women whom most of the Pill enthusiasts in the scientific community did *not* imagine using it—middle-class White women in the mainland United States. The emergence of a technology that made sex without pregnancy possible combined with a women's liberation movement to produce new possibilities for imagining freedom and autonomy. Yet while U.S. women used the Pill in steadily increasing numbers, the feminist movement expressed deep concern. After Congressional hearings on the Pill, Washington Women's Liberation held its own Women's Hearings on the Pill, and suggested that the Pill was a male-produced technology that used women as guinea pigs without even informing them of potentially dangerous effects of the drug. Members of the group complained:

In spite of the fact that it is women who are taking the Pill and taking the risks, it was the legislators, the doctors, and the drug company's [sic] representatives, all men of course, who were testifying and dissecting women as if they were no more important than the laboratory animals they work with every day. (Tone, 1997, p. 235)

This wasn't strictly accurate; in the 1940s and 1950s, as we have seen, feminists associated with PPFA, such as Calderone, McCormick, and Sanger, backed the development and testing of the Pill. Yet the attitude of Washington's Women's Liberation was typical of a new generation of feminists who found themselves very much at odds with the medical and regulatory community's complacence over the side effects of the Pill. In part, this anti-Pill activism emerged out of U.S. women's own experiences with the Pill's side effect, but it also reflected a growing unwillingness by U.S. feminists to take arguments about overpopulation at face value. In subsequent years, a sharp critique of overpopulation arguments as eugenics emerged in activist groups and a new women's studies scholarship (Gordon, 1977; Hartmann, 1995; Mass, 1977).

The thromboembolis crisis was ultimately resolved to the satisfaction of researchers in the 1960s as a statistical artifact of the fact that in this period, North American and British women who took the Pill were disproportionately also more likely to be smokers. Nevertheless, some newer studies continue to show that despite continual changes in dosage and "estrogen" and "progestin" compounding, women who take the Pill continue to show far higher rates—from three to five times higher—of thromboembolism (Drife, 2002). Other researchers argue that these studies show little more than that Pill users are not typical of the general population of women and that these statistics show correlation, rather cause (Ory, 1996). In fact, the shape of the debate has not changed much in the intervening decades. In the long run, whether the Pill is safe remains unclear. Many continue to suggest, much as Satterthwaite did in the 1950s, that the use of oral contraceptives—like hormone replacement therapy—causes increased risk of gynecological and breast cancers (Collins & Schlesselman, 2002). It is certainly less safe than the boldest claims made for it—Pincus at one time insisted that its use in fact *lowered* cancer rates (Reed, 1974). More than anything, however, researchers were simply lucky that it did not cause devastating, widespread ill effects. DES, for example, did. Researchers simply had no way of knowing. What they believed and what they argued, however, was that it was safer than the threat posed by too many Third World bodies, with their penchant for Communism and their poverty.

Notes

1. Although U.S. feminists have often picked up the Nationalist argument that there was a U.S. sponsored mass-sterilization campaign on the island, there seems to be little evidence that this was the case. Clarence Gamble, on hearing of the accusations that this was taking place, twice sent his own researchers to the island to offer to help fund it. They could not find any organized campaign for sterilization, and were discouraged by government and public health officials from starting one. See for example Christopher Tietze to Clarence Gamble, Report 3, September 19, 1946; Report 8, September 25, 1946, Clarence J. Gamble Papers-Countway Library of Medicine, Box 46, Folder 756 and Wilson Wing to Gamble, May 18, 1951, CJGP-CLM, B47, F774. Nevertheless, it seems equally clear that there was also a considerable plurality among physicians who thought sterilization was a good idea for working-class people on the island, and undoubtedly there was improper pressure.

2. Puerto Rican "overpopulation" was everywhere in the news; in fact, it was repeatedly cited as the root cause of all the economic problems of the island. See "Puerto Rico: Problem Island," *New York Times Magazine*, March 7, 1954, pp. 10–11; *Time*, May 2 1949, cover article, p. 33; *Time*, April 23, 1958, cover article, p. 30; "Growing Pains Beset Puerto Rico," *National Geographic Magazine*, April 1951, p. 24.

3. For examples of this narrative, see esp. the popular accounts, Maisel and Vaughan. Pincus and Rock were also constructing a progesterone story; the name of the 1954 project at Rock's clinic was the Pincus Progesterone Project (the PPP, or pee, pee, pee, as it came to be called, for the endless urine collections).

4. This dates back to the earliest studies of "organotherapy" by Charles Edouard Brown-Séquard in the late nineteenth century.

5. Anonymous reviewer for "Enovid, Ortho-Novum, and Thromboembolic Effects," *Medical Letter.* Rockefeller Archive Center, Rockefeller University, Record Group 891, Martin Rizack papers, Box 45, Folder 1.13, March 1963.

6. Ramírez de Arrellano and Seipp, pp. 107–123, report the drop-out rate on the Río Piedras series as 109 women out of 221 participants; 22% of these dropped out because of side effects. For the Ryder series, 32.4% of participants dropped out because of side effects, and 57% total had discontinued after two years. Adaline Satterthwaite, "Experience," p. 476.

7. C. Tietze to M. Snyder, August 15, 1957, CLM-CJGP, B48, F788. Gregory Pincus et al., "Fertility Control with Oral Medication," *American Journal of Obstetrics and Gynecology*, 75 (Aprile 1958): 1333–1346. Oudshoorn criticizes the use of the kind of "woman-years" statistic in the Pill trials in Puerto Rico. However, this statistical device was not unique to these trials, but dated back to the 1930s. Its strength was that it enabled researchers to compare divergent experiences in length of use of a method and made it a simple matter to deduct, for example, 10 months for a pregnancy or 3 months of a sexual partners' absence. Its shortcomings—in overstating researchers' knowledge of a method by making 12 women's experience for one month comparable to one woman's experience for a year—were well-known to researchers, and had spawned a literature of their own, establishing guidelines such as one requiring that at least half of any cases reported in this way involve long-term administration. (See Raymond Pearl in "Contraception and Fertility in 2,000 Women," *Human Biology, 4* (September 1932): 363–407.) Researchers were aware that there was something wrong with the way it was used in the Pill study. Wrote Christopher Tietze, "the aggregate number of person years of

exposure to the risk of pregnancy through Aprile 1957 was 139. Of this total, only 50 years were contributed by women observed 12 months or more, the maximum being 16 months. The proportion of the total exposure contributed by these 'long' cases was only 36%, about half of what is normally considered desirable." C. Tietze to M. Snyder, August 15, 1957. CLM-CJGP, B48, F788.

8. It is possible though by no means self-evident that this oral agent was Max Ehrenstein's synthetic progesterone, derived from the seeds of an African plant. The Belaval-Sanger-Gamble correspondence mentions only that it was from Africa. Ehrenstein's research, however, was not documented until he read a paper before the American Chemical Society in 1944. On Ehrenstein's paper, see Asbell (1995, pp. 108–109).

9. It would be a mistake in this period to speak of FDA "approval"; although the imprimatur of the FDA was often considered in these terms by many in this period, their review of a New Drug Application would be merely to indicate it effective, and to license it for interstate commerce.

10. The first article anywhere—including medical journals—to report the success of Enovid as birth control in clinic trials in Puerto Rico was Albert Q. Maisel's (1957) misleadingly titled "New Hope for Childless Women" and appeared in *Ladies Home Journal*.

11. Anonymous reviewer, March 13, 1963, on "Enovid, Ortho-Novum and Thromboembolic Effects," *Medical Letter*, Rockefeller Archive Center, Rockefeller University, Record Group 891, Martin Rizack Papers, Box 45, Folder 1.

12. Anonymous reviewer reply to "Oral Contraceptives," RAC-RU, RG891, Martin Rizack Papers, B38, F7.

13. Harold Aaron to anonymous reviewer, Aprile 6, 1962. RAC-RU, RG891, Martin Rizack papers, B38, F6.

14. Anonymous reviewer (May or Aprile 1962), reply to "Oral Contraceptives," RAC-RU, RG891, Martin Rizack papers, B38, F6.

15. Anonymous reviewer, July 6, 1962, reply to "Oral Contraceptives," RAC-RU, RG891, Martin Rizack papers, B38, F6.

16. Anonymous reviewer, May 21, 1962, reply to "Oral Contraceptives," RAC-RU, RG891, Martin Rizack papers, B38, F6.

References

Allen, W. M., & Weintersteiner, O. (1934). Crystalline progestin, *Science, 80*, 190.

Asbell, B. (1995). *The Pill: A biography of the drug that changed the world.* New York: Random House.

Briggs, L. (2002). *Reproducing empire: Race, sex, science and U.S. imperialism in Puerto Rico.* Berkeley: University of California Press.

Clarke, A. (1998). *Disciplining reproduction: Modernity, American life sciences, and the problem of sex.* Berkeley: University of California Press.

Collins, J. A., & Schlesselman, J. J. (2002). Perimenopausal use of reproductive hormones: Effects on breast and endometrial cancer. *Obstetrics and Gynecology Clinics in North America, 3*(29), 511–525.

Collins, P. H. (1999). Will the "real" mother please stand up? The logic of eugenics and American national family planning. In A. Clarke & V. Olsen (Eds.), *Revisioning women, health, and healing* (pp. 260–282). New York: Routledge.

Cook, H., Gamble, C., & Satterthwaite, P. (1961). Oral contraception with norethynodrel. American Journal of Obstetrics and Gynecology, 82(2), 437–445.

Diczfalusy, E. (1979). Gregory Pincus and steroidal contraception: A new departure in the history of mankind. *Journal of Steroid Biochemistry, 11*, 3–11.

Djerassi, C. (1992). *The Pill, pygmy chimps, and Degas' horse.* New York: Basic.

Drife J. (2002). Oral contraception and the risk of thromboembolism: What does it mean to clinicians and their patients? *Drug Safety, 25*(13), 893–902.

Fausto-Sterling, A. (1985/1992). *Myths of gender.* New York: Basic.

Fausto-Sterling, A. (2000). *Sexing the body: Gender politics and the construction of sexuality.* New York: Basic.

Gamble, C. (1947). The college birthrate, *Journal of Heredity, 38*, 11.

Goldzieher, A., & Rudel, H. (1974). How the oral contraceptives came to be developed. *Journal of the American Medical Association, 230*, 421–425.

Gordon, L. (1977/1995). *Woman's body, woman's right.* New York: Penguin.

Grant, E. (1985). *The bitter pill: How safe is the "perfect contraceptive"?* London: Elm Tree Books.

Greenfield, N. (1976). *First, do no harm: A dying woman's battle against the physicians and drug companies who misled her about the hazards of the Pill.* New York: Sun River Press.

Gunn, A. D. G. (1987). *Oral contraception in perspective: Thirty years of clinical experience with the Pill.* Carnforth, England: Parthenon.

Hartmann, B. (1987/1995). *Reproductive rights and wrongs: The global politics of population control* (Rev. ed.). Boston: South End Press.

Kevles, D. (1985). *In the name of eugenics: Genetics and the uses of human heredity.* Berkeley: University of California Press.

Kuzrok, R. (1937). The prospects for hormonal sterilization. *Journal of Contraception, 2*, 27–29.

Maisel, A. Q. (1957, August). New hope for childless women. *Ladies Home Journal,* pp. 46–47, 85.

Maisel, A. Q. (1965). *The hormone quest.* New York: Random House.

Makepeace, A. W., Weinstein, G. L., & Friedman, M. H. (1937). The effect of progestin and progesterone on ovulation in the rabbit. *American Journal of Physiology, 119*, 512–516.

Marker, R. E., & Rohrman, E. (1939). Conversion of sarsapogenin. *Journal of American Chemical Society, 61*, 3592.

Marker, R. E., & Rohrman E. (1940). Diosgenin. *Journal of American Chemical Society, 62*, 2525.

Marks, L. (1998). "A cage of ovulating females": The history of the early oral contraceptive pill clinical trials, 1950–59. In H. Kamminga & S. de Chadarevian (Eds.), *Molecularising biology and medicine, 1930s—1970* (pp. 221–47). London: Harwood Academic Publishers.

Mass, B. (1977). *Population target: The political economy of population control in Latin America.* Toronto: Women's Educational Press.

McLaughlin, L. (1982). *The Pill, John Rock, and the Church.* Boston: Little Brown.

Merkin, D. (1976). *Pregnancy as a disease: The Pill in society.* Port Washington, NY: Kennikat Press.

Ory, H. W. (1996). Epidemiology of venous thromboembolic disease and OC use. *Dialogues in Contraception, 5*(1), 4–7, 10.

Oudshoorn, N. (1994). *Beyond the natural body: An archaeology of sex hormones.* New York: Routledge.

Pendell, E. (1956). *Population on the loose.* New York: Funk.

Perone, N. (1994). The progestins. In J. Goldzieher (Ed.), *Pharmacology of contraceptive steroids* (pp. 5–19). New York: Raven.

Pincus, G. (1956). Some effects of progesterone and related compounds upon reproduction and early development in mammals. *Acta Endocrinologica Supplementum, 28,* 18–36.

Pincus, G. (1958). Fertility control with oral medication. *American Journal of Obstetrics and Gynecology, 75,* 1333–1346.

Pincus, G. (1959, August 2). Paradoxical hormone is basis of birth control pill. *Washington Post,* p. E8.

Pincus, G. (1965). *The control of fertility.* New York: Academic.

Ramírez de Arellano, M., & Seipp, C. (1983). *Colonialism, Catholicism, and contraception: A history of birth control in Puerto Rico.* Chapel Hill: University of North Carolina Press.

Reed, J. (1974). Oral history interview with Adaline Pendleton Satterthwaite, MD. *Women's Studies Manuscript Collection of the Schlesinger Library, Radcliffe College, Series 3: Sexuality, Sex Education, and Reproductive Rights; Part A: Family Planning Oral History Project.* Bethesda, MD: University Publications of America.

Reed, J. (1978). *From private vice to public virtue: The birth control movement and American society since 1830.* New York: Basic.

Rice-Wray, E. (1957). Field study with Enovid as contraceptive Agent. In *Proceedings of a Symposium on 19-Nor Progestational Steroids* (pp. 78–85). Chicago: Searle Research Laboratories.

Rice-Wray, E., Schultz-contreras, M., Guerrero, I., & Aranda-Roselli, A. (1962). Long-term administration of Norethindrone in fertility control. *JAMA, 180*(5), 355–361.

Roberts, D. (1997). *Killing the Black body: Race, reproduction, and the meaning of liberty.* New York: Random House.

Rock, J. (1963). *The time has come: A Catholic doctor's proposal to end the battle over birth control.* New York: Knopf.

Rock, J., Celso, R., & Pincus, G. (1957). Synthetic progestins in the normal human menstrual cycle. *Recent Progress in Hormone Research, 13,* 323–346.

Rock, J., Garcia, C. R., & Pincus, G., (1958) Effects of three 19-nor steroids on human ovulation and menstruation. *American Journal of Obstetrics and Gynecology, 75*(1), 82–97.

Satterthwaite, A. (1957, December 12). Personal correspondence with Clarence Gamble. Countway Library of Medicine Clarence J. Gamble Papers (CLM-CJGP), Box 49, File 797.

Satterthwaite, A. (1957–1958) Personal correspondence with Gamble. Countway Library of Medicine Clarence J. Gamble Papers (CLM-CJGP), Boxes 49–50, Files 798–800.

Satterthwaite, A. (1959). Personal correspondence with Clarence Gamble. Countway Library of Medicine Clarence J. Gamble Papers (CLM-CJGP), B50, F820.

Satterthwaite, Adaline. (1965) "Experience with Oral and Intrauterine Contraception in Rural Puerto Rico." In M. Sheps & J. Ridley (Eds.), *Public health and population change: Current research issues* (pp. 474–480). Pittsburgh, PA: University of Pittsburgh Press.

Satterthwaite, A., & Gamble, C. (1962). Conception control with norethynodrel. *Journal of the American Medical Women's Association, 17,* 797–802.

Seaman, B. (1969). *The doctors' case against the Pill.* New York: Wyden.

Sheehan, N. (1988). *A bright shinning lie: John Paul Vann and America in Vietnam.* New York: Vintage Books.

Sturgis, S. H., & Albright, F. (1940). Estrin therapy in dysmenorrhea. *Endocrinology, 26,* 68.

Tone, A. (1997). *Controlling reproduction: An American history.* Wilmington, DE: Scholarly Resources.

Treichler, P. (1992). Beyond Cosmo: AIDS, identity, and inscriptions of gender. *Camera Obscura, 28,* 21–78.

Vaughan, P. (1970). *The Pill on trial.* New York: Coward-McCann.

Vogt, W. (1960). *People! Challenge to survival.* London: Clowes.

Williams, D., & Williams, R. (1978). *Every child a wanted child: Clarence James Gamble, M.D., and his work in the birth control movement.* Boston: Countway Library of Medicine.

8

Biopolitical Media

Population, Communications International, and the Governing of Reproductive Health

RONALD WALTER GREENE & DAVID BRESHEARS
University of Minnesota & University of Texas Austin

SETTING: a village in Tanzania.
CHARACTERS: Mkwaju, a heavy-drinking and promiscuous truck driver who abandoned his family and contracted HIV; Tunu, his wife, who has supported their children since Mkwaju left.

MKWAJU: Tunu, please listen to me.
TUNU: Mkwaju, you cannot trick me anymore. You thought I was a fool, but . . .
MKWAJU: (coughing) I now understand and have come home.
TUNU: Home? Home? You think that this is your home? Your home is at Tila's, your concubine.
MKWAJU: But Tunu, I can't bear life without you.
TUNU: Stupid lies. What about the time you infected me with a venereal disease? (Henderson, 2000)

From July 1993 through the end of 1999, the tumultuous lives of Mkwaju and Tunu were the dramatic centerpiece of *Twende na Wakati*, an internationally acclaimed serial radio drama, broadcast twice weekly throughout Tanzania (Vaughan, Rogers, Singhal, & Swalehe, 2000, p. 86). Produced through the joint efforts of Population Communications International (PCI) and the government, business community, and academic institutions of Tanzania, each half-hour episode attracted millions of listeners, and the show maintained a strong following for the duration of its run (Vaughan & Rogers, 2000, p. 213).[1] *Twende na Wakati* also generated a significant amount of interest among members of the international academic community (Jato et al., 1999; Mohammed, 2001; Rogers et al., 1999; Swalehe, Rogers, Gilboard, Alford, & Montoya, 1995; Vaughn &

Rogers 2000; Vaughn et al., 2000). A program carefully researched and designed to promote the values of gender equality, sexual responsibility, and environmental protection, *Twende na Wakati* became an important case study in the emerging field of entertainment-education (Keyser, 2000) and the template of PCI's approach to mass media public health communication.

This chapter investigates the media production practices of PCI in order to inquire into the role of mass mediated public health campaigns in governing reproductive health. The network of professional expertise represented by PCI media productions often seem "exempt from a critical interrogation of their motives because their communication campaigns are aimed at increasing the social good" (McKinley & Jensen, 2003, p. 183). Perhaps what prevents the critical challenge from gaining traction is the idea that a critical intervention must challenge the *motives* of the participants in these communication campaigns. Rather than focusing on motives, then, our critical intervention challenges the *methods* by which PCI produces soap operas. We interrogate PCI's media production practices to highlight how the governing of female bodies takes place in and through their attachment to specific communicative networks populated by a shifting set of cultural industries, workers, experts, and genres. Specifically, we demonstrate that the governance of women's reproductive and sexual health relies on the ability of biopolitical media industries to transform women into media audiences.

Entertainment Education and the Genres of Governance

The idea that mass mediated communication may function as an instrument of economic and social development has been around for some time. Daniel Lerner's (1958) *Passing of the Traditional Society: Modernizing the Middle East* was an early effort to forge an explicit link between communication research and development strategies. Followed by Wilbur Schramm's (1964) *Mass Media and National Development,* they conceived the mass media as an instrument for the diffusion of development decisions from centralized governing structures to the people "on the ground" Also, in the 1960s Everett Rogers (1962) emphasized the role of the media in the diffusion of innovations necessary to jump-start the change from a traditional society to a modern one. For Lerner, Schramm, and Rogers the goals of development were to be promoted through the interaction of mass media and literacy to generate support for innovations such as birth control technologies associated with modernization. Unfortunately, the optimism associated with the link between development and communication in the 1960s ran into difficulties in the 1970s. Melkote (1991) writes that, "[b]y the seventies it became increasingly clear in Asia and Latin America that socio-economic structural constraints diminished and even eliminated the influence of the mass media in overcoming problems of development" (pp. 172–173). By the 1990s, the assumed good of development had undergone critical interrogation (Dubois, 1991; Escobar, 1995).

Notwithstanding the problems associated with attempts to link communication research to the goals of development, PCI's approach to entertainment-education owes much to this history. However, the fundamental difference between these older attempts and PCI's newer programs is an emphasis on participatory communication strategies. At the heart of these participatory strategies for development and communication is a greater role for the populations affected by the development process. At its most inclusive, participation means that individuals are empowered to "contribute ideas, take initiatives, articulate their needs and problems, and assert their autonomy" (Melkote, 1991, p. 239). Melkote argues that more participatory development and communication strategies opened up the possibility of adding new media options such as "folk media" and indigenous communication channels to the traditional mass media of television, radio, and newspapers. The use of radio and television soap operas to convey ideas about health communication emerged from this interaction between the more participatory discourses on communication and development and the traditional reliance on mass media effects research to evaluate the uptake of new values and behaviors (Meyer, 1981; McCombie, Hornick, & Anarfi, 2002). To assess mass communication's role in stimulating behavioral changes, PCI relies on Albert Bandura's (1977) social learning theory to guide the development of their soap operas. For Bandura behavioral changes are often due to modeling one's behavior on another's behavior. Bandura's value to mass communication is that he expands the range of possible role models to include characters one encounters vicariously through media exposure. For PCI, Miguel Sabido's research on the efficacy of *telenovela's* for promoting family planning and development in Mexico supported the view of soap operas as participatory media. Other organizations, such as the Population Media Center (2004), also echo the Sabido method for using soap operas to promote behavioral change. The popularity of soap operas underwritten by social learning theory and their historical success in Mexico paved the way for entertainment education to emerge as a strategy of health communication.

While not unique, the soap opera genre has become the dominant cultural form of entertainment-education. The rise of entertainment-education as a vehicle for health communication relies on the power of dramatic narrative to frame and supplement the "facts" about public health issues (Myers, 2002). According to entertainment-education writer and broadcaster Pamela Brooke, "Before facts can take root in the human heart, they have to penetrate all the elusive psychological layers that are at work in our interactions with one another. Information is useless to us unless we are able to act on it without severely disrupting family and community norms" (quoted in Myers, 2002, p. 4). PCI argues that "*telenovelas* have often been a 'safe' way to reflect societal changes in a country," including the transformation of popular opinions about family issues such as divorce, remarriage, nonvirgin brides, and acceptance of children from other marriages (Matelski, 1999, p. 28). However, these soap operas do not merely *reflect* societal change—they *promote* it.

Through the construction of "realistic characters" and plot lines that incorporate local beliefs and concerns, PCI asserts that radio soap operas are an effective vehicle for the promotion of healthy behavior. Positive, negative, and transitional characters are variously rewarded and punished for the choices they make, and listeners are encouraged to identify with and emulate these characters' positive choices. According to Myers (2002), "the basic theory underpinning these projects is that audiences develop a strong sense of affective identification with characters and situations, and this kind of identification leads to discussion about issues raised and, eventually, to individual or even collective action" (p. 5). Radio soap operas provide creators and listeners an opportunity to engage health-related social issues to transform attitudes and behaviors. For example, in *Twende na Wakati*, Tunu shows strength and determination by withholding sex from Mkwaju until he has an HIV test (Myers, 2002, p. 4). In a drama from Rwanda, *Urunana*, "a young man learns to recognize the symptoms of an STD, gets it treated at a local health clinic and, while he is there, picks up a supply of free condoms" (Myers, 2002, pp. 4–5). Kenya's *Ushikwapo Shikamana* tackles a variety of issues, including arranged marriages and female circumcision, and India's *Tinka Tinka Sukh* deals extensively with the practice of dowry. Each of these serial dramas provides the audience with an opportunity to identify affectively with positive characters to help transform behavioral practices at the individual level. In Foucauldian language, PCI's radio soap operas are a cultural technology for regulating and fashioning the self (Bennett, 2003; Foucault, 1988).

PCI's radio soap operas express the relation between genre and governance. In the United States, the genres of governance are primarily imagined as forms of political communication: the interview on Sunday morning news programs, the State of the Union address, the tedious

and sometimes spectacular character of Congressional Hearings and/
or Government Accounting Office reports on the budget (Campbell
and Jamieson, 1990). However, the genres of popular culture are also
associated with the problem of governance. As Toby Miller (1998)
writes, "Genres both train the population as readers and agents and
are themselves understood as representative of that population, spatial
markers of governance and resistance" (p. 19). In the case of PCI, the
soap opera becomes a scientifically managed genre aiming to transform
the sexual and reproductive habits of a target population. Popular
genres are economically advantageous because they minimize risk and
innovation as they partake in a "bureaucratically organized regime of
pleasure" (Miller, 1998, p. 20). Thus, PCI's production of soap operas
as a "methodology for social change" is an explicitly bureaucratized
communicative enterprise. At the same time, the use of soap operas
balances the repetition of form with the differences provided by the
cultural attributes and values of distinct and disparate populations.
The point is that the soap opera genre provides a narrative substructure
that can be tweaked with culturally sensitive knowledge about specific
populations in unique geographical locations. PCI relies on other
popular genres besides radio soaps, but the use of radio soap operas
demonstrates how the governance of female bodies increasingly requires
their constitution as media audiences capable of making affective
identifications with the main characters. The close relation between
PCI and the soap operas as a genre of governance suggests the need to
evaluate the role of communication scholars in testing and evaluating
the quantity and quality of the audience for a particular genre.

Communication Expertise and the Governing of Health

Communication research contributes to the governing of female bodies
in and through the discourses of health and medicine. Assuredly, health
communication in the United States and elsewhere has become a growth
industry, generating active networks of scholars and policy makers, and
blending the relation between the two roles. In an era of decreasing
financial support for public education in the United States, for example,
involvement in large-scale mediated health campaigns offer financial
enticements to pull communication research and expertise closer to
the goals and purposes of health-conscious state and international
policy makers. As R. C. Hornick (2002) argues, "many public agencies
assume that public health communication is a powerful tool for behavior
change" (p. xii). For example, in the United States the Office of National
Drug Control Policy spent nearly $1 billion over 5 years on its National

Anti-Drug Media Campaign, while the American Legacy Foundation spent a similar amount to discourage smoking (Hornick, 2002, p. xii). In this context, the financing of PCI's media production requires that numerous international, state, and private donor organizations continue to believe that mass communication is a successful means by which to change behavior.

Established in 1985, PCI is a U.S.-based nongovernmental organization (NGO)[2] dedicated to the promotion of family planning practices, gender equality, environmental protection, and AIDS prevention. With total annual revenues averaging $3,894,809 over the 3-year period between 1997 and 1999, comprised entirely of public grants and private contributions, PCI qualifies as a tax-exempt charity under section 501(c)(3) of the IRS Code, and is eligible to receive tax-deductible contributions (Charities Review Council of Minnesota, 2002). PCI's total annual expenses during this time averaged $3,417,241. Of this amount, 76% of expenses were allocated directly to PCI's programs, 16% to management and general expenses, and 8% to fund-raising. Also during this 3-year period, individual contributions accounted for 23.8% of PCI's annual revenue, with the remaining 76.2% from foundations or organizations (Charities Review Council of Minnesota, 2002). PCI's funding sources for fiscal year 2000 included a $1.8 million grant from the William H. Gates Foundation and a grant from the United Nations Educational, Scientific and Cultural Organization's (UNESCO) International Program for the Development of Communication (IPDC). PCI works in partnership with "government ministries, NGOs, individual radio and television stations, and an assortment of private-sector agencies" in 22 countries across 5 continents. A central element in PCI's media campaigns is the production of "carefully researched and culturally sensitive radio and television soap operas . . . [designed to] motivate individuals to adopt new attitudes and behaviors . . ." (UNESCO, p. 3). Over the past 20 years PCI has become a well-known institutional actor in a global culture industry associated with the design of mass media health campaigns, and as such increasingly relies on experts in media effects research.

Modern forms of government generate a close relation between the production and dissemination of expertise and strategies of rule. Expertise requires the socialization of individuals into the standards of judgment comporting to an ethical and disciplinary code leading to its professionalization (Johnson, 1993). The relation between professional expertise and government is reciprocal. The ability to launch a new health communication campaign requires the languages of human and biomedical sciences to calculate, classify, and categorize reality so that this same reality can be known in a form that makes it amenable to intervention and change. The professions, in turn, depend on the desire to invent, explain, and solve social problems, a demand that not only supplies privileged forms of expertise with grant dollars but guides the formation of disciplinary and professional problematics. What takes place in this reciprocal relation between expertise and governance is the composition of "associations formed between entities constituted as 'political' and the projects, plans and practices of those authorities—economic, legal, spiritual, medical, technical—who endeavor to administer the lives of others in the light of conceptions of what is good, healthy, normal, virtuous, efficient or profitable" (Rose & Miller, 1992, p. 175). The success or failure of professional expertise to garner status as a legitimate knowledge, that is, knowledge capable of speaking truth, increasingly requires the ability of experts to enter into alliances closely associated with activities and agencies of political governance.

Communication scholarship oriented toward investigating the effectiveness of mass mediated public health campaigns partakes in a growing network of organizations (some closer than others to the state) that are becoming increasingly reliant on communicative processes as a field and method for regulating behavior. In the case of entertainment-education, a trend is increasingly visible about what kinds of communicative research and expertise will be given priority. As McKinley and Jensen (2003) note, the impact studies supporting the ability of entertainment-education to change social behavior often reveal negligible "descriptions of media environments," and "very little attention has been devoted to the ethnographic context of the audiences" (p. 185). The growing interactive dependence of public health/development campaigns on the success or failure of communication reveals the need for the description, assessment, and evaluation of these programs to "change reality." McKinley and Jensen (2003) describe the media effects research underwriting entertainment-education as exhibiting the "tenacity of the modernization paradigm lurking beneath the surface of research that aims to measure specific effects as a result of exogamous, strategically launched development communication interventions" (pp. 185–186). Hence, seeing communication scholars such as Everett Rogers (1973), who were once associated with communicating family planning strategies in the 1970s, today evaluating PCI's health communication campaigns in the 1990s (Vaughn & Rogers, 2000), is not surprising. Some forms of communicative expertise are given priority and opportunity due to their ability to translate events, people, and motivations into information that is "stable, mobile, comparable and combinable" (Rose & Miller, 1992, p. 185). In the field of entertainment-education, forms of communicative expertise are increasingly necessary to justify the continued funding of specific programs, a situation that leads McKinley and Jensen (2003) to reasonably ask, "to what extent the choices of communication strategies are driven by the methods by which these strategies will later be evaluated" (p. 186).

What is of utmost importance is not only that one form of communicative expertise is being privileged over another (mass media effects research), but rather the reliance of governing agencies on communicative research and expertise, a situation that has its roots in the development communication campaigns of the 1960s. In this framework, elements within the circuit of communication become sites for transforming populations, values, goals, and programs into a language amenable to communicative expertise. For example, target populations become audiences who provide information for the design of specific media messages so producers may fine-tune the message to better achieve their goals of changing the audiences' knowledge, attitudes, and practices. In this act of translation, the governing of female bodies becomes even more closely attached to a cultural industry whose experts risk, in the words of Horkheimer and Adorno (1944/1997), "not to produce or sanction anything that in any way differs from their own rules, their own ideas about consumers, or above all themselves" (p. 122).

PCI's *Soap Operas for Social Change: A PCI Methodology for Entertainment-Education* outlines the process by which soap operas are conceived and developed as communicative instruments for social change. The project begins with an invitation from "government agencies or NGOs, health personnel, members of the media, or concerned and active citizens" (PCI, 2000, p. 5). In this initial step, an assessment of the broadcast infrastructure and potential partnerships in the host country is undertaken to determine the project's feasibility. Because PCI's approach involves local media providers in both the development and transmission of programs, a country is only viable as a project site if both of these conditions are satisfied. Assuming this is the case, the second phase of program development is initiated.

During this second phase, formative research is conducted in the host country to "identify local attitudes and practices on a range of reproductive health issues, including family size, unmet need for family planning, gender roles, education, and STD/HIV prevention" (PCI, 2000, p. 5). This initial research serves as a guide for the development of messages, characters, and story lines. This formative research involves several steps: identifying research consultants and putting together a research team in each country; reviewing existing literature on the issues involved; conducting in-depth interviews with local experts; and leading focus group discussions with representative samples of the target audience

(PCI, 2000, p. 9). Combined with a country-specific legal and ethical framework "derived from the country's national constitution, relevant national and international laws, and the United Nations documents to which the country is a signatory," this formative research provides "an assessment of health attitudes and behaviors; the status of women and gender relations; media access and uses; and the culture, lifestyle, and social beliefs of various communities within each country" (PCI, 2000, pp. 9–10). This information is then coded into a "values grid," which becomes the actual guide for character and plot development.

In the third phase of program development, a creative team is assembled in the host country, with the task of creating story lines and characters. Radio and television scriptwriters are recruited, among whom are "staff writers at local stations, individuals recruited from university theatre or creative writing departments, or people from the local community" (PCI, 2000, p. 15). Their task is to translate the information contained in the values grid into a "creative and inspiring serial drama" (p. 15). This is not an autonomous project, however. PCI's "professional facilitators" provide training and instruction to these local artistic teams to ensure that program development follows the PCI methodology (pp. 15-16).[3]

Once a soap opera is produced, media partners in the host country take responsibility for broadcasting. This is not the end of the development process, however. The fourth phase involves incorporating audience feedback through monitoring research. By taking into account the audience's reaction to these serial dramas, the dramas are adapted to increase audience share or to enhance the effectiveness of the message. The final phase of PCI's process is not necessarily related to program development, but is instead intended to measure its effectiveness. Impact evaluations, examples of which include the field research on *Twende na Wakati*, function as both a measure of program effectiveness as well as the rationale for reproducing this strategy in other countries (Jato et al., 1999; Mohammed, 2001; Rogers et al., 1999; Swalehe et al., 1995; Vaughn & Rogers, 2000; Vaughn et al., 2000). Indeed, PCI's promotional packet includes full-text copies of two such studies (Law & Singhal, 1999; Rogers et al., 1999), and their promotional literature refers frequently to the positive conclusions of the studies.

Yet, methodological criticisms have been raised concerning the media impact studies of soap operas and education-entertainment (McKinley & Jensen, 2003; Sherry, 1997; Starosta, 1994). In particular, McKinley and Jensen (2003) note that " the continued quest for quantifiable effects of short term media interventions within development communication, particularly health communication, runs counter to contemporary medi-

atcd communication research" (p. 186). As such, different research
methodologies and theoretical literatures are necessary. However,
our point is that while it is an important political struggle to justify
different ways of "being in the true" within the association of experts
and governance, we should not avoid commenting on the will to govern
that permeates much of health communication research. From the
standpoint of governance, recognizing how organizations such as PCI
build associations and constituencies made up of cultural workers, media
professionals, and communication experts is, perhaps, more important.
In other words, the formative and evaluative research methodologies
PCI used belong to the area of media production and PCI should be
studied as a media institution. Such a perspective reveals how the values,
motivations, and the instrumental goals of reproductive health and
gender equality rely on the invention of biopolitical media industries.

Biopolitical Media and the Need for Audiences

Our argument is not that PCI's soap operas promote bad ideological
representations of health and women. Our argument is that health
communication is increasingly associated with the tasks of governing the
reproductive health of women. Moreover, for communication to govern
requires the incorporation of communicative genres and expertise into
institutional partnerships between NGOs such as PCI and the state. We
are less concerned with how soap operas are decoded by an audience.
In fact, research on soap operas in the Middle East suggests soaps can
provide rhetorical and cultural resources for resisting conservative
assumptions about the role of women (Abu-Lughod, 2004). So too
might PCI claim such an effect because it designs its soaps to express
norms of reproductive health consistent with the international human
rights treaties signed by the countries where the soaps are broadcast.
This paper is agnostic on the ideological message being transmitted
and decoded. However, we are interested in what the production story
tells us about the biopolitical governance of female bodies. The argument we pursue is that female bodies are increasingly governed in and
through their attachment to biopolitical media industries. The first step
in our argument concerns the difference between commercial media
and biopolitical media and the "new international division of cultural
labor" (NIDCL).

The NIDCL refers to the possibility that cultural industries, such as
manufacturing, might relocate beyond the borders of the First World.
For Miller (1998), the NIDCL describes how "this could happen at the
level of textual production . . . or in such areas as marketing, information

and high culture, limited-edition work" (p. 172). In other words, the NIDCL refers to how cultural work is done in and across nation-states and how the distribution of the types of work and the value of that work makes a profit possible. The most extensive research on the explanatory value of the NIDCL for understanding the changes brought about by transnational production is the case of Hollywood. For Miller and his coinvestigators, "Hollywood reproduces and regulates the NIDCL through its control over cultural labor markets, international co-production, intellectual property, marketing, distribution and exhibition" (Miller, Govil, McMurria, & Maxwell, 2001, p. 18). The key economic question is "will deindustrial states lose jobs to the periphery, while retaining super-profits for their own ruling elite" (Miller, 1998, p. 173). "Global Hollywood" provides one model by which we can attempt to account for spatial and temporal coordinates of the NIDCL for the production and circulation of value. However, we suggest that PCI provides another model.

In the case of PCI, the NIDCL is associated less with profits and jobs and more with the dissemination and distribution of norms. In our terms, PCI demonstrates the emergence of biopolitical media industries as central actors in the governance of female bodies. We define biopolitical media industries as organizations that produce, disseminate, and evaluate communication programs, practices, and technologies to improve the health and well-being of a population. For Foucault (1990), biopolitics describes how modern forms of governance rely on the promotion of life through the maximization of capacities of individuals and groups to improve their welfare. As such, biopower works by distributing populations around the production of norms more so than the "murderous splendor" of sovereign right (Foucault, 1990, p. 144). Colin Gordon (1991) further remarks that biopolitics concerns itself "with subjects as members of a population, in which issues of individual sexual and reproductive conduct interconnect with issues of national policy and power" (pp. 4–5). While often deployed and organized in terms of national policy, biopolitical media industries work as often above and below the nation-state contributing to the uneven global flow of images and narratives in an effort to attach norms of behavior to new populations. Entertainment-education is one cultural form in which commercial and noncommercial enterprises participate in the creation of a biopolitical media industry.

Biopolitical governance describes how populations learn, train, and promote behaviors and capacities that will make them healthy, virtuous, wise, and economically efficient. Biopolitical media harness the NIDCL to the protection and quality of life. As a model for understanding the NIDCL, biopolitical media industries represent a shifting network of experts, policy makers, NGOs, and social movements dedicated to using communication techniques and technologies to improve the quality of life. These networks work in and across geographical spaces, industries, and welfare services with likely political and economic fissures occurring over the purposes, the design, and implementation of programs. In the case of PCI one has dramatists working on scripts, cultural workers producing value grids relevant to the target populations, and project evaluators in charge of assessing the success or failure of the programs. What we want to emphasize is that biopolitical media industries illustrate how "communication . . . occupies a crucial position in the organization and administration of government" (Innis, 1950/1972, p. 4) by circulating the norms of healthy behaviors and practices.

However, the success or failure of biopolitical media industries is predicated on capturing audiences. Just as commercially focused cultural industries need audiences to turn a profit, so too does a biopolitical media industry require audiences to maximize qualitative and quantitative changes in the welfare of a population. PCI's formative and evaluative research articulates its entertainment-education programs to the search for audiences as a precondition for governing female bodies. This reliance on governing through the creation of audiences owes its history to the interface between marketing, advertising, and public relations in the invention of consumer capitalism in the United States (Mattelart, 2000, pp. 294–295). It is within this horizon that political communication was reimagined as the "engineering of consent" made possible by the help of public opinion surveys contributing to the transformation of the consumer into the citizen (p. 293). The close association between marketing and the new media of the early twentieth century helped to invent the media audience as a particular object of knowledge able to reveal information about its motivations, practices, and values. As Mosco (2003) argues, "the concept of audience was hatched largely out of the marketing departments of companies with a stake in selling products through the media" (p. 342). Similarly, John Hartley (1987) reminds us how the media audience is often a consequence of the representations of institutions that "desire to enter into relations with them" and these representations of the audience serve "institutional needs and purposes" (p. 127). In the case of PCI, soap operas invite women to become media audiences through affective identifications with characters. As media audiences, PCI extracts knowledge from women to better promote the dissemination and distribution of norms.

Biopolitical media industries construct female bodies as objects of knowledge by transforming them into media audiences. Participatory research traditions help biopolitical media industries because they facilitate the production of knowledge about populations. The creation of audiences enables communication research to classify and correct behavior by better modulating media messages. Moreover, the invention of audiences by biopolitical media allows for their supervision regarding the uptake of the norms of healthy behavior within a more general population. Through the constitution and examination of an audience, communication researchers are able to observe how well new behaviors and innovations are being dispersed through the social field. Hence, participatory research does not simply disguise a model of governance based on imposition, but it allows biomedia industries to govern in and through the active involvement of their target populations in creating media programs. Ironically, as communication scholars call for more participatory communication schemes and research methodologies to replace the residual biases left in place by the media effects research dominant in entertainment-education, they are providing a mechanism by which the agency and freedom of media audiences can be better articulated to the normalizing discourses of health. The apparent conflict between human rights of participation and the normalization of society through biopolitical governance is held in check by the emergence of medicine as a "neutral discourse" to arbitrate disagreements (Foucault, 2003, p. 39). Thus, the ability of PCI to articulate the discourses of medicine to human rights shields how health communication transforms women into media audiences as a precondition for attaching them to new global networks of normalization.

Bio-Political Media and the Malthusian Couple

Population Communications International's existence as a biopolitical media industry is closely related to the politics of population control. While PCI's promotional literature fronts several concerns, such as reproductive health, environmental protection, and sustainable development, all of these are ultimately ancillary to the problem of population growth. In *Many Voices, One Vision*, PCI's annual report for 1999, environmental devastation, gender inequality, and the contagion of infectious sexu- ally transmitted diseases are defined principally as concerns related to the problem of population growth. Gender equality, for example, is important because of the role women play in the adoption of family plan- ning practices, as opposed to an end in itself. Likewise, environmental management is to be achieved first and foremost through the adoption of family planning. Both cases illustrate the centrality of population control to PCI's strategy. Malthusian fears about overpopulation have been closely associated with the invention and circulation of biopower (Foucault, 1990, p. 105). Foucault (1990) argues that the nineteenth-century discourses about the "Malthusian couple" helped to put sexuality at the center of modern biopolitics. More recently, Greene (1999) has argued that the location and construction of the Malthusian couple in the Third World as a threat to the global security of the First World was implicated in the invention and composition of the "population apparatus," a global network of power dedicated to improving individual, national, and global welfare by lowering fertility rates.

Of course, alternative social imaginaries exist alongside and apart from the Malthusian modern. One such alternative is the "feminist modern" (Greene, 1999, 2000). The feminist modern emerged on the terrain of international population policy as a counterforce to the Malthusian modern. It is the result of a new consensus put together at the 1994 International Conference on Population and Development (ICPD) shifting priorities away from demographic quotas and timetables to the empowerment of women. Its primary difference with the Malthusian modern is that it takes women's empowerment, health education, and women's rights as the primary building blocks toward a more sustainable vision of development. What marks the feminist modern as modern is the growing emphasis on women as subjects, or active participants, who emerge, often with the help of experts, as capable of challenging cultural norms and practices that limit the choices women need to make to improve their quality of life. While resisting Malthusian forms of modernity, the feminist modern increasingly relies on a Western emphasis on individual action (Wilkins, 1999, p. 63). In her case study of Tanzania's emphasis on women's and girls' education as a development strategy, Vavrus (2003) points out that "women's choices about childbearing, reproductive health, and environmental conservation are shaped by social and political-economic considerations that the independent figure of the feminist modern does not take into account" (p. 41).

Biopolitical media industries, such as PCI, are able to bridge Malthusian and feminist imaginations by linking rights talk with the "neutrality" of medical discourses. However, like its development communication predecessors, such a link often ignores a systematic analysis associated with the structural conditions of women. For example, the rhetoric of "choice" implied by the concept of gender equality PCI employed is often restricted to control over family composition—family size and the spacing of births—rather than "choice" about health care, food, and shelter for self and family. According to Bandarage (1997):

if "choice" is to be expanded to be meaningful for most people, especially poor women, the "new" agenda would have to move far beyond family planning to focusing on poverty alleviation and structural changes in the global political economy. In the absence of such broader social changes required for the empowerment of women and the poor, the "new" reproductive rights approach will become another example of the capitulation of liberal feminism to the Malthusian interest in controlling the number of the poor. (p. 55)

Sonia Correa (1994) calls the rhetoric of reproductive rights "population double-speak," which focuses intervention at the microlevel while ignoring the structural/institutional causes of women's suffering (pp. 62–63). Thus, simply invoking "gender equality" as a goal of program development does not necessarily disarticulate family planning practices and reproductive health concerns from a Malthusian logic of modernity.

Establishing a women's empowerment agenda has radical potential but it is often curtailed by lack of investment in public health and skewed funding priorities that often earmark family planning as the most important health investment (Hartmann, 1995). In the United States, the Clinton Administration supported the ICPD plan of action, while the George W. Bush Administration withheld funding to the United Nations Population Fund due to its alleged complicity with forced abortions in China (Cohen, 2002, p. 13). Thus, while radical critiques of the ICPD make visible the limitations of the women's empowerment agenda, the feminist modern underwriting PCI does circulate reproductive rights in the face of conservative challenges to the women's empowerment agenda of ICPD. PCI's role as a biopolitical media industry provides a specific opportunity for incorporating ICPD's emphasis on women's health, gender equality, HIV/AIDS prevention, and the reduction of maternal mortality as norms embedded in narrative form. PCI's media productions are both feminist and Malthusian. PCI can represent itself as feminist while disguising its Malthusian sensibilities by circulating medical and rights discourses in conservative times. But the "feminism" of PCI is limited to a rather instrumental rationality (women's empowerment to decrease the harms of population growth). If articulating a radical feminist politics to biopolitical media industries is possible, a first step will require the dis-articulation of Malthusian logics from reproductive health and rights. Otherwise, "reproductive rights" and "choice" will mask the oppression inherent in fertility limits and manifested in practices such as forced sterilization, the export of faulty and unsafe IUDs to Third World countries, and forced experimentation on Third World women (Grimes, 1998).

Conclusion

This chapter shows how the governance of female bodies increasingly relies on their transformation into media audiences. To demonstrate this more general claim, we have investigated the cultural work of PCI as a biopolitical media industry dedicated to promoting reproductive health by linking communicative genres, communicative expertise, cultural labor, and media audiences. The need of biopolitical governance to rely on the genres, techniques, and knowledge associated with communication suggests at least three urgent needs.

The first need is to challenge the politics of truth associated with the particular configuration of communicative expertise and media health campaigns. Population Communications International is but one organization among many in the United States and elsewhere increasingly committed to the design of mediated public health campaigns. Yet, certain research traditions and funding agencies are aligning to limit how communication can be imagined within these governing networks. The current "regime of truth" is contributing to a border that defines the value of communication research. High value communication research is research that can enter into an alliance with government agencies and donor organizations, translating communicative expertise into research affiliations and grant dollars. At the same time, communication research loses value when it is unable to directly affiliate with the operations of governing agencies increasingly invested in biopolitical and market governance.

The second need is an honest exploration of communication as a cultural technology of government. The chapter demonstrates how communication emerges as a technique and field of biopolitical governance. Communication is a technique of governance to the extent that it becomes a practical knowledge required for disseminating particular programs, values, and knowledge; and communication is a field of governance to the extent that it is in and through communicative competencies, practices, and vocabularies that the modulation of bodies and souls takes place. Only when we begin to take stock of the ways in which communication makes possible the shift from juridical power to biopower might we begin to appreciate how communication scholars are contributing to the globalization of a "normalizing society" (Foucault, 1990, p. 144).

Finally, we need to investigate the politics of biopolitical media. A radical perspective on biopolitical media requires an appreciation of how biopolitical media thrive in an atmosphere whereby large structural changes are increasingly removed from the social imaginary.

Due to a lack of systematic changes in the world economy, and the dis-articulation of the state from social services, biopolitical media industries are more likely than ever to rely heavily on participatory schemes to better train and incorporate women into the management and governance of themselves and others. Thus, if the creation of a radically feminist biopolitical media industry is possible, such an entity will need to encourage the participation of women and men into new political alliances beyond the globalization of medical discourses and the norms of healthy behaviors.

Notes

1. First aired in 1993, except in the control area of Dodoma. The program received the UNESCO award for Outstanding Rural Communications Program (March 2000) and the Population Institute's prestigious XXI Global Media Award for Excellence in Population Reporting in the category of Best Radio Program" (October 2000). Retrieved May 8, 2002, from http://www.population.org/Pciprog/prog_tanzania.htm. According to Myers (2002), *Twende na Wakati* was the most popular program on Radio Tanzania from 1993 to 1995, and the show regularly reached 5 million people (p. 5).

2. Due to the limitations of space and the interests of clarity, we cannot include an extensive discussion of the role NGOs played in the governance of the "population crisis." In part, the PCI's existence represents the doling out of governmental responsibilities to NGOs. Whereas many critics of statist politics hail the emergence of NGOs as a corrective to centralized decision-making, many reasons exist to view this development with suspicion. NGOs have been characterized as tools for exploitation and a driving force of globalization and the flow of international capital (Puplampu & Tettey, 2000; Stewart, 1997). They have been criticized as ineffective actors when they oppose the interests of ruling elites, functioning merely as "window dressing" for undemocratic governments (Stewart, 1997, p. 31). Owing to their reliance on a business model that privileges the demands of cost-efficiency over other concerns, NGOs are typically organized hierarchically and driven by profit motives (Sogge, 1996). Even southern NGOs suffer from this organizational defect (Mohan & Stokke, 2000; Schuurman, 1993). The hierarchical structure of these organizations is an obstacle to the stated goals of increasing participation by individuals, groups, and communities formerly excluded from the development process (Mohan & Stokke, 2000, p. 254). Additionally, some have suggested that the distinction between "governmental" and "nongovernmental" actors is overstated because even NGOs are incorporated into state structures (Tvedt, 1998). As an example of the limits of this organizational structure, accountability to the state limits the effectiveness of NGO interventions on behalf of women (Kabeer, 1994). While some critics have argued that NGOs fail to incorporate previously marginalized voices (Powell & Seddon, 1997, p. 8), others contend that NGOs actually demobilize indigenous movements pushing for radical change (Arellano-Lopez & Petras, 1994; Tandon, 1996). All of these criticisms suggest that PCI's emergence as a governing institution should be considered more closely.

3. As part of this collaborative process, PCI cosponsors with the University of Southern California (School of Cinema-Television, Annenberg School for Communication, and Population Research Lab) a 3-month Media Leadership

Program for "professionals currently involved in the radio, film or television industries" in one of the following eligible countries: Ethiopia, India, Mexico, Myanmar, Nigeria, Pakistan, the Philippines, or Sudan.

References

Abu-Lughod, L. (2004). *Dramas of Nationhood*. Chicago: University of Chicago Press.

Arellano-Lopez, S., & Petras, J. F. (1994). Non-governmental organizations and poverty alleviation in Bolivia. *Development and Change, 21,* 555–568.

Bandarage, A. (1997). *Women, population and global crisis: A political-economic analysis.* London: Zed.

Bandura, A. (1977). *Social learning theory.* New York: Prentice Hall.

Bennett, T. (2003). Culture and governmentality. In J. Bratich, J. Packer, & C. McCarthy (Eds.), *Foucault, cultural studies and governmentality* (pp. 47–66). Albany: State University of New York Press.

Campbell, K. K., & Jamieson, K. H. (1990). *Deeds done in words: Presidential rhetoric and the genres of governance.* Chicago: University of Chicago Press.

Charities Review Council of Minnesota. (2002). *Annual record.* St Paul, MN.

Cohen, S. (2002). Bush bars UNFPA funding, bucking recommendation of its own investigators. *The Guttmacher Report on Public Policy, 5*(4), 13. Retrieved May 15, 2005, from http://www.guttmacher.org/pubs/tgr/05/4/index.html

Correa, S. (1994). *Population and reproductive rights: Feminist perspectives from the South.* London: Zed.

DuBois, M. (1991). The governance of the Third World: A Foucauldian perspective on power relations in development. *Alternatives, 16*(1), 1–30.

Escobar, A. (1995). *Encountering development: The making and unmaking of the Third World.* Princeton, NJ: Princeton University Press.

Foucault, M. (1988). "Technologies of the self." In L. Martin, H. Gutman, & P. Hutton (Eds.), *Technologies of the self: A seminar with Michel Foucault* (pp. 16–49). Amherst: University of Massachusetts Press.

Foucault, M. (1990). *The history of sexuality. Vol. 1: An introduction.* New York: Vintage.

Foucault, M. (2003). *Society must be defended: Lectures at the College De France 1975–1976.* New York: Picador.

Gordon, C. (1991). Governmental rationality: An introduction. In G. Burchell, C. Gordon, & P. Miller (Eds.), *The Foucault effect: Studies in governmentality* (pp. 1–52). Chicago: University of Chicago Press.

Greene, R. W. (1999). *Malthusian worlds: U.S. leadership and the governing of the population crisis.* Boulder, CO: Westview.

Greene, R. W. (2000). Governing reproduction: Women's empowerment and population policy. In K. G. Wilkins (Ed.), *Redeveloping communication for social change: Theory, practice and power* (pp. 27–38). Lanham, MD: Rowman & Littlefield.

Grimes, S. (1998). From population control to reproductive rights: Ideological influences in population policy. *Third World Quarterly, 19*(3), 375–393

Hartley, J. (1987). Invisible fictions: Television audiences, paedocracy, pleasure. *Textual Practice, 1,* 121–138.

Hartmann. B. (1995). *Reproductive rights and wrongs: The global reproductive politics of population control.* Boston: South End.

Henderson, K. (2000, Fall). Telling stories, saving lives: Hope from soaps. *Ford Foundation Report.* Retrieved May 8, 2002, from http://www.fordfound.org/

Horkheimer, M., & Adorno, T. W. (1944/1997). *Dialectic of enlightenment* (J. Cumming, Trans.). London: Verso.

Hornik, R. C. (2002). Public health communication: Making sense of contradictory evidence. In R. C. Hornick (Ed.), *Public health communication: Evidence for behavior change (pp. 1–23).* Mahwah, NJ: Erlbaum.

Innis, H. (1950/1972). *Empire and communications.* Toronto: University of Toronto Press.

Jato, M. N., Tarasevich. J. M., Awasum, D. N., Simbakala, C., Kihinga,C. N. B., & Ngirwanugu, E. (1999). The impact of multimedia family planning promotion on the contraceptive behavior of women in Tanzania. *International Family Planning Perspectives,* 25, 60–67.

Johnson, T. (1993). Expertise and the state. In M. Gane & T. Johnson (Eds.), *Foucault's new domains* (pp. 139–152). London: Routledge.

Kabeer, N. (1994). *Reversed realities: Gender hierarchies in development thought.* London: Verso.

Keyser, A. M. (2000, Winter). Changing channels. *Perspectives: Research, Scholarship, and Creative Activity at Ohio University.* Retrieved May 15, 2003, from http://www.ohiou.edu/perspectives/0002/profile_channel.htm

Law, S., & Singhal, A. (1999). Efficacy in letter-writing to an entertainment-education radio serial. *Gazette,* 61(5), 355–372.

Lerner, D. (1958). *Passing of the traditional society: Modernizing the Middle East.* New York: Free.

Matelski, M. J. (1999). *Soap operas worldwide: Cultural and serial realities.* Jefferson, NC: McFarland.

Mattelart, A. (2000). *Networking the world, 1794–2000.* Minneapolis: University of Minnesota Press.

McCombie, S., Hornick, R. C., & Anarfi, J. K. (2002). Effects of a mass media campaign to prevent AIDS among young people in Ghana. In R. C. Hornick (Ed.), *Public health communication: Evidence for behavior change* (pp. 147–161). Mahwah, NJ: Erlbaum.

McKinley, M. A., & Jensen, L. O. (2003). In our own voices: Reproductive health radio programming in the Peruvian Amazon. *Critical Studies in Media Communication,* 20, 180–203.

Melkote, S. R. (1991). *Communication for development in the Third World: Theory and Practice.* Newbury Park, CA: Sage.

Meyer. M. (Ed). (1981). *Health education by television and radio.* New York: Saur Munchen.

Miller, T. (1998). *Technologies of truth: Cultural citizenship and the popular media.* Minneapolis: University of Minnesota Press.

Miller, T., Govil, N., McMurria, J., & Maxwell, R. (2001). *Global Hollywood.* London: British Film Institute.

Mohammed, S. (2001). Personal communication networks and the effects of an entertainment-education radio soap opera in Tanzania. *Journal of Health Communication,* 6, 137–154.

Mohan, G., & Stokke, K. (2000). Participatory development and empowerment: The dangers of localism. *Third World Quarterly,* 21(2), 247–268.

Mosco, V. (2003). Citizenship and technopoles. In J. Lewis & T. Miller (Eds.), *Critical cultural policy studies: A reader* (pp. 335–343). Malden, MA: Blackwell.

Myers, M. (2002, February). From awareness to action: Tackling HIV/Aids through radio and television drama. Benfield Greig Hazard Research Center. Unpublished manuscript.

Powell, M., & Seddon, D. (1997). NGOs and the development industry. *Review of African Political Economy, 71*, 3–10.

Population Communications International. (1999). *Many Voices, One Vision. Annual Report.* New York: Author.

Population Communications International. (2000). *Soap-operas for social change: A PCI methodology for education-entertainment.* New York: Author.

Population Media Center. (2004). PMC program fundamentals—Sabido method. Retrieved May 11, 2004, from http://www.populationmediacenter.org/programs/sabido.html

Puplampu, K., & Tettey, W. (2000). State–NGO relations in an era of globalization: The implications for agricultural development in Africa. *Review of African Political Economy, 84*, 251–272.

Rogers, E. M. (1962). *Diffusion of innovations.* New York: Free.

Rogers, E. M. (1973). *Communication strategies for family planning.* New York: Free.

Rogers, E. M., Vaughan, P. W., Swalehe, R. M. A., Rao, N., Svenkerud, P., & Sood, S. (1999). Effects of an entertainment-education radio soap opera on family planning behavior in Tanzania. *Studies in Family Planning, 30*(3), 193–211.

Rose, N., & Miller, P. (1992). Political power beyond the state: Problematics of government. *British Journal of Sociology, 43*, 173–205.

Schramm, W. (1964). *Mass media and national development: The role of information in the developing countries.* Stanford, CA: Stanford University Press.

Schuurman, F. J. (Ed.). (1993). *Beyond the impasse: New directions in development theory.* London: Zed.

Sherry, J. L. (1997). Prosocial soap operas for development: A review of research and theory. *Journal of International Communication, 4*(2), 75–101.

Sogge, D. (Ed.). (1996). *Compassion and calculation: The business of private foreign aid.* London: Pluto.

Starosta, W. J. (1994). Communication and family planning campaigns: An Indian experience. In A. A. Moemeka (Ed.), *Communicating for development: A new pan-disciplinary perspective* (pp. 244–260). Albany: State University of New York Press.

Stewart, S. (1997). Happy ever after in the marketplace: NGO's uncivil society. *Review of African Political Economy, 71*, 11–34.

Swalehe, R. M. A., Rogers, E. M., Gilboard, M. J., Alford, K., & Montoya, R. (1995). *A content analysis of the entertainment-education radio soap opera, Twende na Wakati (Let's Go With the Times) in Tanzania.* Albuquerque: University of New Mexico.

Tandon, Y. (1996). An African perspective. In D. Sogge (Ed.), *Compassion and calculation: The business of private foreign aid* (pp. 179–184). London: Pluto.

Tvedt, T. (1998). *Angels of mercy or development diplomats? NGOs and foreign aid.* Trenton, NJ: Africa World Press.

Vaughan, P. W. & Rogers, E. M. (2000). A staged model of communication effects: Evidence from an entertainment-education radio soap opera in Tanzania. *Journal of Health Communication, 5*, 203–227.

Vaughan, P. W., Rogers, E. M., Singhal, A., & Swalehe, R. M. (2000). Entertainment-education and HIV/AIDS Prevention: A field experiment in Tanzania. *Journal of Health Communication, 5*, 88–100.

Vavrus, F. (2003). *Desire and decline: Schooling amid crisis in Tanzania.* New York: Lang.

Wilkins, K. G. (1999). Development discourse on gender and communication in strategies for social change. *Journal of Communication, 49*(1), 44–64.

9

Disciplining the Ethnic Body

Latinidad, Hybridized Bodies
and Transnational Identities

ISABEL MOLINA GUZMÁN & ANGHARAD N. VALDIVIA
University of Illinois

IN RECENT YEARS, as the number of Latina and Latinos living in the United States have increased, Latinidad—the cultural state and process of being, becoming, or appearing Latina or Latino—has become not only a widely culturally intelligible identity but also a culturally desirable ethnicity, style, and corporeal practice. Recently and historically, the construction and transformation of Latinidad has been produced and mobilized primarily, though not exclusively, through mass mediated discourse and other modes of public culture. This chapter examines the popular culture narratives and symbolic strategies surrounding the signification of Latina bodies against the background of contemporary and public discourses about Latinas to interrogate the tensions of policing and producing racialized and gendered bodies. In particular, we focus on Latina women with widely circulated media representations and analyze these popular narratives by engaging with Foucault's concept of normalization as an instrument of power and discipline to theorize through the tension between racial and ethnic hybridity/multiplicity and racial and ethnic homogenization/fragmentation. Given the way mass communication is both informative and informed by the contemporary U.S. discursive formation about race, ethnicity, gender, and identity, we conclude by contextualizing our analysis within the terrain of public talk about Latina health and bodies.

Decades of research on ethnic, racial, and feminist studies demonstrate that active mediation and production of racialized and ethnicized bodies are traversed by gendered power relations. In other words, the sign of "woman" often functions as a stand-in for objects and concepts ranging from nation to beauty to sexuality, and in contexts that often relegate feminized images, bodies, and the objects to which they are connected, to less powerful positions than their masculinized counterparts. As a result, the body that becomes both racialized *and* feminized is the product of a double-edged construction of "otherness." For example, if *Latino* bodies can be said to be generally devalued and feminized, then *Latina* bodies are doubly displaced in that they fall beyond the margins of both *Latino* culture generally, and the mainstream of femininity and beauty. Additionally, the culturally powerful discourses of border crossing contamination and excessive sexual reproduction singles out Latina bodies as symbolically impure and dangerous bodies requiring state-sanctioned inspections and medical interventions. This is the contemporary context for the study of gender and Latinidad in the United States and in the many places across the globe where U.S.-produced cultural products circulate.

This chapter draws on feminist media theories and Latina and Latino Studies to explore recent writing surrounding the representational politics of hybridized bodies and transnational identities. Through an exploration of the politics of Latinidad the chapter investigates the dual processes of producing and policing the Latina body and alternative forms of corporeal beauty. Furthermore, we investigate how these public and spectacularized bodies are traversed and disciplined by homogenizing European narratives of origin and binary racialized prescriptions of the body, such as those that surround Latina migration, immigration, and health. At the same time, the chapter explores how the hybridized body (i.e., the Latina body) characterized through discourses of multiplicity connects to broader transformative notions of transnational bodies and identities to put these European and racialized narratives into question and to push beyond them. Drawing on Shohat's and Stam's (1994) notion of "ethnicities in relation," this chapter explores the relational construction of gender, nation, race, and class. At the same time, the chapter engages the Foucauldian (1979) concept of "normalization" as an instrument of power and discipline to theorize the contemporary tensions between hybridity/multiplicity and homogenization/fragmentation to address the useful formation of new and productively globalized corporeal practices toward the manufacture of alternative embodiments and identities.

Contextualizing Latinidad in U.S. Public Culture

Recent historical shifts, including global economic transformations, geographical migrations and diasporas, and newly forming global identities have brought previously minoritized cultures to the foreground. In particular, demographic and cultural changes in racial and ethnic diversity mean there is both an empirical and representational growth in Latina and Latino bodies. Recent increases in population, market power, and cultural influence demand that the U.S. Latina and Latino population be acknowledged in its richness, complexity, and multiplicity. According to the 2000 U.S. Census, "Hispanics" have increased their share of the total population by 38.8% from the last census, resulting in major population shifts in some parts of the United States. In the summer of 1996 Latinos surpassed Blacks as the second largest ethno-racial group in U.S. classrooms, for example.[1] While 1971 was the last year Anglo Americans reproduced at a rate to replace their proportion of the total population (Hacker, 2000), the proportion of the population that calls itself Hispanic or Latina and Latino is increasing at a rate 5 times faster than other populations (Davis, 1999). As of early 2003 the U.S. Census officially declared "Hispanics" the largest U.S. minority.

The "browning of America" has forced the U.S. government and corporations to rethink fixed hierarchical constructions and classifications surrounding U.S. populations and notions of citizenship while simultaneously mobilizing industry to reconfigure approaches to marketing and consumption in terms of particular formations of bodies, populations, and consumer communities. Although the entertainment industry recognized decades ago the need to rearticulate their products to accommodate shifting domestic terrain of racial, ethnic, linguistic, and economic heterogeneity, this most recent formulation and strategy is quite distinct in its intensity, strategy, and broad cultural legitimacy (Dávila, 2001; Halter, 2000). A historical approach to the study of Latinidad suggests that this is not the first time that Latinidad has been represented as a highly marketable commodity in the United States—the 1940s, for example, also saw such a period. Yet, the most recent proliferation of Latina and Latino bodies in public culture, along with the particular demographic trends and marketing developments that connect to its current mobilization, demands that the contemporary formation and marketability of Latinidad be addressed as a novel historically and culturally specific phenomenon.

As a sign that constructions and organizations of the contemporary notion of the U.S. Latina and Latino population have changed over time, marketers acknowledge their purchasing power and conceptualize this target audience quite differently that in the past. Nonetheless, traces of a previous approach remain because the Latina and Latino population is considered one of the last "unified" or homogenous target markets in the United States.[2] Prior to the 1990s, the entertainment industry perceived and addressed U.S. Latina and Latino audiences as ethnically undifferentiated, racially non-White, Spanish-dominant, socioeconomically poor, and most often of Mexican origin (Rodriguez, 1999). Such a construction had very specific effects: Throughout the 1970s and 1980s, this market framework promoted the development of Spanish-language narrow-casting via networks such as Telemundo and Univisión and encouraged the exclusion of Latinas and Latinos from mainstream English-language network programming.

However, beginning in the mid-1980s Latina and Latino industry officials worked diligently to reframe dominant marketing discourses about the U.S. Latino audience: by highlighting projected increases in U.S. Latina and Latino population; the commercial profits from dual-language marketing; and, the existence of more than 1 million Latina and Latino households with incomes of more than $50,000 living in the United States, Latina and Latino industry officials effectively redefined mainstream industry perceptions about the economic importance of the Latina and Latino consumer audience while still using homogenizing constructions of Latinas and Latinos to differentiate them as a market (Dávila, 2001; Rodriguez, 1999; Sinclair, 1999). In the overall global economic climate that includes the identity-making practice of "shopping for ethnicities," advertising trade magazines and marketing research corporations increased spending levels on "Hispanic" marketing in the late 1980s (Goodson & Shaver, 1994, p. 192; Halter 2000). If marketing strategies function as a Foucauldian form of discourse, "as a set of practices which support particular forms of knowledge or ways of knowing" (Foucault quoted in Rabinow, 1984, p. 54), then the ruptures and discontinuities within the marketing and global entertainment industry texts point to potentially resistant moments of transformations.

Within this particular historical context, strong demand from Latin American audiences for U.S. programming, as well from U.S. Latina and Latino audiences for more inclusive programming have increased the production of film and television shows and marketable stars that appeal to audiences across a matrix of race, ethnicity, gender, and class throughout the late 1990s. Warner Brother's 1997 *Selena* starring Jennifer Lopez specifically targeted Latin American audiences, U.S. Latina and Latino audiences, and young U.S. girls across all ethnic categories (Hindes, 1997). Celebrities Shakira and Thalia both began their cross-over attempts without English fluency yet that did not stop the marketing apparatus from widely promoting them in the United States. Currently the commodification of Latinidad relies primarily of Latina bodies.

Multiplicity and Homogeneity
in the Discourse of Latinidad

The tendency to classify and describe U.S. Latina and Latino bodies and populations as "Latina and Latino" is quite recent. Whereas previous formulations of the U.S. study of populations originating from Latin American included Chicano Studies to refer to Mexican origin populations and Boricua Studies to refer to Puerto Rican origin populations, the current usage of the category "Latina and Latino" represents an attempt to broaden the concept to include a comparative ethnic and Latina perspectives—in short, it is a response to and recognition of both material and symbolic changes—and the complex multiplicity of the U.S. Latina and Latino population. For example, Dominicans are quickly outnumbering Puerto Ricans in New York City; Nicaraguans are outnumbering Cubans in Miami; Los Angeles is the second largest Mexican, Salvadorian, and Guatemalan city in the world. Given that the largest Mexican city, Mexico City, numbering 25 million people is the largest city in the world, being the second largest is demographically and symbolically significant. In fact, clusters of Latina and Latino populations live in almost all major cities, despite the fact that the bulk of Urban Studies and indeed the U.S. imaginary continue to circulate the binary discourse of the city as Black and suburbs as White, a binary that obscures the demographic diversity of the U.S. population and leaves Latina and Latinos and others in the margins, in some unspecified undetermined space (Davis, 1999). Consider, for instance, the Levi's jeans ad in the 2002 Super Bowl where a digitally enhanced Mexican man danced through a downtown street intersection in Mexico City. Despite the productive inclusion of Latinidad in the hyperexpensive and usually unreachable universe of Super Bowl ads, this ad placed the Latino body outside the boundaries of the United States and thus underscored and supported the construction of U.S. urban space as Black and the location of Latina and Latinos as somewhere beyond the boundaries of U.S. cities and suburbia. As well dominant narratives situate Latina and Latinos bicoastally although the fastest growing region for Latina and Latinos is the Midwest. Contrary to popular homogenizing constructions, the U.S. Latina and Latino population is geographically dispersed throughout and beyond the states; racially, culturally, linguistically diverse; and multiple, dynamic, and perpetually transforming.

The same can be said of the concept of Latinidad, which remains a dynamic, diverse, and changing set of attributes, styles, tendencies, and personas (much like the bodies and cultures that are assembled and organized under the category). Latinidad is something constructed from without and within. Thus, it becomes inescapably dynamic, celebratory and contested—and functions simultaneously as multiplicity, as singularity, and as organized similarity. As Juan Flores (2000) describes, nearly every Latina and Latino individual traces his or her identity to a particular country—that is, Latinidad is nearly-always a subjectivity that is only ever partially completed such that one is identified always as a multiple: a Mexican American Latina or a Chilean Latina or a Puerto Rican/Dominican Latina. María Lugones (2003) argues that such multiplicities or impurities of identity become a point of resistance because it vexes governmentality through its unclassifiable nature. Governmentality depends not on blood and violence for its power, but on its ability to perpetuate and normalize classificatory discourses that "qualify, measure, appraise and hierarchize" (Foucault, 1979, p. 266). Consequently, bodies that rupture hierarchical classifications expose disciplining binary logic and exploit essentialist divisions to problematize the norm.

Nevertheless, despite the hybrid and multiple nature of Latina and Latino identity, as a U.S. collective we share a colonial past, the formation and construction of a syncretic ethnic culture, and a life connected to the homogenizing categories constructed and mobilized through mainstream culture (Aparicio, 2003). Moreover, Achy Obejas (2001) proposes that a growing proportion of Latinas and Latinos ethnically classify themselves primarily and exclusively as Latinas and Latinos, an identity that is a potentially homogenous panethnic category and as a result more susceptible to data collection and government surveillance. For most government policing agencies and agents, such as law enforcement officials, no or little differentiation exists among Latinas and Latinos or within Latinidad—just the normalizing discourses of Latinas and Latinos as potentially illegal immigrants, diseased border crossers and, more recently, terrorist threats (Saldivar, 1997). The normalizing discourse places Latinas and Latinos on the social and moral margins making them more vulnerable to government disciplining through surveillance activities such as racial profiling. These two discursive strategies (Latina and Latino hybridity/multiplicity and Latina and Latino homogeneity/fragmentation) productively illustrate a long-standing Latina and Latino presence in the United States as well as the complicated inflections, background, and affiliations that contribute to the formation of collective identities. As such, Latinidad epitomizes and emblematizes contemporary formations of bodies and selves as the product of real and imagined mobility, as global, hybrid, and multiple.

The Cultural Disciplining of Latina and Latino Bodies

Latina and Latino bodies are brought into the normalizing discourse through the gendered and racialized tropes of Latinization, more specifically tropicalism, in U.S. mainstream culture. Aparicio and Chávez-Silverman (1997) define *tropicalism* as "the system of ideological fictions with which the dominant (Anglo European) cultures trope Latin American and U.S. Latina and Latino identities and culture" (p.1) As a typology and classification system, one might expect the concept of tropicalism to apply only to those bodies deemed to have Caribbean origins. Yet the usage extends to bodies from Latin America and, more recently, to bodies in the United States, which are said to have Caribbean and Latin American origins. Tropicalism as a trope erases corporeal specificity and assembles all that is "Latin" and "Latina and Latino" into one homogeneous classification (e.g., López, 1991; Perez Firmat, 1994). According to Lugones (2003), homogenous classifications are implicitly grounded in notions of purity and become forms of social control. Thus, she argues such classifications are "attempts at control exercised by those who possess both power and the categorical eye and who attempt to split everything impure, breaking it down into more pure elements . . . for the purposes of control" (p. 123). Not only is this mechanism of control exercised by formal government structures such as the legal system, but it is also used by the informal structures of governmentality such as the media and popular culture. Under the homogenizing category of "tropicalism," previously mentioned attributes such as brown or olive skin contribute to some of the most enduring characterizations of Latinas and Latinos. However, as the "non-Hispanic White" phrase used by the U.S. Census Bureau suggests, the hybridity of Latinas and Latinos threatens to rupture the normalizing discourse U.S. racial hierarchies through the hypervisible display of White Latina bodies, such as Cameron Diaz and Christina Aguilera, who are continuously circulated through the popular media. "Latina and Latino," then, encompasses a diverse range of bodies and racial formations. Brown eyes, therefore, or any other phenotypic characteristic, are merely a conventionalized attribute that is identifiable and locatable and that can be mobilized toward the construction, assemblage, and policing of corporeal boundaries—part of the typological apparatus that functions toward the organization of an otherwise unwieldy and dispersed heterogeneous population.

Within globally commodified media narratives gendered aspects of "tropicalism" include the dominant male Latin lover—macho, dark haired, mustachioed—and the submissive female Latina—hot, red lipped and seductively dressed, curvaceous (read, bootie), long brunette hair beauty with hoop earrings. Sexuality plays an important role in the tropicalization of Latinas and Latinos,[3] and Latinas are frequently constructed in the popular media as sexually available, sexually proficient, and sexually excessive (Valdivia, 2000). In contradiction, though in keeping with a binary modern logic and historically effective typologies, U.S. Latina and Latinos are often constructed as predominantly Roman Catholic and are linked to associated signifiers, such as a cross pendant, the crucifix on the wall, candles, and divinely ordained virgins (especially the Virgin of Guadalupe, who although of great importance to the Mexican imaginary, is not the only revered virgin icon across the Americas). Latinas and Latinos are also often coded as family oriented with the obvious associated signifiers of large loud extended families and Latina and Latino characters unable or unwilling to leave home. Thus, Latinas and Latinos are often positioned as thoroughly embedded in a traditional and nostalgic past as opposed to the postmodern subject that actively forges brave new worlds. Finally, the use of Spanish, Spanglish, or accented English is attributed to Latina and Latino bodies both as a way of marking a general exotic otherness but also as a way of reiterating the perennial status of Latina and Latino bodies as outside of the law and susceptible to illegal border crossings (both material and discursive). Furthermore, tropicalism as trope contributes to the normalizing discourse by erasing the historical knowledge that in many parts of the U.S. Latina and Latino territorial presence and residence predates both the Anglo and African American populations. Overall use of words such as "hot," "energy," and "motion," often connected to red and yellow images of fires and suns add to the tropical, nearly combustible feel of Latina and Latino bodies and selves. Mobilized in isolation or in combination, these characterizations are the components of the "tropicalization" of U.S. Latina and Latino bodies and populations, a process that organizes, homogenizes, and polices an otherwise dynamic, heterogeneous, and multiple "Latinidad."

Rupturing the Normalizing Discourse
Through Latina Iconicity

Culturally dominant and intelligible constructions circulated through globally commodified media narratives of Latinidad and Latinas provide a useful case study for investigating the tensions between multiplicity and homogeneity inherent in contemporary formations of gender, ethnicity, and race. The remainder of this chapter explores the contradictions, oppositions, and continuities of "Latinidad" as a trope formed and mobilized through public Latina bodies, including those of Salma Hayek, Jennifer Lopez, and other representationally significant Latinas. More specifically, we explore how a particularly *gendered* "Latinidad" is produced and mobilized by and through contemporary public culture, and how this gendered Latinidad is implicated in both organizing and policing the Latina body, and in actively producing alternative and multiple embodiments of corporeal beauty—embodiments that productively push beyond narrow European prescriptions of normative corporeality.

We begin with Jennifer Lopez, often characterized as a "sex goddess" of the screen, pop music, cosmetic, perfume, and fashion worlds. That she is considered a "sex goddess" is itself indicative of "tropicalization" and the mobilization of a gendered and sexualized Latinidad. Not only has Jennifer Lopez (as known as La Lopez or J-Lo) become the highest paid Latina performer in Hollywood, simultaneously commanding $11 million per film and gaining a certain level of agency in terms of the roles she plays, but she has also released three highly successful albums making her a rare film/music/dance sensation. Lopez has already negotiated a development deal with Telemundo to produce a sitcom loosely based on her life and is continuing negotiations with the NBC networks. Her increased visibility on television combined with recent cosmetic, fashion, and negligee deals make "La Lopez" one of the most powerful multimedia mogul. Although she has lost considerable weight and inches since her entry into the cultural mainstream (Winter 2003), Jennifer Lopez continues to busily participate in the (re)formation of ideal of beauty through the marketing of her "shapely," "womanly," or "posterior" beauty. Thus, she has shaped public narratives about the bootie and the Latina body even as her own body is reshaped by the disciplining discourse of contemporary Anglo European standards of thinness and beauty.

More than a decade ago another Latina body, Rosie Perez, was asked to reduce the size of her "bootie," after already trimming down to 103 pounds for her Oscar-nominated role as supporting actress in *Fearless* (1993). Perez, in a moment of unruliness, resisted prescriptive ideals when she told producers that she would not lose more weight, nor could she drop her Spanish accent, despite extensive voice coaching. Although Perez never became the phenomenon that is Jennifer Lopez, her location in the U.S. cultural landscape remains significant toward the production and reproduction of Latina and Latino culture (Valdivia, 2000). Among Perez's recent activities are the full-length films *Dance with the Devil* (1997), *Somebody to Love* (1997), and *24-Hour Woman* (1999); a stage role in the *Vagina Monologues*; and the voice of the vamp in DreamWorks animated feature-length film *El Dorado* (2000). Few people are likely to have heard of Perez's latest movies, as she appears to be relegated to the dustbin of flash-in-the-pan Latina actresses whose careers dwindle to unremarkable movies and increasingly typified and small roles.[4] A case in point is Perez's character in *Riding in Cars with Boys* (2001), starring Drew Barrymore. At the movie's conclusion, Perez circulates as the body of excess: loud, ugly, insensitive, controlling, and drug-addicted, as opposed to Barrymore's role of contained and successful rebellion; she is unlike Lopez or Hayek whose bodies are less racialized because of their ability to perform ethnic ambiguity. Ironically, the less marketable Perez has used her celebrity body to discipline the political discourse rather than the discourse of global commodification. She is a spokesperson for the scholarship foundation the Hispanic Fund, and a vocal activist for research and funding for HIV/AIDS in the United States (Latinas and Latinos are one of the communities hardest hit by the epidemic).

Salma Hayek is another prominent global figure contributing to the popular constructions of Latinidad. As her fame in the mainstream has increased, her identity and physical body have been equally disciplined through the normalizing discourse of whiteness. For instance, Hayek's hair, which was stereotypically curly and "big" when she premiered in a 30-second stint as the jealous ex-girlfriend in Alison Ender's *Mi Vida Loca*, has become progressively straighter and more controlled. Her border crossing from Mexico to the United States, from the imagined margins to the romanticized mainstream, has yielded more complex supporting and leading roles, including *Wild Wild West* (1999), *Dogma* (1999), *Fools Rush In* (1997), and *Frida* (2002). While not quite as high profile as Jennifer Lopez, Hayek's public body has nevertheless participated in both affirming and disrupting long-held cinematic constructions of the Latina body. Indeed, Hayek's role in *Fools Rush In* challenges normative notions of bodily coupling when, at the conclusion of the film, her character remains alive and happily married to her wealthy Anglo husband. Historically, such couplings within popular narratives have resulted in estrangement or even death. Additionally, Hayek's art house role in the innovative aspects of *Frida* explored bodily pleasure and pain as well as challenged heteronormative visions of romantic couplings (Guzmán, 2007). Hayek continues to push the corporeal limits usually assigned to Latina actresses in Hollywood while performing the idealized hourglass shape.

Within the television landscape there is Jessica Alba, star of James Cameron's apocalyptic series *Dark Angel* and *Honey (2003)*. Most reviews about the series singled out Alba as the reason to watch the show. Selected from thousands of applicants, Jessica Alba was virtually the only prominent Latina presence on U.S. mainstream television in 2001, a year in which Latinas and Latinos comprised less than 2% of the total leading or supporting characters on U.S. television (Children Now, 2002). In fact, until *American Family* entered the winter 2002 lineup on PBS (after CBS turned down the pilot), the only other leading role for a Latina in U.S. television was the "bilingual" and "interactive" Dora in Nickelodeon's Saturday morning's animated show *Dora the Explorer.* More recently, the television landscape is a dynamic one with subtle traces of Latinidad and Latinas in several shows, including *Lizzie McGuire* on the Disney Channel and NBC's *Scrubs* in addition to the Latino family sitcom shows, such as the *George Lopez Show.*

Destabilizing the Sexualized Latina Body

From Dolores del Río, Lupe Velez, and Carmen Miranda, to Charo, Raquel Welch, Maria Conchita Alonso, Gloria Estefan, and then to the many Latina bodies addressed in this chapter, a historical and continuous trend is the production of difference and hierarchical fragmentations through the normalized sexualization of Latina bodies. During the era of classic Hollywood cinema, formal codes restricted sexual images of White women resulting in the displacement of a generalized female sexuality onto the bodies of working-class women and women of color. Many scholars describe the hyperritualized construction of del Río, Vélez, and Miranda as produced within a system of differentiation that demanded Latina bodies to be either sexual spitfires or virgins (Beltrán, 2002; Fregoso, 1993; López, 1991; McLean, 1993; Rodriguez, 1997). Carmen Miranda, in particular, emblematizes the "tropicalized" body because she was produced through a hyperbundance of fruits, energy, and sexuality.

Of course, there has always been an "invisible presence" of Latinas whose hybrid bodies could not be read through the normalizing discourse of U.S. racial binaries. Prominent Latinas who passed as White include the late Rita Hayworth and Raquel Welch, who has recently embraced and publicized her Latinidad through her (still sexualized) role in PBS's *American Family.* We can only hypothesize about the number of Latina actresses who eluded racial categorization and remain unidentifiable as ethnic subjects. Contemporary constructions of Latinas range from hypercoded Latinas such as Charo to more ambiguously coded Latinas such as Christina Aguilera, Cameron Diaz, and Mariah Carey. Actors born and trained in Spain are also treated and included in academic and popular culture articles, Web sites, and discussions about Latinas and Latinos as illustrated by the inclusion of both Antonio Banderas and Penélope Cruz within the amorphous space of Latinidad. In fact,

Dávila (2001, p. 1) begins her book on Latinos and marketing with an anecdote in which Banderas speaks for Latinos on behalf of the Spanish television network, Telemundo. Historical and contemporary Latina and Latino bodies in popular culture span media, genres, typologies, and levels of visibility.

As an ethnicity paradigm, Latinidad sometimes celebrates a socially constructed singularity that erases nation-specific, historical, socioeconomic, and cultural differences. It is a paradigm simultaneously based on the concepts of cultural assimilation and cultural pluralism (Aparicio, 2003; Omi & Winant, 1986). Some scholars argue that by highlighting the strength of collectivity, Latinidad as a panethnic identity (even if site-specific and contingent) increases the productive assemblage and political and cultural efficacy of Spanish-speaking peoples living in the United States (Padilla, 1982). Although the category Latina and Latino covers more than 30 nationalities, these national distinctions are rarely represented in U.S. public culture. Consequently, the particular Latinidad that circulates in U.S. films is often homogenized, stereotypical, and contained within the geographical spaces of Cuba, Puerto Rico, and Mexico. As Shohat and Stam (1994) argue, "dominant cinema is fond of writing 'dark' or Third World people into substitute others, interchangeable units who can 'stand in' for one another" (p. 189). Contemporary Latina bodies represent a significant departure from Hollywood's practice of casting Anglo actresses to play Latina characters, yet they still exist in tension with the continuing investment in narrow, bounded identity categories characterized by fragmentary notions of purity and the presumption of ethnic interchangeability.

Public and spectacular Latina bodies inherit traces of that contested history. Jennifer Lopez has repeatedly said she wants it all: the career, the fame, the knight in shining armor, the kids, and the trademark perfect Latina posterior (reportedly insured for $1 billion). The magazine *GQ* reminded its readers that Lopez herself acknowledges that "the American public knew my butt before they knew my name." Although Lopez clearly uses her body and sexuality to produce agency for herself, like other Latina bodies under popular surveillance she still remains exoticized and sexualized. Whenever she appears in the popular press, whether a newspaper, a television news magazine, or *People*, Lopez's behind (judged to be gorgeous) is discussed not only as the "Other" but also as a viable entity onto itself. Even the September 2002 cover of *Redbook* magazine, not generally known for its sexual explicitness, linked its cover star and story to the butt through the discourse of exercise—you too can have J-Lo curves if you do these exercises. Chris Rock jokes that Lopez's butt needs its own zip code. Celebrity Death Match on Comedy Central network aired a Jennifer Lopez vs. Dolly Parton match with J-Lo's butt battling against Dolly's breasts. Lopez's buttocks function within a system of differentiation, a system predicated on and traversed by racialized and gendered difference. At the same time, this difference is classified as fascinating yet "abnormal" and "irregular."

As such, the objectification of Lopez's body exists in relation to a longer history of technologies of the body that have scrutinized, judged, and disciplined the bodies of racialized Others. Beginning with the medical discourse surrounding the Hottentot Venus, the bodies of women of color—specifically their genitals and buttocks—are excessively sexualized, exoticized, and pathologized (Gilman, 1985). Like other U.S. constructions of the exotic, this cultural construction of the Latina focuses primarily on the lower body (Beltrán, 2002; Desmond, 1997; Guzmán & Valdivia, 2004), a corporeal site with great cultural overdeterminations: Within the Eurocentric mind/body dualism, culture is associated with the higher functions of the mind/brain, and it is separated and differentiated from the physiology and movement of the lower body, including hips, legs, sexual reproductive organs, and orifices of excrement and waste. Such a taxonomy and associations of upper and lower bodily strata contribute to discourses of dominant and nondominant peoples respectively, and actively reconstitute systems of differentiation and separation: high/low, mind/body, culture/nature, Anglo/Latina, human/animal, civilized/primitive, control/chaos. Thus, Lopez and her lower body remain commodified, exoticized, and sexualized as part of the ambivalent desire for the Other, and, as such, she reproduces classifications and typologies that fragment Latinas into exotic and sexual and "Others." Simultaneously she is located beyond whiteness but short of blackness ultimately reinscribing the unacceptability of the Black corporeal particularity.

Examples of such sexualizations include Lopez's roles in the film noirs *Blood and Wine* (1996) and Oliver Stone's *U-Turn* (1997). In both of these films, Lopez's body and sexuality is represented in animalistic and primitive terms that are irresistibly dangerous to the Anglo American males in their lives. Lopez's body is cinematically sliced into objectified parts and sexually consumed by the male protagonists and the cinematic spectator. For example, in *U-Turn*, Lopez's character Grace McKenna, a half-Anglo/half-Navajo woman, is explicitly fetishized through visual montages of her eyes, lips, and breasts linking her highly sexualized body to the hot, dry Arizona desert/nature. Indeed, the narrative falsely climaxes in the final sex scene, when Grace, with the fresh blood of her own body and that of murdered father/husband, has sex with her accomplice in front of the dead body and is visually made to resemble her

Navajo mother, who is depicted as a mentally unstable savage alcoholic. Similar to Hayek's portrayal of Satanico Pandemonium in *From Dusk Till Dawn* (1996), Lopez's characters in these two films construct the Latina as a temptress with insatiable sexual appetites that eventually consume her and whose sexual excess is eventually contained by the male protagonists. In these cinematic narratives, feminine Latinidad is normalized into preexisting racial hierarchies by constructing it as a source of sexual contamination, a foreign and uncontrolled substance that is usually punished and ultimately tamed by the Anglo male characters. In these films, Latinas who cross racial boundaries to pursue Anglo men are disciplined for their social transgression and eventually repositioned within the social margins.

Rupturing U.S. Racial Discourses

Due to the ambiguity of their phenotypic characteristics, Hayek and Lopez possess physical markers that allow their bodies to circulate across a field of ethnic categories. Both actresses have brown, full-bodied hair, brown eyes, somatically light skin, and a range of more or less European facial features. Physically they are "every-woman" (to the extent that any of us could fantasize about resembling highly made-up and digitized models and actresses we see in media representations) with only a slight physical suggestion of exotic Otherness. Indeed, these actresses have portrayed characters whose ethnic identities escape existing typologies and thus remain undetermined and peripheral to their role, text, and narrative action. In *Dogma, Out of Sight* (1998), and *Gigli* (2003),[5] Hayek and Lopez play characters whose ethnic and racial identity are absent from the character description, plot, and narrative theme. In *Dogma* Hayek portrays the ethnically, racially, and sexually undetermined supernatural character Serendipity, and in *Out of Sight* Lopez portrays the ethnically unspecified character Karen Sisco.[6] Within these ethnically ambiguous representations, racial Otherness is visually displaced and replaced with an exotic connotation of Ethnic-Otherness often communicated through dialogue, costuming, mise-en-scène and sound (Guzmán, 2001).

In several films, Hayek and Lopez are also cast in ethnically ambiguous roles suggesting, but not explicitly signifying, an Otherness without a specific racial or national identity. In three films, Hayek's *54* (1998) and *From Dusk Till Dawn* and Lopez's *Anaconda* (1997), the Latina ethnicity of the character is only subtly referenced through contextual codes such as the character's name or splices of Spanish dialog. The ethnicity of the characters is often so secondary, that in interviews Lopez has stated that she had to fight for her character, initially cast as an Anglo woman, in *Anaconda* to have a Spanish surname. Within films featuring ethnically commodified bodies, spatial signifiers play an important role in establishing an ethnic context. For instance, the film *From Dusk Till Dawn* implies that Hayek's character Satanico Pandemonium, a supernatural demon, is of Latina origin only because the film references that the narrative action occurs south of the U.S.–Mexico border. Only through indirect narrative information is the audience made aware that in *Anaconda* Lopez's character, Terri Flores, is a "home girl from the Southside of L.A.," the Mexican quarter of the city. Likewise, although the audience is never explicitly told their ethnic identity, we discover that the characters in *54* and *Anaconda* both have Spanish-sounding names, Anita and Terri Flores respectively. Of these three characters, Anita is the only who speaks any dialogue in Spanish. These contextual clues contribute to the implicit communication of ethnic difference.

Lopez's cross over roles in *Enough* (2002), *The Wedding Planner* (2001), and *Maid in Manhattan* (2002) further exploit the physical liminality that allows her mobility across historically fragmented and essentialist racial fields. In *Enough* and *Wedding* once again she plays a working-class ambiguously Italian American role, reversing the Hollywood tradition of having Italian American actresses such as Marissa Tomei play Latina roles. Yet in the highly publicized *Maid* Lopez plays the role most identifiable as Latina since *Selena*. Envisioned as Lopez's *Pretty Woman*, *Maid* was not as successful as its Cinderella story counterpart but nonetheless maintained her position as Hollywood's reigning Latina. Nevertheless, Lopez movement through a bevy of racial roles problematizes the normative binary racial schema in the U.S. and demonstrates a shift in the discursive formation of race and ethnicity.

Contesting Latina Authenticity, Producing Multiplicity

Because of the dominant homogenizing constructions of Latinidad and Latina ethnicity circulated through global popular culture, the actresses themselves have sometimes engaged in a battle over corporeal ethnic authenticity—debating over which actress is the true, pure, or authentic Latina in order to win coveted roles. Jennifer Lopez and some of her roles exemplify this rift. In three of the five films Lopez released between 1995 and 1999, she plays characters outside of her ethnicity. Although Lopez was born in the United States, her parents are of Puerto Rican origin, and she alternates between identifying herself as Puerto Rican and Nuyorican. Nevertheless, in *Selena* Lopez portrays the legendary Mexican American music star; in *Mi Familia* Lopez portrays the Mexican immigrant Maria Sanchez; in *U-Turn* she portrays a Native American, and in *Out of Sight* and *The Wedding Planner* she plays an Italian American.

The selection of Lopez was highly criticized by Mexican-American activists who wanted a Mexican-American actress cast in the role of Selena. The public debate between understanding of Latina identity as multiplicity and Latina identity as fragmented singularity continues in the scholarship as exemplified by Aparicio (2003) and Gaspar de Alba (2003). More recently, the conflict over the Frida Kahlo biopic highlights the tension between hybridity/multiplicity and purity/fragmentation as embodied in the exchange between Lopez as an U.S. Nuyorican and Hayek as a Mexican woman. Whereas Lopez, whose body and commodified performances depend on multiplicity, refused to engage in the discussion over the limits of Latina authenticity, Hayek explicitly argued that she, as the "true" and pure Mexican, should be the one to portray Frida's life. In an interview foregrounding the debate over authenticity, Hayek (2001) stated:

> I don't believe in the so-called Latino explosion when it comes to movies. Jennifer Lopez doesn't have an accent. She grew up in New York speaking English and not Spanish. Her success is very important because she represents a different culture, but it doesn't help me. I grew up in Mexico, not the U.S., and the fact is that there just aren't any parts for Latin actresses. I have to persuade people that my accent won't be a problem.

Of course, Hayek's corporeal formation and cultural identity is itself complicated. Her father is a Lebanese businessman and her mother is Spanish, making her barely a first-generation Mexican. Frida herself was half Mexican, half Hungarian, and decidedly Jewish.[7] Lopez's portrayals across racialized and ethnic bodies have productively—if inadvertently—opened up a Pandora's box surrounding the question of corporeal and ethnic authenticity.

Latino Studies interrogates this vexed notion of corporeal authenticity or purity based on physical phenotype, country of origin, and language. The fact is that second, third, and fourth generations of Latinas and Latinos born in the United States have never visited their parents', grandparents' or great-grandparents' nation of birth. As the U.S. Census 2000 documents Latinas and Latinos identify as both Black and White and a growing number identify as more than one race. Not all, nor necessarily most, U.S. Latinas and Latinos can speak Spanish. For example, Christina Aguilera toyed with the idea of taking the "h" out of Cristina to more explicitly articulate her Latinidad through a traditional

Spanish spelling of her name. Mariah Carey considered recording in Spanish even though it would mean learning a new language for her. Jennifer Lopez's much awaited Puerto Rican concert broadcast on U.S. television in December 2001 demonstrated a less than facile use of the Spanish language. The experiences of Jennifer Lopez, Mariah Carey, and Christina Aguilera as U.S. Latinas is not atypical in that none of them speak Spanish fluently, and it illustrates the difficulty in defining (not to mention actually locating) a person of pure racial or ethnic authenticity. Even if finding such authenticity were possible, the Latino populations would certainly not be the place to look for racial or ethnic purity. Although Cherríe Moraga and Gloria Anzaldúa may not exactly have had this productive hybridity in mind when they edited *This Bridge Called My Back* (1989), Latin American women have historically chosen or been forced to engage in mixed-race relationships, further engendering complicated racial formations. Feminists' recastings of La Malinche (e.g. Alarcón, 1994) have reframed the masculinist framework of sexual and cultural prostitution, of selling one's body and culture, in terms of a more progressive and redeeming narrative of the mother of a new hybrid, cosmic race and intercultural translator.

Jessica Alba, Hayek, and Kahlo are themselves manifestations of this corporeal and cultural hybridity and multiplicity of identities. Alba, whose father is Mexican and whose mother is Canadian/French-Dutch, was cast in the role of Max precisely because James Cameron wanted an unidentifiable hybrid heroine for his show with potential appeal to a broad range of audiences—a Tiger Woods of television if you will. Apparently, Cameron's instinct proved successful because Alba has appeared on the cover of *TV Guide, Teen Latina, Allure,* and *Maxim,* to name a few and has gone on to star in major Hollywood films. Because some Latinas, such as Alba and Lopez, are liminal subjects who super-sede racial origins and categorizations, and who exist in the malleable in-between, that Latinas are often placed in the position of racial and ethnic bridge roles is not surprising. In this sense, they are indeed globally iconic (Guzmán & Valdivia, 2004). The culturally dominant narratives of Latina corporeality and sexuality are articulated through a complex but normalizing matrix of race, class, gender, and geography. Whereas Black-White relationships were until recently sexually taboo, the Western genre has copious examples of border Latina women mixing with Anglo heroes. The reverse is not equally true—that is, Latino men have rarely been portrayed as mixing with Anglo frontier women. In fact, as Shohat (1991) outlines, a political economy of gender mixing is shown on the Hollywood screen. Shohat argues that White bodies can only desire other White bodies, yet these same White bodies are consistently desired by the bodies of racialized Others. Consequently, a relationship between a White male body and a female body of color, such as Latinas, is always consensual because under this particular political economy of sexuality a woman of color would desire a White man. However, a White woman cannot desire the racialized Other, so these relationships are nearly always portrayed as sexually violent and nonconsensual. Within this discursive formation, Latino men do not generally interact sexually with Anglo women unless it is to threaten or enact forced sexual violence or rape, as in the Pancho Villa films. This common representational practice affirms the social order by disciplining Latina bodies as a symbolic site through which culture is biologically and symbolically negotiated, contested, opposed, and eventually homogenized through global commodification (Beltrán, 2002; Guzmán, 2005).

Moreover and significantly in relation to Frida Kahlo—narratives of authenticity and Latinidad more often than not hark back to the mother continent, to Latin America. As such, U.S. Latina and Latinos are never quite authentic, anywhere, because the boundaries of the body are policed by multiple cultures. Thus Frida Kahlo functions as a powerful signifier of identity because she is often articulated within the narrative of "The Motherland." Within the narrative of the motherland, Eurocentric discourses of authenticity, which erase indigenous, African, and other non-White populations, hark back to Spain, a place often constructed as the site of whiteness despite its history of African Moorish occupation. Not coincidentally, Penélope Cruz is identified in surveys of U.S. Latina and Latinos as *more* Latina, more authentic, and more beautiful than either Hayek or Lopez. Somewhat oppositionally, compared to Lopez whose body is articulated as raw natural energy, Cruz is linked to civility and sophistication (Valdivia, 2007). These narratives of authenticity and origin privilege a mythical nostalgic racially pure Spain that, in a discursively productive manner, proves to be untenable and like other discourses of purity produces hierarchies of essentialist fragmentation.

Governing Racial-Otherness in Popular Culture

Despite their ability to destabilize racial categories, Latina bodies are traversed, mobilized, and eventually normalized by the interconnected discourse of fear and desire. At the level of fear and disciplinarity, the imagined hypersexuality and hyperfertility of Latina (not Latino) bodies function as a threat to racially grounded definitions of national identity. At the level of desire and surveillance, Latina bodies are purveyed and sought as the sexually proficient exotic other. Furthermore, Acosta and Kreshel (2002) stress the contradictory nature of this racialized and gendered Othering. Latina beauty and sexuality is marked as Other, yet it is that Otherness that also marks Latinas as desirable. Similarly, Jessica Alba, Salma Hayek, Jennifer Lopez, and Rosie Perez all circulate as sexually desirable bodies but their desirability is produced through a complicated ambivalence toward racialized, exotic Otherness.

With the exception of Lopez's roles in *Blood and Wine* and *U-Turn*, Salma Hayek is most often sexualized and objectified in cinematic representations. Given the more racialized articulations of Hayek's and Perez' bodies, the hypersexualization of their bodies is not surprising. Although Lopez is the professional singer and dancer, it is Salma Hayek who is most often depicted sexually gyrating to music in *54, Dogma, Dusk Till Dawn*, and *Wild Wild West*. As mentioned previously, dance, bodily expressivity, and the lower bodily stratum have been historically linked to the popular construction of Latinidad. However, dance itself, especially the type involving movement below the waist, is marked as Other within mainstream U.S. culture and both gendered and racialized (Desmond 1997). The bifurcation of the body reifies the preexisting U.S. system of informal governmentality where notions of racial purity are used to hierarchically classify bodies of gendered and racial difference. Through this system of informal governmentality, Lopez's ability to perform racial and ethnicity ambiguity and multiplicity allows her to occupy more easily the privileged space of acceptable White sexuality, while Hayek's racializing accent continually pushes her toward the margins of aberrant sexual excess. Like Jessica Alba, Lopez's English-language fluency and absence of clearly identifiable Spanish accent allows her to circulate through and among a range of cinematic narratives that are generally unavailable to Hayek and Perez. For example, Lopez has portrayed characters ranging from a psychologist (*The Cell*, 2000) to an independently wealthy Italian American FBI agent (*Out of Sight*). Despite her racial and ethnic multiplicity, Lopez's agent still had to convince the producer of *The Wedding Planner* that she could play a non-Latina character. The role was first cast as Eastern European, and the producer did not want to recast it as a Latina. More so than Hayek and Rosie Perez, Lopez has effectively tapped into her ability to perform the hybrid Latina body to meet Hollywood's demand for the commodified exotic Other.

Conclusion: New Corporealities

What is important to remember about constructions and classifications of Latinidad and Latina identity within globally commodified U.S. popular culture is that it is often disembodied from the lived experiences of most Latina and Latinos. One can buy, wear, and perform this corporeality without ever encountering actual Latina and Latinos or Latina and Latino bodies or culture. Moreover, given the contradictions and globalization of the capitalist marketplace, few Latina and Latinos and even fewer Latin American men and women can afford to buy these globally commodified artifacts of Latinidad, even though many of them take part in their production. Investigating the production and mobilization of a gendered Latinidad as implicated in the global marketing and the manufacture of global corporealities is important. Contemporary discourses of Latinidad draw on historical types and classifications of Latina bodies through a system of difference even while it engages Latinidad to sell products in the global marketplace through standardization. While this contemporary proliferation of Latina bodies may open spaces for new formations, vocality, and action, they nevertheless build on a history of "tropicalization," exoticization, racialization, and sexualization of Latina bodies—of Latina bodies as foreign, out of control, and threatening to social order, the body politic, and the health of the country.

The fictional representations of Latina sexual excess and bodily contamination often reaffirm public health discourses. Maria Ruiz's work (1996, 2000) analyses the overlap between Hollywood film and U.S. health concerns, especially as demonstrated through health pamphlets and videos aimed at the Latina and Latino population. Contemporary hysteria about immigrants and migrant workers often single out the potentially infectious pathogens carried by "illegal" border crossers. Marie Leger and Maria Ruiz (in press) warn that "the symbolic and material convergence of blood, borders, and bodies in the context of Latino cultural commodities and movement across national borders . . . highlight contradictions in the contemporary status of Latinos in the U.S." Thus, while Latina and Latino bodies are commodified and desired within mainstream cultural products, they are simultaneously labeled as dangerous to the stability of U.S. national identity and as a result Latinas and Latinos are politically and economically marginalized through federal, state, and local government policies.

Consequently public policy discourses often position the Latina and Latino population as mostly immigrant, inherently diseased and sexually uncontrollable, a discourse of bodily pathology that affirms many of the Hollywood representations discussed in this chapter. Not coincidentally, the demographic increase in the Latina and Latino population is often framed as a public health problem. Indeed Ruiz (2000) documents that the Latina population is often constructed as a threat to dominant U.S. national identity because of the relatively high birth rate of Latinas as compared to other segments of the U.S.

population. Often cited within this discourse of bodily pathology are undocumented, migrant, poor, and working-class Latinas living in urban areas. During the early 1990s conservative politicians targeted African American and Latina women, suggesting that all women on public assistance be required to use Norplant, a surgically implanted long-term birth control device. Within this discourse Latinas are pathologized as reproducing out of control and in need of sexual self-regulation. Reifying the narrative of feminine pathology, road signs U.S. Interstate 5 on the U.S.-Mexican border visually warn motorists to slow down by foregrounding a Latina woman dragging a child across the freeway (Ruiz, 1996).

Another example of the discourse of pathology that marks Latina and Latino bodies is the fast growth in HIV infection rates among the Latina and Latino population during a time when the general HIV infection rate in the United States is decreasing. Currently, HIV/AIDS cases in the Black and Latino gay male population outnumber those in the White gay male population (Centers for Disease Control, 2000). Although the HIV/AIDS infection rate does not necessarily support border hysteria or the century-old pathologization of the border (Inda, 2002; Stern, 1999), it does highlight the systematic regulation of access to health care for a growing number of dangerous health conditions facing the Latina and Latino community. More than 32% of U.S. Latinas and Latinos lack health insurance, and Latinas and Latinos account for one quarter of the nation's 44 million uninsured (American Health Line, 2000; Hargraves, 2002).

The contemporary global visibility of Latinidad in popular culture shares a discursive space with the public discourse. Both contribute to the production of a normalizing discourse about ethnic, racial, and national identity grounded in the gendered and racialized narratives of fear and desire circulated through the commodified hypervisibility of Latina bodies and the public discourse regarding the growth in the Latina and Latino population in general (Inda, 2002; Ruiz, 2000). These oppositional and complimentary representations point to the ongoing need to remain critical and vigilant about the multipronged forces of global commodification, corporeal (re)configuration, and spatial and territorial reconstitution. Latina and Latino bodies whether on film, television, magazines, the news, or other forms of mass communications circulate as ambivalently desired, commodified, consumed, marginalized, and feared. Nevertheless, the dual representational forces of fear and desire have the potential for reconstituting fragmentary divisions *and* simultaneously disrupting the terrain for a more egalitarian cultural politics. The study of Latinidad as a gendered and racialized practice promises to productively intervene in cultural politics, social movements, and public policy (Guzmán, 2005). The development of a dynamic construction of Latina identity Latinidad is resistant in its potential to produce new corporealities, bodily practices that exceed familiar categorizations yet does not merely end with the "hybrid" but, rather, begins at the hybrid toward a complex multiplicity with culturally and politically resistant implications.

Notes

1. Yet it is important to remember that the United States has always been a multiracial and multicultural society. Promising (or threatening) Census Bureau demographic projections predict a "brown America" and a dwindling non-Hispanic White population by midcentury. These projections are apt to be misleading, however, because of a lack of realistic assumptions regarding intermarriage and the increasingly dynamic formation of racial and ethnic identities. Indeed, the Census Bureau assumes no intermarriage and that all children inherit the racial and ethnic identities of their parents. These assumptions are challenged by estimates that upwards of 25% of Hispanics and Asians marry a person from a different racial or ethnic group. Although African American intermarriage rates are much lower, the last 30 years have seen an upward trend (Russell Sage Foundation Call for Papers, 2002).
2. Dávila (2001) documents the positioning of all three major minorities in this "unique" way. In other words, Latina and Latinos, Asian Americans, and African Americans all market themselves as the last unified segment of the U.S. market. Halter's work supports Dávila's with myriad data from the many ethnic markets and identities available in the U.S. marketplace.
3. Incidentally, sex tourism is one of the major industries in the Caribbean.
4. An Internet search for Rosie articles or images only yields (as of March 2002) links to nude photograph Web sites.
5. Here we draw on film reviews rather than personal analysis of the movie because it was out of theatrical distribution before we were able to see it.
6. Sisco being the Anglo version of the Spanish surname Cisco.
7. To make matters more complicated, a recent poll suggests that Penélope Cruz, the Spanish-born actress who has recently taken Hollywood by storm, is considered to be more authentically Latina by a majority of Latina and Latino audiences.

References

Acosta, C., & Kreshel, P. (2002, May). *Who gets to be an American girl?* Paper presented at the International Communications Association Conference in Acapulco, Mexico.

Alba, A. Gaspar de (2003). The Chicana/Latina dyad, or identity and perception. *Latino Studies, 1,* 106–114.

Aparicio, F. (2003). Jennifer as Selena: Rethinking Latinidad in media and popular culture. *Latino Studies, 1*(1), 90–105.

Aparicio, F. R., & Chávez-Silverman, S., Eds. (1997). *Tropicalizations: Transcultural representations of Latinidad.* Hanover, NH: University Press of New England.

Beltrán, M. C. (2002). The Hollywood Latina body as site of social struggle: Media constructions of stardom and Jennifer Lopez's "cross-over butt." *Quarterly Review of Film and Video, 19*, 71–86.

Centers for Disease Control. (2000). *Morbidity and Mortality Weekly Report.* Atlanta, GA

Children Now. (2002). *Fall colors: Prime time diversity report.* Oakland, CA: Children and the Media Program.

Dávila, A. (2001). *Latinos inc.: The marketing and making of a people.* Berkeley: University of California Press.

Davis, M. (2000). *Magical urbanism: Latinos reinvent the US city.* London: Verso.

Desmond, J. C. (Ed.). (1997). *Meaning in motion: New cultural studies of dance.* Durham, NC: Duke University Press.

Flores, J. (2000). *From bomba to hip hop: Puerto Rican culture and Latino identity.* New York: Columbia University Press.

Foucault, M. (1979). *Discipline and punish: The birth of the prison.* New York: Vintage.

Fregoso, R. L. (1993). *The bronze screen: Chicana and Chicano film culture.* Minneapolis: University of Minnesota Press.

Gilman, S. (1985). *Difference and pathology: Stereotypes of sexuality, race, and madness.* Ithaca, NY: Cornell University Press.

Goodson, S., & Shaver, M. A. (1994). Hispanic marketing: National advertiser spending patterns and media choices. *Journalism Quarterly, 71*, 191–198.

Guzmán, I. M. (2001, April). The commodification of Latinidad: A cinematic analysis of Jennifer Lopez and Salma Hayek in films from 1995 to 2000. Paper presented at the American Studies Association/Popular Culture Association Annual National Conference, Philadelphia, Pennsylvania.

Guzmán, I. M. (2005). Gendering Latinidades: Racializing US Cuban women in the Elián González news coverage. *Latino Studies, 3*, 179-204.

Guzmán, I. M. (2007). Salma's *Frida*: Latinas as transnational bodies in U.S. popular culture. In Myra Mendible (Ed.), *From bananas to buttocks: The Latina in popular film and culture* (pp. 117–128). Austin: University of Texas.

Guzmán, I. M., & Valdivia, A. (2004). Brain, brow or bootie: Latina iconicity in contemporary popular culture. *Communication Review, 7*(2), 203–219.

Hacker, A. (2000, November 30). The case against kids. *New York Times Review of Books*, pp. 12–17).

Halter, M. (2000). *Shopping for identity: The marketing of ethnicity.* New York: Shocken.

Hargraves, J. L. (2002). The insurance gap and minority health care, 1997–2001. Center for Studying Health System Change. Retrieved February 13, 2003, from www.hschange.com/CONTENT/443.

Hayek. S. (2001). Personal quotes. Internet Movie Database. Retrieved April 20, 2003, from http://www.us.imdb.com/?Hayek,+Salma

Hindes, A. (1997). WB betting on appeal of Selena. Retrieved March 17, 2002, from http://www.variety.com.

Inda, J. X. (2002). Biopower, reproduction, and the migrant woman's body. In A. J. Aldama & N. H. Quiñones (Eds.), *Decolonial voices: Chicana and Chicano cultural studies in the twentieth-first century* (pp. 98–112). Bloomington: Indiana University Press.

Leger, M. C. & Ruiz, M. V. (in press). "Hot-blooded": Latino bodies and politics of health and disease. In M. Garcia, M. C. Leger, & A. N. Valdivia (Eds.), *Geographies of Latinidad: Latina and Latino studies into the twenty-first century.* Durham, NC: Duke University Press.

López, A. M. (1991). Are all Latins from Manhattan? Hollywood, ethnography, and cultural colonialism. In L. D. Friedman (Ed.), *Unspeakable images: Ethnicity and the American cinema* (pp. 404–424). Urbana: University of Illinois Press.

Lugones, M. (2003). *Pilgrimages/peregrinajes: Theorizing coalition against multiple oppressions.* New York: Rowman & Littlefield.

McLean, A. L. (1993). "I'm a cansino": Transformation, ethnicity, and authenticity in the construction of Rita Hayworth, American love goddess. *Journal of Film and Video, 44*(3–4), 8–26.

Obejas, A. (2001, September 21). Carving out a new American identity: Nationalism is an obsolete idea as Latinos outgrow labels. *Chicago Tribune*, sect. 2, pp. 1, 6.

(Eds.), *Cultural Politics in Contemporary America* (pp. 111–122). London: Routledge.

Omi, M, & Winant, H. (1986). *Racial formation in the United States: From the 1960s to the 1980s.* London: Routledge.

Padilla, F. (1982). On the nature of Latino ethnicity. *Social Science Quarterly, 65,* 651–664.

Perez Firmat, G. (1994). *Life on the hyphen: The Cuban-American way.* Austin: University of Texas Press.

Rabinow, P. (1984). *The Foucault reader.* New York: Pantheon.

Rodriguez, A. (1999). *Making Latino news: Race, language, class.* Thousand Oaks, CA: Sage.

Rodríguez, C. E. (1997). *Latin looks: Images of Latinas and Latinos in the U.S. media.* Denver, CO: Westview.

Ruiz, M. V. (1996, May). *Latinas and border crossing.* Paper presented at the Annual International Communication Conference, Chicago, IL.

Ruiz, M. V. (2000, June). *Latinas, health and the media.* Paper presented at the Annual International Communication Conference, Acapulco, Mexico.

Russell Sage Foundation Call for Papers. (2002, February). Retrieved 2003, from http://www.russellsage.org/programs/proj_reviews/immigprop. htmimmigratio n.htm.

Saldivar, J. D. (1997). *Border matters: Remapping American cultural studies.* Berkeley: University of California Press.

Shohat, E. (1991). Gender and the culture of empire: Toward a feminist ethnography of cinema. *Quarterly Review of Film & Video, 131,* 1–2.

Shohat, E., & Stam, R. (1994). *Unthinking Eurocentrism: Multiculturalism and the media.* New York: Routledge.

Sinclair, J. (1999). *Latin American television: A global view.* New York: Oxford University Press.

Stern, A. M. (1999). Buildings, boundaries, and blood: Medicalization and nation-building on the U.S.-Mexico border, 1910–1930. *Hispanic American Historical Review, 79*(1), 40–81.

Valdivia, A. (2000). *A Latina in the land of Hollywood.* Tucson: University of Arizona Press.

Valdivia, A. (2007). Is Penélope to J-Lo as culture is to nature? Eurocentric approaches to "Latin" beauties. In M. Mendible (Ed.), *Bananas to buttocks: The Latina body in popular culture* (pp. 129–148). Austin: University of Texas Press.

PART IV
Science, Nature and Gender

10

"Doing What Comes Naturally . . ."

Negotiating Normality in Accounts of IVF Failure

KAREN THROSBY

University of Warwick

THE NEW REPRODUCTIVE and genetic technologies constitute a broad and dynamic technosocial domain within which new social relations are produced. Implicit in this process of the forging of new relations is the production of new bodily norms and regulatory practices. Writing from a Foucauldian perspective about the new reproductive technologies, and particularly in vitro fertilization (IVF), Jana Sawicki (1991) identifies these new technologies as disciplinary techniques, which operate by "creating desires, attaching individuals to specific identities and establishing norms against which individuals and their behaviors and bodies are judged and against which they police themselves" (p. 68). While the new reproductive and genetic technologies provide new forms of knowledge and opportunity, they also function to govern the body in novel ways. Carlos Novas and Nikolas Rose (2000) have described this governance in terms of "somatic individuality," where, for example, knowledge of genetic risk produced through the availability of genetic testing produces new responsibilities around the body and the self. Individuals, according to Novas and Rose, are not rendered passive by the diagnosis of disease (or the risk of future disease), but rather are produced as new types of subjects, becoming "skilled, prudent and active, an ally of the doctor, a proto-professional" (p. 489). Paul Rabinow (1996), elaborating Michel Foucault's (1978) concept of biopower, articulates these new social relations and obligations in terms of "biosociality," where identity groupings are formulated in relation to biomedical and technological knowledge and practices, and new forms of identity in turn produce their own norms and responsibilities in relation to bodily governance and health practices.

In this work on the new forms of bodily governance emerging out of the rise of the new reproductive and genetic technologies, however, the gendering of bodies and practices is often lost, and little attention is paid to the differential productions of biosocial responsibilities. The work of Rayna Rapp, Deborah Heath, and Karen-Sue Taussig (2001) provides an important exception to this. In an article describing a range of U.S.-based genetic support and activist groups, they show that "in most genetic support groups, the kinship activists are disproportionately wives and mothers" (p. 397). Briefly discussing the history of health activism, they suggest that over the course of the twentieth century, "health activism became increasingly marked as the domain of female volunteerism" (p. 398). Many of the local and national genetics-related groups they studied were founded by women, usually mothers of children with genetic problems, who they describe as "staking public claims on the turf of family health" (p. 398). This finding suggests that the active bodily management practices of the somatic individual are not necessarily carried out by the individual themselves, but may become the responsibility of others, disproportionately women, for whom the work of caring is easily naturalized and therefore rendered invisible as work. The prime site for exploring these issues further is IVF because although the "couple" has emerged as the "patient" in fertility treatment (van der Ploeg, 2004), the treatment itself focuses almost exclusively on the female body, even in the case of male factor infertility, rendering women not only as objects of substantial medical intervention, but also producing significant responsibility for women in relation to treatment and its outcomes.

Importantly, the exclusion of women from IVF narratives is not simply a matter of representational oversight, which could be rectified by "adding in" women. Instead, the dominant representations of IVF are in fact predicated on this exclusion, through the prevailing construction of IVF as "giving nature a helping hand." The work of IVF, then, becomes an extension of the "natural" reproductive labor of "normal" (normative) femininity. This understanding is central to the construction of IVF as a "normal" and mainstream technology, and constitutes a primary rhetorical means, for both patients and treatment providers, of distinguishing the IVF "miracle baby" from its more socially contentious sibling, the "designer baby." The need for this discursive work highlights not only the extent to which the (un)reproductive female body is subject to surveillance and discipline, but also the widely held unease about the use of technology for reproduction—an unease that is readily apparent in the voracious media appetite for stories about "designer babies" or cloning. These stories draw on a wide repertoire of fears of "meddling with nature," with each new announcement or scientific development seen as (potentially, at least) undermining what it means to be human (see Fukuymama, 2003; Gosden, 1999; Silver, 1999). For IVF to be "normal," then, the engagement with it must necessarily be located within the domain of "natural" reproduction. When treatment is successful, the presence of a reassuringly "natural" baby performs much of the work of alleviating anxiety about "meddling with nature," with the "natural" order restored through reproduction. However, the reality of IVF in the United Kingdom is that almost 80% of all treatment cycles started are unsuccessful, leaving those for whom treatment is unsuccessful to negotiate not only what it means to have technologized the "natural" reproductive process, but also to be living either without children or without the desired number of children.

Those for whom IVF fails and who subsequently stop treatment find themselves ambiguously and liminally located in relation to reproductive norms: they have tried to conceive, but have been unable to; they desire (genetic) children, but are no longer actively pursuing that desire through IVF, and they have brought technology into the reproductive process without the counterbalancing "natural" baby. This liminal location is what Elspeth Probyn (1996) has described as one of "outside belonging"—a state of "ongoing inbetweenness" (p. 6) that is full of both possibility and risk. As Rosi Braidotti (1994) observes, "it is crowded at the margins, and nonbelonging can be hell" (p. 20). The patients, and particularly the women, have to do the work of negotiating the "ongoing inbetweenness" of their experiences. This burden of work can be described as the "negotiation of normality" (Throsby, 2002, 2004) and is performed through a panoply of profoundly gendered disciplinary techniques, which extend both temporally and spatially beyond the confines of the clinical encounter. This multiplicity of "techniques for achieving the subjugation of bodies" (Foucault, 1978, p. 140) can be seen as a manifestation of biopower, which Foucault describes as "everywhere; not because it embraces everything, but because it comes from everywhere" (p. 93), emerging through disciplinary practices over individual bodies and regulatory practices over populations (p. 140). In the engagement with IVF, women's bodies become the intense focus of medical and social surveillance, which is matched by women's rigorous policing of their own bodies, constituting a panoptical "trap" (p. 200) whereby the individual "who is subjected to a field of visibility, and who knows it, assumes the responsibility for the constraints of power . . ." (p. 202). The material-discursive work of locating the self as natural/normal, post-IVF, then, is ongoing, and the achievement of watchful docility is hard work.

Drawing on a series of interviews with 15 women (whose male partners chose not to participate) and 13 couples, and using discourse analysis (Gill, 1996, 2000; Potter & Wetherell, 1987; Wood & Kroger, 2000), this chapter explores the ways in which the participants both deployed and resisted discourses of nature and the gendered body in relation to the engagement with IVF to locate themselves as "normal." The participants had all had IVF unsuccessfully at least once with their most recent cycle having failed and having taken place at least two years prior to the interviews. The participants were recruited through the dormant patient records at a specialist fertility unit in a large National Health Service (NHS) teaching hospital. However, importantly, a relative paucity of NHS funding for IVF means that approximately 80% of all IVF cycles in the United Kingdom are self-funded by the patients, either in NHS units or within the private sector. There are long waiting lists for funded treatment, and patients, therefore, commonly undergo treatment in several clinics, moving between the private and the public sector (as was the case for many of the participants in this study). The number of cycles undergone ranged from 1 to 13, and the amount of money spent on treatment ranged from nominal amounts up to well in excess of $30,000. The participants were predominantly (although by no means exclusively) White, middle class, and educated to degree or professional level—an outcome that has been well-documented by other studies in this field (Daniluk, 1996; Franklin, 1997; Sandelowski, 1993).

This chapter is divided into two sections: the first section argues that IVF produces an imperative to engage with it, but that this can be mobilized, post-IVF failure to produce a new, technologically mediated, legitimized form of childlessness; the second section looks at the ways in which women surveilled and disciplined their own bodies to maximize their chances of treatment success and minimize their own sense of responsibility for its failure. The analysis explores the ways in which this discursive work is both produced by, and productive of, gendered bodily governance in ways that impact deleteriously, but asymmetrically, on both men and women. The chapter concludes by arguing that IVF, for all its rhetorical "newness," is predicated on deeply entrenched problematic discursive resources and practices around the gendered body, motherhood, and nature, which are both resisted and deployed by women in the management and negotiation of IVF failure.

'Our consciences are clear'

The rise of IVF as a relatively mainstream reproductive technology has been swift and widespread. In the 31 years since the birth of the first

IVF baby, Louise Brown, IVF has long been supplanted by "designer babies," preimplantation genetic diagnosis (PGD; see Braude, Pickering, Flinter, & Ogilvie, 2002), stem cell research, and cloning as the focus of tabloid reproductive horror stories. Indeed, patients, doctors, and the public increasingly attach the epithet "normal" to IVF to mark a distinction between the mainstream fertility treatment and those newer, more controversial technologies to which the laboratory technique of IVF is central. In the United Kingdom alone, 72 clinics are licensed to perform IVF, treating well in excess of 20,000 women a year,[1] and in May 2005, as part of a scientific conference on preimplantation genetics, a concert was held in London to celebrate the lives of the estimated 2 million babies worldwide who have been conceived using IVF.[2] The increasingly mainstream status of IVF, and its normalization in relation to other more socially controversial technologies, produces a strong imperative to engage with treatment. This imperative is given a particular dynamic in the United Kingdom because of two key factors. First, fertility treatment in the United Kingdom is subject to one of the strictest systems of regulation in the world, under the aegis of the Human Fertilization and Embryology Authority (HFEA). This governance at the national level provides legitimacy for individual engagements with IVF:

> ANGELA: But I would say that probably because you know that the HFEA is spoken about, you know that it's being controlled. You know you're not, you know, there's not some wacky doctor doing, you know . . . you know that you are in a controlled environment, that it is regulated, they're not allowed to put more than three embryos back in and all that sort of thing.

The second normalizing factor is the provision of treatment within the NHS, which is subject to significant funding constraints, and consequently, debates about what constitutes a treatment priority are a recurrent feature of health discourse in the United Kingdom. A 2001 report by the British Medical Association (BMA), for example, categorized fertility treatment alongside tattoo removal, gender reassignment, and drugs for baldness and impotence as draining resources away from essential services, and therefore as potential candidates for exclusion from NHS provision.[3] However, on August 26, 2003, the National Institute for Clinical Excellence (NICE)[4] issued the second draft of the clinical guidelines on the assessment and management of fertility problems. The draft guidelines propose the provision of three "fresh" IVF cycles for women. In response to these guidelines, in February 2004, Health Secretary John Reid announced that all women younger than

40 will be entitled to a single funded cycle, with no timetable given for the full implementation of the NICE recommendations.[5] This move confirms the status of IVF in the United Kingdom as a necessary and effective medical treatment, further normalizing both the technology and the engagement with it.

Fundamentally, from the patients' perspective, the imperative to undergo IVF stems from the need, which participants frequently cited, to have "done everything possible" to get pregnant before becoming reconciled to the prospect of a life without children. Indeed, for the participants in this study, the engagement with IVF was experienced as a precondition to being able to even begin to accept childlessness. IVF, then, even when it fails, functions as a means of distinguishing the self from those who would be candidates for treatment but who have chosen not to undergo it, as well as from those who have chosen to live without children—a life choice widely assumed a priori to be indicative of selfishness.[6] This, in turn, produces a novel, legitimized form of childlessness:

> CLAIRE: . . . I can say, "At least I tried." So there can be no stage in the future when I might say to myself, "Oh well, if only I'd tried, it could have been different." Erm . . . it's almost like I can say to society, "Look, I tried to be the typical female, I tried to be the mother, you know, but it conspired against me, so I now have the right to go off and spend my money on nice holidays or whatever and don't need to feel guilty."

Having undergone IVF serves not only to preempt Claire's own potential future regrets, but also performs a silencing function toward others—"society"—who might choose to evaluate her negatively because of her life without children. IVF takes on a public, confessional dimension (Foucault, 1978, p. 62) through which the intention and desire to parent is made clear, in spite of the absence of a child. As Tim noted in an interview with him and his wife, Katy, "our consciences are clear." Indeed, for Claire, only by trying IVF is the "right to go off and spend my money on nice holidays . . ." earned—an understanding that reflects the powerful association of certain kinds of consumption with the presumed "selfishness" of childlessness. Several other women repeated this sentiment, expressing concern that overseas holidays, a new car, or new soft furnishings might be misread by others as indicative of being too "selfish" to be a parent, causing them either to conceal their consumption, or to spread out purchases to make them less noticeable to others. This highlights the extent to which IVF, while conventionally represented as a private practice between a couple (and their doctors), is a surveilled public practice whose meanings have to be negotiated and managed in the public domain. Furthermore, that this discursive work is necessary highlights the extent to which reproduction, particularly for women, is normatively prescribed, and the failure to do so always has to be accounted for; those who do not engage with treatment are potentially "guilty" and their consciences cannot be clear. Voluntary childlessness, then, is rendered the discursive Other against which the conformity—or normality—of those experiencing IVF failure can be defined. This is important in the context of the NICE recommendations discussed earlier because in the face of free treatment, the decision not to have IVF risks becoming an act of "refusal," denoting a voluntary element to the life without children. Where IVF is seen as an extension of the "natural" reproductive process, those women who "refuse" free treatment risk being evaluated by others as "too selfish" to perform the reproductive labor of normative femininity. Therefore, the nonmother who "refuses" treatment is rendered as lacking the self-sacrificial qualities of normative ("natural") womanhood/motherhood.

However, in itself, an engagement with IVF does not unproblematically constitute "doing everything possible" because the technology remains one of seemingly endless possibility, always offering the "maybe-next-time" promise of success that postpones the end of treatment. What constitutes "everything," then, is never clear, and when treatment fails, can only be determined retrospectively and discursively. One of the primary strategies through which this is endpoint is discursively achieved is through the mobilization of a discourse of desperation, and in particular, the figure of the "desperate infertile woman." The desperate infertile woman is a rhetorical figure, much beloved of media representations of IVF and its associated technologies, signifying immoderation and irrational excess; she is "obsessed" with treatment, even to the point of financial ruin and relationship breakdown, and is willing to go to any lengths to have a genetic child. While the epithet "desperate" clearly signifies the intense desire to have a child—a desire that is normatively prescribed as "natural" in women—it also signifies an unsuitability to be a parent. The "desperate infertile woman," then, is not only a nonmother, but her excess and immoderation renders her a "bad mother" (May, 1998), and therefore constitutes an identity that has to be strongly repudiated by the women in the accounts:

SUSAN: I didn't want to be one of those women that you saw on television, that are sort of in their 50s, that have had sort of like hundreds and hundreds of it. And it does take over your life. I didn't

want to be . . . I mean, we did get obsessive, but I didn't want to be
one of these completely obsessive people that that's all they live for.
And we had to have some sort of . . . reality. You know, we had to
have some sort of life. Although it did take over, that sort of three
seemed . . . I don't know. Three just seemed a good control number,
a good sort of, you know, that's your best shot.

The hyperbolic caricature of the aging woman doggedly pursuing
endless cycles of treatment featured regularly in the accounts, and
her rhetorical function here is as the irrational, out-of-control Other
against which Susan's moderation can be defined. Importantly, what
actually constitutes desperation is indefinable in objective terms;
instead, what matters is the discursive mobilization of the excessive "not
me." Therefore, for some of the participants, three was posited as excessive and desperate; for another of the participants, Katy, on the other
hand, her plan to undergo six cycles was a sign of strength, not
weakness, describing herself as "not a giver-upper," with far higher
numbers of cycles signifying desperation. Desperation, then, constitutes a discursive resource through which the participants were
able to construct their own engagement with treatment as enough,
but not too much—a fine balance to strike, and one that is not at
all stable, requiring constant maintenance and negotiation. That this
discursive work is necessary highlights the surveillance and discipline
to which the women were subjected to, both by themselves and by
others.

The number of treatment cycles was not the only site for this discursive work, and particular kinds of treatment were also mobilized as
signifying desperation, leading to an unnatural degree of intervention.[7]
In this context, "designer babies," sex selection for social reasons,
large multiple births, and the use of IVF by postmenopausal women
constituted abnormal uses of the technology, which were perceived to
be sullying their own more "normal" uses of it:

ROBERT: It was natural . . . it was just the mechanics of it that were
assisted. It wasn't like cloning a sheep, or growing ears on the backs
of mice, or things like that.

Tim complained that the more newsworthy cases "give us IVF-ers a
bad name," laying claim to a biosocial community of "normal" users of
IVF to shore up the construction of his and his wife Katy's own engagement with IVF as normal, natural, and morally unproblematic.

Importantly, no male counterpart correlates to the desperate infertile woman, although she does have female counterparts in other contexts; the "scalpel slave" or "surgery junkie" of cosmetic surgery is another rhetorical incarnation of the same irrational excess (Davis, 1995), as is the kleptomaniac "lady" shopper (Ableson, 2000), the shopaholic, or the "obsessive" dieter. These are all sites that are constructed as constituting normative femininity—beauty practices, shopping, weight control—but that require a comparable balancing act of doing enough, but not too much. Writing of the feminized domain of shopping, Rachel Bowlby (2000) argues that periodic madness in relation to consumption—for example, in the sales—is constructed as a facet of normal femininity, in contrast with the stability of male sanity and reason (p. 124). This parallels the understanding of the female hormonally regulated body as cyclically (dis)ordered, in comparison with male hormonal stability (Oudshoorn, 1994, p. 146). This contrast between the disordered normality of femininity and the rational normality of masculinity was duplicated explicitly in the accounts via a discourse of the hormonal reproductive drive:

> MARTIN: I think it's been a bit of a burning desire for Nancy to have a child. But if I'm honest with myself, I'm very much . . . I was very much, if it happens, it happens. If it doesn't, it doesn't.

> BRIAN: Why go with all that stress? Be happy with what you've got, which was always what I said. Obviously, you have to, erm, put that against the maternal instincts, and so on. . . .

Women are conventionally understood as hormonally driven (Oudshoorn, 1994), both toward reproduction and toward erratic and irrational behavior; in both of these examples, the male partners are witnesses to the natural drives, not subject to them. The hormonal discourse provides a strongly normalizing justification for the use of technology for reproduction because it retains the dominance of the natural in the reproductive endeavor with technology simply serving as a "helping hand." In Lisa's case, her doctor also confirmed the irrepressibility of the maternal drive:

> LISA: I remember that first meeting, he [the consultant] was very sympathetic, and he said, "I do understand that secondary infertility is actually more distressing than being infertile, because your body is screaming out, because the hormones have already been through the process of being pregnant and having a child. Your body wants to do it again.

Lisa's body, according to the consultant, is literally demanding to
be pregnant, embodying the traditional biomedical view that women
are controlled by their bodies, rather than the other way round as
is assumed to be the case with men (although this fails to take into
account discourses of irrepressible male sexual drives, for example,
or male violence). Lisa's body is credited with volition and voice, and
its "screaming out" for a baby is to be taken seriously, although this
acquiescence to the presumed demands of the body is notably absent in
other areas of women's lives, such as diet or sexuality, where pressure to
control and silence the unruly female body is more commonplace. In the
face of the "natural/normal" demand of the female body to reproduce,
the engagement with IVF is rendered an equally "natural/normal"
response, making the act of IVF "refusal" one of going against nature.
Therefore, while this discursive strategy is useful as a justification for
engaging with treatment and for normalizing that treatment, it also
leaves in place the potent equation of womanhood and motherhood,
and reproduces the imperative to engage with IVF.

'It might make all the difference'

But the degree of bodily governance that IVF produces extends far
beyond the imperative to engage with treatment (within reason), as
discussed earlier. Instead, in the public practice of IVF at the everyday
microlevel, the gendered panoptical nature of the experience of IVF
and its failure becomes fully apparent.

In the course of IVF treatment women's "performance" as patients
is closely surveilled both by themselves and others. One participant,
Liz, for example, described seeing the words "poor performer" written
across the top of her medical records, following her first cycle, where a
very small number of eggs had been collected:

> Liz: I thought, well . . . I was just sitting there thinking . . . gosh, they
> can't . . . I feel labeled! You sort of . . . like a school report—could do
> better, you know.

Many of the women for whom the hormonal treatment had not
produced the desired results expressed the failure as belonging to
themselves. Jane commented that she never "did that well with the eggs,"
and others described themselves as producing "crap eggs" (Stephanie),
or being "rubbish at producing eggs" (Jenny). The medical technology
itself remains unblemished in these accounts, and the participants drew
instead on the discourse of failed productivity within themselves—a

discourse that already has considerable currency in accounts of menstruation and the menopause (Martin, 1989, 1990). The fear of a "poor
performance" led women to subject themselves to careful disciplinary
surveillance in the implementation of the IVF process, and particularly
in the administration of the hormonal drugs, on which the production
of multiple egg follicles is dependent:

> Katy: Yeah, I'm very, very focused in that I'm disciplined but I have to
> have everything just so. So, as long as everything's just so. So the fact
> that, you know, . . . getting the ampoule out and making sure there's no
> air in the needle, if a little spurt spurted out I'd be horrified. Whereas,
> subsequently, you know, they'd sort of you know, spurt out the end
> and I said "Oh!" [horrified] and they said, "It's alright, they allow
> factors of, you know, loss." And I'd been doing everything sort of [all
> laughing]—mustn't lose anything. It might make all the difference.

Katy's vigilance in relation to her meticulous preparation of the
hormonal drugs is self-deprecatingly told in terms of her lack of medical
knowledge about the built-in excess, but her story also highlights the seriousness with which she approached her responsibilities in the treatment
process and particularly her attention to detail—a precision in which she
exceeds that of the medical professionals and that reflects the "proto-
professionality" of somatic individuality. Writing of the "body work" of
women at aerobics classes, Deborah Gimlin (2002) argues that rather
than aiming at a bodily ideal per se (for example, the "beautiful" body),
the women she observed sought to "neutralize the moral significance of
flawed bodies in favor of more positive indicators of strength, capability
and determination" (p. 145). The same kind of "body work" can be seen
in Katy's case; unable to demonstrate the "ideal" reproductive body, she
instead demonstrates her commitment, skill, and self-discipline, which
show her to have both "done everything possible" to make the cycle
successful and as having many of the qualities that would have made her
a good mother. However, this need for absolute precision also reflects the
responsibilities she feels—"it might make all the difference"—and while
claiming an expertise demonstrates the meeting of those responsibilities,
it also leaves the burden of responsibility unchallenged.

But for the women, the disciplining of the body to maximize the
chances of treatment success extended far beyond the specific requirements of the injections into every aspect of their daily lives. In the
context of reproduction, this is utterly in keeping with bombarding
women with messages from both the alternative and conventional
medical fields about the importance of preconceptual and antenatal

nutrition, environmental hazards, and other practices with regard to fertility, conception, and early pregnancy. It is also concordant with the potent contemporary discourse of "helping yourself" in relation to health care—a key feature of "somatic individuality." Consequently, the vast majority of the female participants in this study disciplined themselves closely throughout the treatment process (and often for years prior to that), drawing on common-sense knowledges of the importance of rest, relaxation, and diet in achieving and sustaining a pregnancy, as well as specific (alternative) therapeutic regimens of nutrition, stress management, detoxification, homeopathy, acupuncture, hypnosis, or herbs, alongside the close monitoring of the body for signs of fertility or pregnancy that was habitual to many of the women after years of trying to conceive.

Responding to the commonly held fear on the part of the women that they would "wash away" the transferred embryos if they went to the toilet, one of the doctors I spoke to routinely told patients that they could go bungee jumping and it would make no difference to implantation. However, the majority of the participants disregarded these assurances and focused instead on the measures that they perceived as potentially effective in maximizing their chances of conception, for example, by taking time off work for the two-week period following embryo transfer, or eating certain foods and avoiding others. This was reinforced by the women's partners and other friends and relatives, who would chastise them for "doing too much" or for failing to be positive. This highlights the extent to which women are subject to the disciplinary surveillance of others throughout their treatment, and therefore, that the disciplinary techniques that they employ serve not only to preempt future feelings of guilt about treatment outcome, but also demonstrate to others that everything possible has been done.

This rigorous policing by both the self and others implies that a successful outcome may be within the remit of the individual woman. Arthur Frank describes this assertion of control as characteristic of the disciplined body—that is, where the body is perceived as dissociated from the self, and as something to be managed and controlled to assert predictability (Frank, 1995, p. 41). Interestingly, Frank describes disciplined bodies as making good patients (p. 42), although in this case the patients clearly disregarded medical assurances that those measures would make no difference. However, this deviation from medical advice could only take place because none of the measures taken were perceived by the doctors as actually endangering a successful outcome. Instead, they were simply regarded as having no proven positive value, and therefore, the participants saw themselves as having nothing to lose and everything to gain. In this sense, they are still being good patients, even by disregarding medical advice because they are doing more than is required.

The management of stress emerged as a common site of disciplinary surveillance for the women. This draws on a very long tradition of assumptions that women can influence the outcome of pregnancy by the force of their imagination, mood, or state of mind. Women's dreams or imaginings were traditionally believed to be the cause of deformity or "monstrosity" in babies (Braidotti, 1996; Stonehouse, 1994), for example, and in contemporary discourse, stress is widely held to inhibit conception (although no evidence exists to support this):

MARTIN: . . . because all the way through it, you get the people who do know [about their infertility], like your friends, your boss . . . my boss—"Take her on holiday," "Get her drunk," "Make her relax."
NANCY: And you think, I've been there, done that.
MARTIN: "Tell her to stop work" was a big one.
KAREN: Really?
NANCY: And we did consider that, but I didn't [stop work].
MARTIN: But I did. I told you to pack up work, because . . . she wasn't in a management position of any description, but she seemed to be somewhat stressed. And er . . . I just felt, well, let's find out. Let's give it a year and find out. But Nancy's answer to that was, "What's the bloody point?" Because we could end up without a job, without a year's salary, and without a baby."

Conventional values of masculinity converge to make Martin responsible for resolving the "relaxation" issue, by getting her drunk, or taking her on holiday—strategies that have their echoes in discourses of seduction, rather than reproduction. Nancy's decision to keep working, however, closes the discussion, and Martin is torn between his suspicion that his work colleagues may be right about the need for Nancy to stop working and his need to respect Nancy's decision.

Significantly, although some of the male partners accepted responsibility with regard to overcoming what were seen as female problems of stress management, even where male infertility was implicated, few cases were found where the connection between behavior and fertility was made and acted on by men. Several of the men were recommended to take simple steps to improve sperm count and quality, such as wearing loose underwear, not taking hot baths, abstaining from alcohol and tobacco, and taking supplements. However, the compliance rate was very low (see also, Lee, 1996, p. 20), which contrasted sharply with the women who policed their own behavior (and were policed by others) rigorously even where there was doubt as to whether it made any difference to the outcome, as this quote illustrates:

> ALICE: And [the doctors said] don't have hot baths, which he loves, so he still has hot baths. And erm . . . they talked about sort of putting a bag of frozen peas on appropriate areas [both laugh]. And he did try a dash of cold water once, and he said, "Never again!" I won't show him this transcript! But he does . . . Still, I think . . . sometimes he'll come out of the bath and say, "Cor, boiling hot, that was !" And I say, "Don't tell me!" Because to me, that's like saying, "You won't get pregnant in 6 weeks' time." And I said to him a couple of times, and he was going, "No, no, no, the doctor doesn't know what he's talking about."
>
> KAREN: Was he just disregarding the advice? He just didn't believe the advice?
>
> ALICE: No, and he didn't see why he should change, just on the doctor's say-so. Even though it's come up in programs since, but he just doesn't change anything, so I just think, "Well, it's down to me then." You know, "I'm the one that's got to do everything—you just carry on as you were before."

Importantly, this lack of compliance should not be read as the male partners not caring about the outcome of treatment; indeed, the men in this study undoubtedly experienced the grief of childlessness and IVF failure profoundly—a grief that normative gender relations and the assumptions of reproduction as the "natural" domain of women render inexpressible. To use Bernadette Susan McCreight's (2004) term, writing in relation to male experience of pregnancy loss, this is "a grief ignored" and one about which very little research has been done to date.[8] Instead, this lack of compliance can be seen as a product of normative (and naturalized) gendered social relations. In particular, the disinterest on the part of the men in engaging in sperm improvement regimens can be explained by two key factors: first, the evaluation of sperm quality according to fertilization capacity; and second, the normative association of virility, fertility, and masculinity in popular culture.

Irma van der Ploeg (2004) highlights the ways in which IVF discourse produces "the (normal) oocyte as a troublemaker" (p. 165), with eggs providing obstacles to sperm, which are represented as "the active agents in fertilization" (p. 166), even in cases of male factor infertility. However, once male fertility has been confirmed by fertilization (or predicted by a positive sperm count), the focus falls onto the female body in the case of treatment failure. The presumption of male fertility (as shown either in testing or facilitated by micro-manipulation techniques)[9] is exemplified by Sandra Leiblum and Dorothy Greenfield (1997), who describe one of their studies as involving "an infertile couple where the *wife* is diagnosed with "unexplained infertility" (p. 91; my emphasis). Ultimately, only reproduction itself can confirm female fertility. Consequently, the engagement with IVF tends to confirm male fertility, even when it fails, while continuing to locate reproductive failure within the female body. With their fertility either confirmed (or enabled) by technology, male partners have little incentive to engage in sperm improvement regimens, while the unruly unpredictability of the female body continues to require constant management. As van der Ploeg (2004) argues, "[no] matter how infertile, it seems, a man is never really infertile, provided all 'external conditions' (other bodies, that is) are made conducive to letting his body function" (p. 167).

The second explanation for the relative absence of pressure on men to modify their behavior in relation to sperm quality is the enduring association of fertility and virility in men; a sperm improvement regimen, therefore, can be seen as a direct challenge to masculinity. Male fertility, then, becomes evaluated in popular discourse through a very different kind of "performance" (the ability to perform sexually) to the performance of female fertility (the ability to respond appropriately to the drug regimen):

> BETH: I sent [partner] a card on Valentine's Day last year, saying "to the world's greatest lover" and there's a friend of mine in here, who actually has 4 children . . . and her boyfriend said "Oh, how come I didn't get a card saying, "Greatest lover"?" and she said, "You've got children to prove you are."

The study revealed some moments of quite shocking cruelty and insensitivity toward men in relation to their fertility, including finding pots of seedless jam or bags of Jaffa (seedless) oranges on their desks, or being subjected to offers to "stand in" or "come round and see your wife." From this perspective, while within the framework of normative femininity, the women must be seen to be doing everything possible to have a child through the careful disciplining of the body, normative masculinity can be seen to be working to the opposite effect, constraining men from engaging in sperm improvement regimens, which might cast their own fertility/virility/masculinity into doubt. This is a construction in which both partners are often complicit—a finding Russell Webb and Judith Daniluk (1999, p. 13) also supported—with male factor infertility being relocated within the "couple." Angela, for example, described her and her husband as "a pair of old duffers," even though the fertility problem appeared to lie with her husband's low sperm count. Ann Woollett (1992) also notes that in the treatment context, men experiencing fertility problems are repeatedly assured by doctors and their partners that their infertility does not reflect on their masculinity, although no such assurances are offered to women who are infertile in relation to their feminine identity (p. 169).

Conclusion

In this brief discussion, I have demonstrated some of the ways in which the unsuccessful engagement with IVF produces new forms of governance of the female body. The very availability of IVF produces an imperative to engage with it because it offers the possibility of a novel, technologically mediated form of socially authorized childlessness that is (morally) distinct from that which is chosen. However, this drive toward treatment reflects a more pervasive assumption that women, in particular, should "do everything possible" to have a child. This, in turn, produces an imperative to engage in an array of bodily disciplinary practices oriented not only toward maximizing the chances of a positive outcome, but also toward demonstrating to others that "everything possible" (although not too much) has been tried. These practices are profoundly gendered, with the responsibility falling primarily to the female partners.

Importantly, however, this analysis is not intended to constitute a case against IVF; on the contrary, it demonstrates clearly the extent to which IVF is replete with both risks and possibilities for those engaging with it, and that those undergoing treatment are active (if always constrained) agents—or users (Saetnan, Oudshoorn, & Kirejczyk, 2000)—in the production of IVF and its meanings. Instead, the critical argument here is that for all its "newness," IVF is both produced by, and productive of, perniciously familiar discourses about the female body as "naturally" reproductive, and unpredictable and liable to failure. This construction results not only in the female body being rendered as an object of medical surveillance and intervention in ways that are easily made invisible through the naturalization of those interventions, but it also means that the female body can be held responsible for the failure of those interventions. This burden of responsibility becomes lost in the construction of "the couple" as the IVF patient—a construction that is sustained by assumptions of reproductive labor as a "natural" part of femininity. This, argues Irma van der Ploeg (2004), is a necessary site of ongoing resistance:

In the face of technology's new body ontologies and redefinition of biological processes, we can insist on invoking justice and fairness in their construction. In a context where there is not much that is natural about the nature of reproduction anyhow, we can try for a more socially just definition of "nature." There, we certainly can contest technologies, knowledges and ontologies that structurally presuppose and biologize female embodiment as angelic selflessness. (p. 178).

One of the unifying features of feminist writing on the new reproductive and genetic technologies, in all its diversity, is the placing of women at its centre (see Throsby, 2004, chap. 2). Importantly, however, this feminist work does not simply restore women to the list of actors, but rather, it has the potential to disrupt the naturalization of women's reproductive labor on which IVF is predicated. By rendering visible the construction of "natural" embodied femininity, and particularly from the liminal location of IVF failure,[10] new spaces (potentially) can be opened up from which to contest, and reconfigure, the normative reproductive categories on which IVF, and the new forms of bodily governance that it produces, are reliant.

Notes

I am very grateful to Celia Roberts, who provided key readings, interesting insights, and encouragement. Paula Saukko was also very supportive (and patient), and her insightful comments on earlier drafts were extremely helpful. This chapter draws on work from my doctoral research on IVF failure, which has recently been published by Palgrave (2004), titled *When IVF Fails: Feminism, Infertility and the Negotiation of Normality*. The chapter also draws on an article written with Ros Gill (Throsby & Gill, 2004), titled, "'It's Different for Men': Masculinity and IVF," and a paper published in *Narrative Inquiry* (Throsby, 2002), titled "Negotiating 'Normality' When IVF Fails.".

1. See www.hfea.gov.uk, retrieved February 7, 2001.
2. Sixth International Symposium on Pre-implantation Genetics (May 19–21, 2005), Queen Elizabeth II Conference Centre, London (www.pgdlondon. org). The organizers also celebrated the birth of "thousands" of PGD babies and released a CD of "International Lullabies.".
3. See www.guardian.co.uk, retrieved February 7, 2001.
4. NICE provides recommendations to the NHS on treatment and care (www. nice.org.uk).
5. See www.guardian.co.uk, retrieved February 25, 2004.
6. For a more detailed discussion of the experience of voluntary childlessness, see Campbell, 1999; Lisle, 1999; 2000; May, 1995; Morell, 1994.
7. Other sites that were identified as potentially indicative of desperation, and through which "normality" could therefore be expressed, included the use

of alternative therapies, the amount of money spent on treatment, the use of counseling services (see Throsby, 2004), and adoption.

8. While male infertility has received some attention (e.g., Imeson & McMurray, 1996; Lee, 1996; Mason, 1993; Webb & Daniluk, 1999), the male experience of fertility treatment, particularly where male factor infertility is *not* implicated, has received very little research attention (although, see Meerabeau, 1991; Throsby & Gill, 2004).

9. For example, intra-cytoplasmic sperm injection (ICSI), where a single sperm is injected into an egg.

10. The edited collection by Layne (1999) argues that this kind of reconfiguration becomes possible precisely from the "fringes" of motherhood.

References

Ableson, E. S. (2000). Shoplifting ladies. In J. Scanlon (Ed.), *The gender and consumer culture reader* (pp. 309–329). New York: New York University Press.

Bowlby, R. (2000). *Carried away: The invention of modern shopping.* London: Faber and Faber.

Braidotti, R. (1994). *Nomadic subjects: Embodiment and sexual difference in contemporary feminist theory.* New York: Columbia University Press.

Braidotti, R. (1996). Signs of wonder and traces of doubt: On teratology and embodied differences. In N. Lykke & R. Braidotti (Eds.), *Between monsters, goddesses and cyborgs: Feminist confrontations with science, medicine and cyberspace* (pp. 135–152). London: Zed.

Braude, P., Pickering, S., Flinter, F., & Ogilvie, C. M. (2002) Preimplantation genetic diagnosis. *Nature Review Genetics, 3*(12), 914–953.

Campbell, A. (1999). *Childfree and sterilized: Women's decisions and medical responses.* London: Cassell.

Daniluk, J. C. (1996). When treatment fails: The transition to biological childlessness for infertile women. *Women in Therapy, 19*(2), 81–98.

Davis, K. (1995). *Reshaping the female body: The dilemma of cosmetic surgery.* London: Routledge.

Foucault, M. (1981). *The history of sexuality. Vol. 1: An introduction.* Trans. M. Hurley. Harmondsworth, England: Penguin. (Original work published 1978).

Frank, A. W. (1995). *The wounded storyteller: Body, illness and ethics.* Chicago: University of Chicago Press.

Franklin, S. (1997). *Embodied progress. A cultural account of assisted conception.* London, Routledge.

Fukuyama, F. (2003). *Our posthuman future: Consequences of the biotechnology revolution.* London: Profile.

Gill, R. (1996). Discourse analysis: Practical implementation. In J. T. E. Richardson (Ed.), *Handbook of qualitative research methods for psychology and the social sciences* (pp. 172–190). Leicester, England: BPS Books.

Gimlin, D. L. (2002). *Body work: Beauty and self-image in American culture.* Berkeley: University of California Press.

Gosden, R. (1999). *Designer babies: The brave new world of reproductive technology* London: Phoenix.

Imeson, M., & McMurray, A. (1996). Couples' experiences of infertility: A phenomenological study. *Journal of Advanced Nursing, 24,* 1014–1022.

Layne, L. L. (Ed.). (1999). *Transformative motherhood: On giving and getting in consumer culture.* New York: New York University Press.

Lee, S. (1996). *Counselling in male infertility*. Oxford, England: Blackwell Science.

Leiblum, S. R., & Greenfield, D. A. (1997). The course of infertility: Immediate and long-term reactions. In S. R. Leiblum (Ed.), *Infertility: Psychological issues and counseling strategies* (pp. 83–100). New York: Wiley.

Lisle, L. (1999). *Without child: Challenging the stigma of childlessness*. London: Routledge.

Martin, E. (1989). *The woman in the body: A cultural analysis of reproduction*. Milton Keynes, England: Open University Press.

Martin, E. (1990). Science and women's bodies: Forms of anthropological knowledge. In M. Jacobus, E. F. Keller, & S. Shuttleworth (Eds.), *Body/politics: Women and the discourses of science*. London: Routledge.

Mason, M. (1993). *Male infertility—Men talking*. London: Routledge.

May, E. T. (1995). *Barren in the promised land: Childless Americans and the pursuit of happiness*. Cambridge, MA: Harvard University Press.

May, E. T. (1998). Nonmothers as bad mothers: Infertility and the "maternal instinct." In M. Ladd-Taylor & L. Umansky (Eds.), *"Bad" mothers: The politics of blame in twentieth-century America* (pp. 198–219). New York: New York University Press.

McCreight, B. S. (2004). A grief ignored: Narratives of pregnancy loss from a male perspective. *Sociology of Health and Illness, 26*(3), 326–350.

Meerabeau, L. (1991). Husbands' participation in fertility treatment: They also serve who only stand and wait. *Sociology of Health and Illness, 13*(3), 396–410.

Morell, C. (1994). *Unwomanly conduct: The challenges of intentional childlessness*. London: Routledge.

Morell, C. (2000). Saying no: Women's experiences with reproductive refusal. *Feminism and Psychology, 10*(3), 313–322.

Novas, C., & Rose, N. (2000). Genetic risk and the birth of the somatic individual. *Economy and Society, 29*(4), 484–513.

Oudshoorn, N. (1994). *Beyond the natural body: An archaeology of sex hormones*. London: Routledge.

Potter, J., & Wetherell, M. (1987). *Discourse and social psychology: Beyond attitudes and behaviour*. London: Sage.

Probyn, E. (1996). *Outside Belongings*. London, Routledge.

Rabinow, P. (1996). Artificiality and enlightenment: From socio-biology to biosociality. In P. Rabinow (Ed.), *Essays on the anthropology of reason* (pp. 91–111). Princeton, NJ: Princeton University Press.

Rapp, R., Heath, D., & Taussig, K. (2001). Genealogical dis-ease: Where hereditary abnormality, biomedical explanation, and family responsibility meet. In S. Franklin & S. McKinnon (Eds.), *Relative values: Reconfiguring kinship studies* (pp. 384–412). Durham, NC: Duke University Press.

Saetnan, A. R., Oudshoorn, N., & Kirejczyk, M. (Eds.). (2000). *Bodies of technology: Women's involvement with reproductive medicine*. Columbus: Ohio State University Press.

Sandelowski, M. (1993). *With child in mind. Studies of the personal encounter with infertility*. Philadelphia: University of Pennsylvania Press.

Sawicki, J. (1991). *Disciplining Foucault: Feminism, power and the body*. London: Routledge.

Silver, L. (1999). *Remaking Eden: Cloning, genetic engineering and the future of humankind*. London: Phoenix.

Stonehouse, J. (1994). *Idols to incubators: Reproduction theory through the ages*. London: Scarlet.

Throsby, K. (2002). Negotiating "normality": When IVF fails. *Narrative Inquiry*, *12*(1), 43–65.

Throsby, K. (2004). *When IVF fails: Feminism, infertility and the negotiation of normality*. London: Palgrave.

Throsby, K., & Gill, R. (2004). "It's different for men": Masculinity and IVF. *Men and Masculinities*, *6*(4), 330–348.

van der Ploeg (2004) "Only angels can do without skin": On reproductive technology's hybrids and the politics of body boundaries. *Body & Society*, *24*(2–3), 153–181.

Webb, R., & Daniluk, J. C. (1999). The end of the line: Infertile men's experiences of being unable to produce a child. *Men and Masculinities*, *2*(1), 6–25.

Wood, L. A., & Kroger, R. O. (2000). *Doing discourse analysis: Methods for studying action in talk and texts*. London: Sage.

Woollett, A. (1992). Psychological aspects of infertility and infertility investigations. In P. Nicolson & J. Ussher (Eds.), *The psychology of women's health and health care* (pp. 152–174). London, Macmillan.

11

Feminism's Sex Wars
and the Limits of Governmentality

BARBARA MENNEL
University of Florida

GOVERNMENTALITY, MICHEL FOUCAULT'S (1978/2000) concept that enables us to theorize the linkage between governing and power, on the one hand, and power and subjectivity, on the other, has received limited reception by feminists, even though particularly the latter concern, the relation between gendered (state) power and gendered subjectivity, centrally shapes feminist projects. In general, the productivity of Foucault's work for feminists remains controversial. Feminist responses to his work include a wholesale import of his theoretical and methodological framework, concessions of partial productivity, accusations of blind spots, and outright rejection.[1] Feminist engagements with Foucault tend to focus on disciplinary technologies, biopower, resistance, and the techniques of the self, while "theoretical debates on the usefulness of governmentality for feminism are in relatively short supply" as Catriona Macleod and Kevin Durrheim (2002) rightly point out. Pragmatically, Macleod and Durrheim suggest that "this ellipsis is possibly due to the fact that his lectures on governmentality were unpublished until the 1990s, and are available largely from secondary sources" (p. 42).

Yet, I suggest that Foucault's intellectual interests and the political and theoretical trajectory of the feminism moved into opposite directions during the late 1970s and early 1980s: Foucault moved outward from his interest in micropower to theorizing governmentality, including the state, whereas feminism shifted its attention from the power of the state and institutions to female sexuality, desire, and subsequently subjectivity. Ulrich Bröckling, Susanne Krasmann, and Thomas Lemke (2000) add a regional and disciplinary dimension to the account of the reception of Foucault's work in general, and governmentality studies in particular, by claiming that primarily social and political sciences engage in a broad reception of Foucault. They claim that especially in Anglophone academia Foucauldian concepts, such as biopower, discourse, and techniques of the self shape cultural, anthropological, feminist, and minority studies, all of which the authors separate from governmentality studies.[2]

Governmentality, according to Foucault's (1978/2000) lecture of the same title, emerges with the development of the state. Foucault locates a specific interest in "the government of oneself, that ritualization of the problem of personal conduct" at the end of the eighteenth century (p. 201). The discourse on governmentality resulted from a cross-over of "the establishment of the great territorial, administrative, and colonial states" and the Reformation and Counter-Reformation, which "raises the issue of how one must be spiritually ruled" (p. 202). Foucault locates the origin of the question "how to be ruled, how strictly, by whom, to what end, by what methods" in the historical shift from the singularity of the prince to a dispersion of power in the form of the state (p. 202). In the model of governmentality, the family occupies a privileged site; thus "three fundamental types of government [exist]: the art of self-government, connected with morality; the art of properly governing a family, which belongs to economy; and, finally, the science of ruling the state, which concerns politics" (p. 206). Governmentality ensures continuity between self, the family, and the state.

Mitchell Dean (1999) defines Foucault's term *governmentality* as "conduct of conduct," which refers to "our behaviors, our actions and even our comportment" (p. 10). Discussions about conduct, therefore, according to Dean, "are almost invariably evaluative and normative," assuming that it is "possible to regulate and control that behavior rationally, or at least deliberately, and that there are agents whose responsibility it is here to ensure that regulation occurs" (p. 10). Different forms of knowledge and expertise, such as medicine, criminology, social work, therapy, and pedagogy produce "truth," define their objects of study, and codify appropriate ways of dealing with them. According to Foucault one cannot be free from governmentality even if one uses a discourse of emancipation because it often implies "a normative framework, largely inherited from certain forms of critical theory" (p. 35).

The prevalence of essays on nursing, female adolescent sex education, genetics, and the legal discourse within the limited feminist reception of governmentality bespeaks the applicability of governmentality to precisely those constellations in which interests of the state are waged in seemingly invisible ways on women and girls' bodies and subjectivities (see, e.g., Macleod & Durrheim, 2002; but also Fullagar, 2003; Ruhl, 1999; Weir & Habib, 1997). In these cases, the concept and approach of governmentality enables authors to uncover the connection between micro- and macrolevels of power that transform individuals into docile bodies. For example, Macleod and Durrheim's (2002) convincing study of sex education of adolescent girls exemplifies the "intimate knowledge of the individual" (p. 47), the "disciplinary technology," "hierarchical observation," and "normalizing judgment" (p. 48) of those involved in educating young women about sex and the "internalized surveillance" (p. 49) of the young women, which are all part of biopower.

A more complex relation between feminism and governmentality needs to be mapped out for feminist projects emerging in the 1980s and 1990s and that exist in an antagonistic relation to the patriarchal state and its institutions but that ground themselves in feminist discourses around desire and the female body. The topic of this chapter—feminism's so-called sex wars—not only opens up the internal conflicts and contradictions in feminism, but also points to the limits of Foucault's model of governmentality. What has since been labeled the sex wars began in April 1982 when the Scholar and Feminist IX Conference "Towards a Politics of Sexuality" at Barnard College in New York became the stage for opposing feminist groups (see Duggan & Hunter, 1995). New York's Women Against Pornography (WAP) wore T-shirts exclaiming "For Feminist Sexuality" and "Against S/M," whereas the Lesbian Sex Mafia, a support group of "politically incorrect sex," held a speak-out. The polarized debate about sexuality, which seemed to tear feminism apart for years to come, focused on the two related topics of pornography and lesbian s/m; the latter became a focal point for feminism's internal controversy. The conflicts about lesbian s/m and pornography were symptomatic for disagreements over political and theoretical positions regarding notions of sexuality and power. Far from having been resolved, the conflict has dissipated with a new generation of women shaped by and shaping popular culture that has long since appropriated the style of s/m in fashion, cinema, and music (see, e.g., Rosenfeld, 2000–2001).

This discursive explosion was not the first time that sexuality and power was prominently featured in the second women's movement. On the contrary, the pairing of sexuality and power is constitutive of the feminist movement, which established itself with a claim of discrimination that found its most extreme expression in violence against women through sexual abuse, domestic violence, and rape. Yet, the forceful articulation of the pro-s/m lesbians and pro-pornography activists created a caesura in feminist discourse, a caesura that recast the discourse on sexuality and power in relation to pleasure in ways that cannot be undone. The conflict over lesbian s/m in the early 1980s, while circling precisely around the issues of power and (feminist) subjectivity, is marked by conflict between two positions that equally claim to represent a feminist stance but are utterly—and presumably for the women at the time painfully—at odds with each other. Applying Foucauldian concepts, including governmentality, to the divergent arguments of pro-s/m lesbians and anti-s/m feminists allows me not only to unlock theoretical and political impasses between these two positions but also to take Foucault's model of governmentality to task.

Presupposing a clearly demarcated feminist movement, Macleod and Durrheim (2002) list as the "points of convergence" between Foucault and feminism the focus on sexuality, social domination as an aspect of the political, a critique of humanist and scientific "truth," and a concern for personal relationships and everyday life (p. 42–43). But how can those "points of convergences" be mapped onto a feminist project when feminists disagree with each other precisely over the nature of sexuality in personal relationships and everyday life in a framework of patriarchal domination? The lesbian s/m debate is of interest for a discussion of Foucault precisely because the issues negotiated are central to Foucault's own theoretical thinking: power, sexuality, and (self) knowledge. The sex wars' two opposing positions seem to be easily summarized: s/m lesbians argued that employing the signifiers of power to create pleasure among women represents subversive and liberating appropriation of regimes of dominance. Anti-s/m feminists argued that the signifiers of s/m reference violent oppression and their erotic investment is thus juxtaposed to the feminist project of a utopian vision of nonhierarchical sexuality. Foucault (1978/2000) understands power as neither held by one person or group, nor operating from a center: "power relations are rooted deep in the social nexus, not a supplementary structure over and above 'society' whose radical effacement one could perhaps dream of" (p. 222). However, anti-s/m feminists conceptualize power as something that one can resist by opposing it and positioning oneself outside of it. To put it in simple terms: while s/m lesbians claim to transform power, anti-s/m feminists claim to reject it. Even though both positions rely on the centrality of the absolute significance of gender, community, and a political vision of resistance and change, notions that are either absent in Foucault's theoretical model (gender and community) or questioned (resistance and change), both positions offer conflicting interpretations of these notions.

Thus, the positions of anti-s/m feminists and s/m lesbians pose a conceptual problem in relation to Foucault's model of power, generally, and governmentality, specifically. Can one accuse anti-s/m feminist of misreading power or does their absolute rejection of signifiers of patriarchal power model a form of agency based on an ethics of resistance? But what if the individuals to be governed create their own regime of practices and what if those practices solely function to produce pleasure? Does the insistence on s/m during the early 1980s foreground and simultaneously deconstruct the process of governmentality by investing the governing of bodies with unproductive pleasure or does the governing of the body in s/m solely recreate the pleasures of governmentality otherwise associated with normative heterosexual patriarchy? How does the debate relate to older discourses on masochism and sadism put in place by nineteenth-century sexology, such as by Richard von Krafft-Ebing (1946)? What narratives emerge from the contemporary discourse of sadomasochism and feminism?

Two collections from the early 1980s exemplify the two positions. *Coming to Power: Writings and Graphics on Lesbian S/M*, edited by members of SAMOIS (1981/1987), a lesbian/feminist S/M organization, takes an explicit pro-lesbian s/m stance, and *Against Sadomasochism: A Radical Feminist Analysis*, edited by Robin Ruth Linden, Darlene R. Pagano, Diana E. H. Russell, and Susan Leigh Star (1982),takes an explicit position against s/m. The two collections *Coming to Power* and *Against Sadomasochism* articulate the positions at the most polarized point of the controversy. *Coming to Power* was the second publication by SAMOIS, and includes fantasies, interviews, confessionals, and political essays. *Against Sadomasochism* is a collection of theoretical and political essays that articulate positions explicitly against s/m. Thus, both collections intend to persuade and convince feminists in general but are also aimed at each other.

A cursory reading of the juxtaposition of Foucauldian thinking and the feminist position against s/m could lead us to suggest that those feminists were simply wrong in their understanding of power. In contrast, however, Monique Deveaux (1994) points to "the tendency of a Foucauldian conceptualization of the subject to erase women's specific experiences with power; and the inability of the agonistic model of power to account for, much less articulate, processes of empowerment" (p. 224). Deveaux traces the feminist reception of Foucault through three waves to recent feminist theorists who have taken up his emphasis on discourses of sexuality in a process of subjectifying (p. 223). Deveaux concludes:

> If we agree with Hartsock's suggestion that feminists need to envisage a nondominated world, we should not slip into fatalistic views about the omnipresence of power. This means rejecting Foucault's assertion that absolutely no social or personal relations escape permeation by power. (p. 233)

Like the anti-s/m feminists, contemporary discourse on lesbian s/m also poses a problem for a concept of governmentality because lesbian s/m offers an exaggerated performance of negotiations of micropower on the body in antagonistic relation to the state. Lynda Hart (1998), in her book *Between the Body and the Flesh: Performing Sadomasochism,* poses the question "*why* lesbian s/m has become the marginal center, the paradoxical *place* around which much of this controversy has circled" (p. 4; emphasis in original). Her own answer suggests that this is the case "because it is the masochistic sexual desire that most profoundly signifies a destabilization of 'self' that feminism so jealously guards" (p. 60). Judith Butler's (1990) influential emphasis on the performative in gender formations seems to echo the significance that lesbian s/m achieved both in the feminist movement, as well as in feminist and queer theory in the early 1990s.[3] Lisa King's (2003) essay, "Subjectivity as Identity: Gender Through the Lens of Foucault," outlines Judith Butler's reliance on Foucault's understanding of "power as productive" to "reveal the contingency of what she terms the 'heterosexual matrix,' the confluence of gender and sexuality in a way that excludes and thereby oppression women and sexual minorities" (p. 337).

The emphasis on performativity in s/m exaggerates iconic acts that function in the production of power. Foucault (1980) explains his project as:

> . . . a study of power in its external visage, at the point where it is in direct and immediate relationship with that which we can provisionally call its object, its target, its field of application, there—that is to say—where it installs itself and produces its real effects. (p. 97)

However, lesbian s/m does not produce "real effects," but pleasure. Like Foucault's (1982) claims about power, that it "incites, it induces, it seduces," s/m lesbians recirculate the signifiers of power and thereby foreground the ways that power becomes (re)articulated in its physical, bodily, psychological, and libidinal dimensions (p. 341). According to Suzanne Gearhart (1995) in "Foucault's Response to Freud: Sadomasochism and the Aestheticization of Power," Foucault considers power to be "productive of *pleasure,*" meaning that inequality, subordination, humiliation, or pain inherent in power can be converted from displeasure into pleasure (p. 391; emphasis in original).

Since s/m, however, borrows the signifiers of power for its performance, it produces a paradox, which Anne McClintock (1993) described in "Maid to Order: Commercial S/M and Gender Power":

At first glance, then, S/M seems a servant to orthodox power. Yet, on the contrary, with its exaggerated emphasis on costume and scene S/M performs social power as scripted, and hence as permanently subject to change. As a theater of conversion, S/M reverses and transmutes the social meanings it borrows, yet also without finally stepping outside the enchantment of its magic circle. In S/M, paradox is paraded, not resolved. (p. 208)

"Girl Gang" (Bailey, 1981), a short story in *Coming to Power*, for example, restages a paradigmatic heterosexist pornographic scene, in which several men sexually and violently circulate a woman in gang rape, as an s/m fantasy among women. "Girl Gang" borrows from traditional heterosexual pornography a structure steeped in the power relations of heterosexism and sexism and rewrites it for lesbian pleasure.

According to Julia Creet (1991), feminism is accorded a central role in lesbian s/m fantasies. Creet offers a psychoanalytic reading of the casting of feminism in lesbian s/m scenarios in her essay "Daughter of the Movement: The Psychodynamics of Lesbian S/M Fantasy." Creet suggests that s/m lesbians staged themselves in an antagonistic relationship to feminism casting feminism as dominant mother "within the economy of a lesbian s/m fantasy" (p. 136). She suggests:

Charges on both sides of the "sex wars" are strikingly similar: both the charge of repression (by the "pro-sex" side) and the charge of replicating masculine desire (by the "anti-sex" side) carry with them the symbolic weight of the father.... We are afraid of collapsing into the very system from which we struggle to liberate ourselves.... Although Lacan could only imagine an order created by a symbolic father, what I propose in this paper is that, within the economy of the contemporary lesbian s/m fantasy, feminism acts as a kind of symbolic mother. (p. 138)

Her suggestion allows us to read another short story in *Coming to Power*, "Passion Play" (Alexander, 1981), in which the dominant partner Carole humiliates her friend Meg after she has attended a National Women's Studies Association (NWSA) Conference where she delivered a paper entitled "The Redefinition of Community as a Trend Toward Exclusion" (p. 230). Meg's sexual humiliation consists of Carole turning her into a "girl" when Carole commands her to put on pink lace, ribbons, silk, and frilly garters. In Foucauldian terms, the narrative is motivated by converting the governing of the feminine body into pleasure. "Passion Play" thus subverts processes of governmentality.

On an extratextual level, the story also humiliates feminism by parading the perverse pleasure found in the construction and performance of femininity. The story confronts feminism with its inability to circumscribe the boundaries of its ideology by controlling its membership. Meg's NWSA presentation positions Meg as part of feminism by relying on a feminist vocabulary to address a feminist topic to be presented at the NWSA Conference, a vortex of institutional feminism in the United States. What could be imagined as self-critical feminist analysis from within the feminist community functions as an unacknowledged justification for the action that is to follow in the narrative. The narrative development positions Meg and Carole outside of standard feminist paradigms, but Meg's prior lecture title functions retroactively to blame feminism for that exclusion. Thus, the story relies on yet another paradox: the lesbians engaged in s/m in that story claim agency for rewriting the script of feminization. At the same time, however, they disavow their agency by invoking feminists as disciplinarians who control the boundaries of feminist identity via an implied injunction against perverse pleasure. In Creet's (1991) Lacanian terms, feminism appears as symbolic mother who thus has to be humiliated.

The staging of an alternative familial constellations solely among women contrasts with the normative family scenario that underwrites Foucault's concept of governmentality, in which state, family, and self are linked coherently via the pater familias. Even though Foucault's definition of *governmentality* presupposes a continuity of patriarchal institutions, Gearhart suggests that Foucault's view of Sigmund Freud's (1961) account of masochism implies "a clear and powerful challenge to Freud's patrocentrism," precisely because Foucault does not take gender into account in his model of sadomasochism (p. 394). Gearhart (1995) explains Foucault's gender neutral account of sadomasochism:

Foucault makes no attempt here to distinguish a masochistic from a sadistic manner of mixing pleasure and power. On the contrary, he stresses the interchangeability of the dominant and subordinate positions in the *"spirals of power and pleasure,"* with the result that both pleasure and power are exchanged freely between them. It is not just that these spirals place the subject in differing positions, some of which are sadistic and others masochistic. Instead, each position in the spiral is indeterminately sadistic and masochistic, both sadistic and masochistic at the same time, because attached to each position is a certain pleasure and a certain power. (pp. 391–392; emphasis in original)

Freud defines *masochism* as "feminine," even though he finds it primarily in men, which Gearhart correctly interprets as Freud's understanding of masochism as "essentially feminine" (p. 394). At the same time she points out that Freud sees the real problem of a masochistic relationship taking place between son and father. Freud (1961) reads the desire to be beaten by the father as a desire "to have a passive (feminine) sexual relation to him," which, in turn, sexualizes the father (p. 169). Gearhart argues that sadomasochism undermines patriarchal authority "because it undercuts the desexualization at the basis of that authority" but because Foucault does not take up the gendered model of masochism, he, in turn, questions the Freudian assumption of patrocentrism (p. 393).

Since in the s/m fantasy of "Passion Play" (Alexander, 1981) the father is absent, neither the Freudian nor the Foucauldian model of sadism and masochism can account for the conversion of power between women that structures the s/m scenario. The Freudian gendered structure of sadism and masochism relies on the specificity of gender that ascribes essential qualities onto femininity and masculinity, whereas Foucault's understanding of masochism does not capture the specific transgressive nature of s/m lesbianism and the implications for a relationship between women (and ultimately the community of feminists) because Foucault does not take gender into account. Even though governmentality, when applied to gender, enables us to carve out normalizing forces, the term itself, as Foucault's reception of sadomasochism, does not take into account the specific ways in which normalcy is produced as gender.

Foucault, however, despite his distrust for libratory movements to escape governmentality, gave (lesbian) s/m practices a singular status in an interview with *The Advocate* in 1984, the year of his death:

Well, I think what we want to speak about is precisely the *innovations* that those practices imply. For instance, look at the S/M subculture, as our good friend Gayle Rubin would insist. I don't think that this movement of sexual practices has anything to do with the disclosure or the uncovering of S/M tendencies deep within our unconscious, and so on I think that S/M is much more than that; it's the real creation of new possibilities of pleasure, which people had no idea about previously. The idea that S/M is related to a deep violence, that S/M practice is a way of liberating this violence, this aggression, is stupid. We know very well what all those people are doing is not aggressive; they are inventing new possibilities of pleasure with strange parts of their body—through the eroticization of the body. I think it's a kind of creation, a creative enterprise, which has as one of its main features what I call the desexualization of pleasure. (pp. 27–28)

Foucault idealizes s/m as a new invention of the late twentieth century. Yet, the practices of s/m, and hence of masochism and sadism are not inventions by subcultures in the late twentieth century. Instead, Richard von Krafft-Ebing (1946) defined *masochism* and *sadism* as nongenital and nonprocreative bodily pleasures in his *Psychopathia Sexualis* in 1890, and thus imbricated in the definitions of normal and perverse sexuality in governmentality.[4]

The psychoanalytic discourse, beginning with the turn-of-the-century sexologist Krafft-Ebing (1946) and later Freud (1961) defined *masochism* as essentially female but only of interest to psychoanalytic discourse when it afflicts men. Krafft-Ebing focused on the male masochist, casting him as pathological. Normalcy exists for Krafft-Ebing when femininity is aligned with masochism and masculinity with sadism. Perversion, which is the condition for psychoanalytic discourse, occurs only when the roles are reversed in the male masochist. The male masochist does not necessitate a female sadist, but instead a woman who performs dominance. Krafft-Ebing's case studies, except three, are about men who visit dominant women. Krafft-Ebing addresses "Masochism in Woman" only in a later section, the fourth section in his chapter on masochism (pp. 195–200). That section's opening paragraph spells out the essentialist nature of women's masochism, based on the biological role of women:

> In women voluntary subjection to the opposite sex is a physiological phenomenon. Owing to her passive role in procreation and long-existent social conditions, ideas of subjection are, in women, normally connected with the idea of sexual relations. They form, so to speak, the harmonics which determine the tone-quality of feminine feeling. (p. 195)

Thus, while Krafft-Ebing (1946) privileges the discussion of male masochism, female masochism is integral to his explanation of the nature of masochism because he sees female masochism as an extension of specific female traits:

> Thus it is easy to regard masochism in general as a pathological growth of specific feminine mental elements—as an abnormal intensification of certain features of the psycho-sexual character of women—and to seek its primary origin in that sex. It may, however, be held to be established that, in woman, an inclination to subordination to man (which may be regarded as an acquired, purposeful arrangement, a phenomenon of adaptation to social requirements) is to a certain extent a normal manifestation. (p. 196)

Masochism in women is pathological only to the extent that it exaggerates their natural qualities, which, in turn, result from adaptation to social conditions of patriarchy. Krafft-Ebing's discussion of female masochism is, however, caught in a contradiction. He claims that cases of female masochism should occur frequently, yet they are difficult to document because women suppress the articulation of perversion (p. 197). While masochism is an extension of feminine characteristics, it is, in turn, female "modesty" and "custom" that hinder women's expression of perversion. Therefore Krafft-Ebing claims that only three cases of female masochism are known.[5]

The discourse by Krafft-Ebing (1946) in which he defines masochism and sadism as pathology exemplifies the workings of governmentality through the institution of sexology. The underlying principle of normativity privileges genital sexuality and hence reproduces gender norms and the patriarchal family. Krafft-Ebing's liberal discourse defines the normative vis-à-vis pathological behavior while articulating the liberal tolerance for such pathological behavior. Pro-s/m lesbians deconstruct and question those gender prescriptions that fossilize women as masochistic for biological reasons and men as potential sadists without an explanation. Sadomasochistic lesbians claim that women can take on flexible gender roles. Thus, it would seem as a albeit politically questionable—transgression of psychoanalysis's gender configuration to imagine women as possible sadists. Yet, while women take on the dominant role in s/m among lesbians, their accompanying discourse takes pain to clarify that those lesbians are not sadists. Performing as the dominant woman when the woman is not a sadist has been inscribed into the definition of masochism from the beginning of the sexologists' discourse on masochism.

The emphasis on the performativity inherent in the role play of s/m seems to lend itself to an argument against essentialism, yet the writers of *Coming to Power* articulate a decidedly essentialist argument in favor of lesbian s/m. According to them, the fact that s/m takes place among women situates it in an essentially different realm than heterosexual and gay male s/m. Despite the s/m lesbians' explicit critique of traditional concepts of femininity, several essays base the difference between lesbian and heterosexual s/m on the goodness and kindness of women: "They ask my permission first, and are loving and gentle in their manner," claims J. in "Proper Orgy Behavior" (Lucy, 1981, p. 42). Juicy Lucy's essay "If I Ask You to Tie Me Up, Will You Still Want to Love Me?" differentiates between lesbian s/m and "prick violence & pornography":

> The distinction here is that lesbian S/M is consensual, bringing
> pleasure & strength. Porn & violence bring pain mutilation fear &
> death. It's the difference between being powerful & loved & being a
> hated victim. (p. 39)

Thus, the violence in male pornography is accorded the status of the
real: men enact power to victimize women, whereas women reenact power
for the consensual and pleasurable play with each other embedded in
a discourse of care.

The paradoxical status accorded to "care" in lesbian s/m discourse
warrants revisiting the theorization of "care" in Foucault's model of
governmentality. Macleod and Durrheim (2002) contextualize "care"
in Foucault's model of governmentality in a system of regulation, which
"becomes self-regulation as the person subjects him/herself to an internalized surveillance" (p. 48). The authors rely on Nikolas Rose (1996)
who outlines "three forms of self-technologies—relating to the self
epistemologically (know yourself), despotically (master yourself) and
attentively (care for yourself)" (pp. 48–49).[6] The emphasis on lesbian
s/m writing on care in a lesbian s/m relationship reproduces discursively
constructed femininity, even though the setting for care differs from the
examples provided by Macleod and Durrheim (2002), who investigate a
setting of what Foucault termed "pastoral techniques," which "are linked
to the macro-strategies of government through guidance and care,
rather than surveillance and normalizing judgment as in disciplinary
technology" (Macleod & Durrheim, 2002, p. 51).

Because the s/m lesbians claim that masochism and sadism among
women are essentially different than their counterparts, they negate
any significance of Sacher-Masoch's or Sade's work because they were
men. Kitt (1981), in her essay "Taking the Sting out of S/M" argues:

> The strong, negative reaction to S/M is due in part to the fact hat we
> have hand-me-down words, still clothed in many layers of patriarchal
> connotations. (Both the words sadist and masochist are derivatives
> of the male authors' names who wrote about these sexual practices:
> Count Donatien de Sade, 1740–1814, and Leopold von Sacher-Masoch,
> 1835–1895). Many members of the women's community, as outsiders,
> see only the hurting in the S/M experience, never the touching of
> the fine line between pleasure and pain to heighten pleasure. They
> see the acting out of power, never the demonstration of consensuality.
> They see the pain or humiliation, never the sharing, concern, and
> love. (p. 61)

The essentialism in this passage, representative of the volume, ties the gender of the writers to the respective qualities of masochism and sadism. Patriarchy and heterosexual life are defined as emotional sadism and masochism and thus real violence. The pragmatically and theoretically troubling essentialism of the division between heterosexual s/m and lesbian s/m takes sexual orientation and gender of those engaging in s/m as its only point of reference, which allows s/m lesbians to discard an ethical or political imperative for an engagement with the signifiers of their actual s/m scenarios. It freezes a discussion of the s/m act in relation to the identity of the actors, also freezing the actors' identities as lesbian or straight. While identity is performative in relation to the roles enacted in s/m to be the dominant or the submissive—it is fixed in relation to the identity of those who perform the game lesbian or straight, woman or man.

The reliance on a rhetoric of feminine identity goes hand in hand with rhetoric of victimization that connects both positions and that warrants a closer reading on the introduction to *Coming to Power* and *Against Sadomasochism*. Even though the two collections are ideologically juxtaposed to each other, they share an unacknowledged rhetoric of victimization expressed in each their "Introduction." Since the "Introduction" frames the collected essays, it functions to align victimization with a moral entitlement to speak. In each introduction the narrator herself embodies victimization through a personal narrative to portray the victimization of the position expressed in the book. The s/m lesbians accord the public sphere of feminism an oppressive quality and the anti-s/m feminists project an oppressive function onto the gay male public sphere. Both authors construct a position of victimization by claiming that their desire to participate in that public sphere was rejected and oppressed. In the "Introduction" to the pro-s/m collection *Coming to Power* Katherine (SAMOIS, 1981/1987) argues:

> Few of us have been able to admit to anyone our interest in S/M or have been able to talk about the content of our fantasies. Some of us could not even admit those fantasies to ourselves. Social and political costs run very high. In the public arena of the lesbian, feminist, and gay press, positive feelings about S/M experiences have been met for the most part with swift negative reaction and authoritative reprimands. In this context, trashing has been renamed "feminist criticism," honest dialogue has been submerged by wave after wave of ideological censure calling itself "debate," and those of us who continue to resist this treatment are accused of being contaminated by the patriarchy. (p. 7)

Davis claims internalized oppression as a result of the reprimand in the feminist public sphere. The victimization of the s/m lesbians is described through detailed accusations of the abuse committed by feminist "authoritative reprimands," "trashing," "censure," and "treatment." Thus, the paradigmatic tables of feminist analysis are turned and feminists are cast as perpetrators of discursive violence against women who practice s/m.

Robin Ruth Linden (Linden, Pagano, & Russell, 1982), the author of "Introduction: Against Sadomasochism" of the collection *Against Sadomasochism,* claims a victim position vis-à-vis the visible signs of s/m in the gay area of San Francisco, the Castro:

> I live in the Castro district of San Francisco, a gay quarter of the city. Almost every day I walk the short distance to the heart of Castro Street, down the foothills of Twin Peaks, to shop or do errands. . . . As a woman alone, I feel like a visitor to a foreign country. It's not that gay men necessarily are hostile to women; actually, they are more or less oblivious. This invisibility can be a blessing in disguise; it lends a sense of safety when I'm walking after dark, freedom from the fear of threat: nameless, amorphous. The passion is cold, at times almost macabre.
>
> It is commonplace to see men with black leather collars and leashes around their necks to indicate they are sexual "slaves"—masochists; men with padlocks clasped around their throats, another sign of sexual "enslavement"; men in military uniforms sometimes bearing swastikas; men with color-coded handkerchiefs neatly folded in their hip pockets, indicating their preferred sexual role and practices. After several years I have become accustomed to seeing men wearing the paraphernalia of sadomasochism: studded black leather belts, handcuffs dangling from pockets, black leather gloves, chains, devices I don't recognize flanking the hips of passersby. But recently, there is an occasional woman in similar dress. (pp. 1–2)

Linden sets the stage for her description of s/m by positioning herself in a state of vulnerable womanhood: a woman alone at night among men. Despite the qualifying reference to gay men's obliviousness toward women, the "nameless, amorphous" "threat" to femininity rhetorically foreshadows the threat of sadomasochism.

The rhetorical positioning vis-à-vis the otherwise marginal public sphere of feminism and male gay culture turns the position of the narrator into one of victimization, which, in turn, entitles the narrator to a moral position. In both cases, the rhetoric of victimhood relies on implicit understandings of femininity constructed as defenseless vis-à-vis public discourse and public space. While both volumes construct an unacknowledged victim position in the "Introduction," they explicitly articulate resistance to women's victimization and argue against masochism understood as women's desire to suffer. Both volumes rely on a structure of disavowal, denying the existence of their own psychic investment in victimhood that frames their argument, which, in turn, argues explicitly against women's victimization.

The claim to victimization and its accompanying gender essentialism goes hand in hand with the preferred genre of the volume, the coming-out narrative, traditionally based on a notion of a coherent self. When the pro-s/m lesbians create coming-out narratives around s/m identity, according to Foucault (1984), they only reinstate coherent notions of identity, falling behind their own practice of fluctuating gender and sexual power positions. Foucault explains:

> But if identity becomes *the* problem of sexual existence, and if people think that they have to "uncover" their "own identity," and that their own identity has to become the law, the principle, the code of their existence; if the perennial question they ask is "Does this thing conform to my identity?" then, I think, they will turn back to a kind of ethics very close to the old heterosexual virility. (p. 28)

According to Foucault, neither anti-s/m feminists nor pro-s/m lesbians can ultimately escape governmentality because their rhetorics rely on liberal discourse, which folds back into disavowed concepts of femininity.

We are still left with the fact that these individuals who constitute the subculture of pro-s/m lesbians, situate themselves as abject, outside the family, outside the economy, outside the proper state, outside heterosexual reproduction, and, at that historical juncture, outside of feminism. The fact that their discourse can be accounted for by governmentality that reproduces itself in biopower but that they are simultaneously radically juxtaposed to the interest of the state and the family points to the entrenchment of Foucault's concept of governmentality in a notion of normativity. It is thus productive to analyze counterinstitutional practices and sites of abjection where narratives of sexuality, power, and desire emerge, in addition to feminist projects that study women's and girls' bodies and subjectivities under the regime of governmentality. Even though the narratives of pro-s/m lesbians in many ways fall back onto notions of coherent identity, configurations of essentialist femininity, projections of domineering feminism, and sexologist definitions of masochism and sadism, their discourse nevertheless complicates our accounts of power and sexuality with perverse pleasure. And while anti-s/m feminists project a reductive vision of sexuality beyond patriarchal power, governmentality is unable to provide a framework to account for the utopian vision and agency that attacks institutions perpetuating the sexualization of gendered violence. Foucault aides us to see the production of power even in discourses outside traditional institutions of the state, such as the government and the family, yet those discourses also serve to highlight Foucault's own idealizations and historical blind spots.

Notes

1. Diamond and Quinby's (1988) work includes several important essays on the topic and a substantial selected bibliography. Deveaux (1994) offers an insightful historical account of the feminist reception of Foucault. I will engage with several feminist writers on Foucault in the course of this chapter.
2. The translation from the German is mine.
3. Despite the fact that a use of Butlerian (1990) argument seems to be applicable to a theory based on the performative aspects of lesbian s/m, she is included in the volume *Against Sadomasochism*.
4. Between 1886 and 1903, Krafft-Ebing edited fourteen editions of *Psychopathia sexualis*, two under the title *Neue Forschungen auf dem Gebiet der Psychopathia sexualis* (*New Research in the Field of the Psychopathia Sexualis*). He continuously added new case histories and sometimes new perversions. In 1890, Krafft-Ebing introduced masochism in conjunction with sadism in *Psychopathia sexualis*, which appeared under the title *Neue Forschungen auf dem Gebiet der Psychopathia sexualis*. My quotes and page numbers follow the English edition cited in the References.
5. The German edition states three and lists three cases. The English edition states that "two cases of masochism in woman have been scientifically established," (197) yet then goes on to list three cases (197-200).
6. They reference Rose (1996).

References

Alexander, M. (1987). Passion play. In SAMOIS (Ed.), *Coming to power: Writings and graphics on lesbian s/m* (pp. 230–244). Boston: Allyson. (Originally published in 1981)

Bailey, C. (1987). Girl gang. In SAMOIS (Ed.), *Coming to power: Writings and graphics on lesbian s/m* (pp. 141–147). Boston: Allyson. (Originally published in 1981)

Bröckling, U., Lemke, T., & Krasmann, S. (2000). Gouvernementalität, neoliberalism und selbsttechnologien. Eine einführung [Governmentality, neo-liberalism, and technologies of the self: An introduction.]. In U. Bröckling, S. Krasmann, & T. Lemke, *Gouvernementalität der gegenwart: Studien zur ökonomisierung des sozialen* [*Governmentality of the contemporary: Studies of the economization of the social*] (pp. 7–40). Frankfurt: Suhrkamp.

Butler, J. (1990). Gender trouble: Feminism and the subversion of identity. New York: Routledge.

Creet, J. (1991). Daughter of the movement: The psychodynamics of lesbian s/m fantasy. *Differences, 3*(2), 135–159.

Davis, K. (1987). Introduction. In SAMOIS (Ed.), *Coming to power: Writings and graphics on lesbian s/m* (pp. xx–xx). Boston: Allyson. (Originally published in 1981)

Dean, M. (1999). Governmentality: Power and rule in modern society. London: Sage.

Deveaux, M. (1994, Summer). Feminism and empowerment: A critical reading of Foucault. *Feminist Studies, 20*(2), 223–247.

Diamond, I., & Quinby, L. (Eds). (1988). *Feminism and Foucault: Reflections and resistance*. Boston: Northeastern University Press.

Duggan, L., & Hunter, N. D. (1995). *Sex wars: Sexual dissent and political culture*. New York: Routledge.

Foucault, M. (1978/2000). Governmentality. In J. D. Faubion (Ed.), *Michel Foucault: Power. Vol. 3. Essential Works of Foucault, 1954–1984* (pp. 201–222). New York: New Press.

Foucault, M. (1980). Two Lectures. In C. Gordon (Ed.), *Power/knowledge: Selected interviews & other writings, 1972–1977* (pp. 78–108). New York: Pantheon.

Foucault, M. (1982/2000). The subject and power. In J. D. Faubion (Ed.), *Michel Foucault: Power. Vol. 3: Essential Works of Foucault, 1954–1984* (pp. 326–348). New York: New Press.

Foucault, M. (1984, August 7). An interview: Sex, power, and the politics of identity. *Advocate*, pp. 26–30, 58.

Freud, S. (1961). The economic problem of masochism. In J. Strachey (Ed.), *The standard edition of the complete psychological works of Sigmund Freud* (pp. 159–170). London: Hogarth.

Fullagar, S. (2003, March). Governing women's active leisure: The gendered effects of calculative rationalities within Australian health policy. *Critical Public Health, 13*(1), 47–60.

Gearhart, S. (1995, Fall). Foucault's response to Freud: Sado-Masochism and the aestheticization of power. *Style, 29*(3), 389–403.

Hart, L. (1998). Between the body and the flesh: Performing sadomasochism. New York: Columbia University Press.

King, L. (2003). Subjectivity as identity: Gender through the lens of Foucault. In J. Z. Bratich, J. Packer, & C. McCarthy, *Foucault, cultural studies, and governmentality* (pp. 337–352). Albany: State University of New York Press.

Kitt. (1987). Taking the sting out of s/m. In SAMOIS (Ed.), *Coming to Power: Writings and graphics on lesbian s/m* (pp. 60–63). Boston: Allyson. (Originally published in 1981)

Krafft-Ebing, R. von. (1946). *Psychopathia sexualis*. New York: Pioneer.

Linden, R. R. (1982). Introduction. In R. R. Linden, D. R. Pagano, D. E. H. Russell, & S. L. Star (Eds.), *Against sadomasochism: A radical feminist analysis* (pp. 1–15). San Francisco: Frog in the Well.

Linden, R. R., Pagano, D. R., Russell, D. E. H., & Star, S. L. (Eds.). (1982). *Against sadomasochism: A radical feminist analysis*. San Francisco: Frog in the Well.

Lucy, J. (1987). If I ask you to tie me up, will you still want to love me? In SAMOIS (Ed.), *Coming to power: Writings and graphics on lesbian s/m* (pp. 29–40). Boston: Allyson. (Originally published in 1981)

Macleod, C., & Durrheim, K. (2002). Foucauldian feminism: The implications of governmentality. *Journal for the Theory of Social Behaviour, 32*(1), 41–60.

McClintock, A. (1993). Maid to order: Commercial s/m and gender power. In P. C. Gibson & R. Gibson, *Dirty looks: Women, pornography, power* (pp. 207–231). London: British Film Institute.

Rose, N. (1996). Identity, genealogy, history. In S. Hall & P. du Gray (Eds.), *Questions of cultural identity* (pp. 128–150). London: Sage.

Rosenfeld, K. (2000, December–2001, January). S/M chic and the new morality. *New Art Examiner,* pp. 27–31.

Ruhl, L. (1999, February). Liberal governance and prenatal care. *Economy and Society, 28*(1), 95–117.

SAMOIS (Ed.). (1987). *Coming to power: Writings and graphics on lesbian s/m.* Boston: Allyson. (Originally published in 1981)

Weir, L., & Habib, J. (1997, Spring). A critical feminist analysis of the final report of the Royal Commission on New Reproductive Technologies. *Studies in Political Economy, 52,* 137–154.

12

Beyond X-X and X-Y

Living Genomic Sex

INGRID HOLME

University of Stirling

IN THIS FINAL CHAPTER OF *Governing the Female Body*, I reflect on how in a Foucauldian sense we are formed as sexed "agents with particular capacities and possibilities of action" (Dean, 2004, p. 29). Feminist theorists have been successful in problematizing the sex-gender and social-natural binaries, with biological knowledge playing a critical role in their discussions. For example, Elizabeth Grosz (1994) has challenged the notion of the female and male bodies as fixed and concrete substances, while Judith Butler (1990, 1993) and Anne Fausto-Sterling (2000) have problematized sex as a biological and hence natural category. Building on Butler's idea of gender performance, the perception of genetic sex, as a fixed and static entity, plays an important role in the governmentality of sex-gender performance. Drawing on the new field of genomics, which is currently contained within the binary sex-gender framework, this chapter demonstrates the potential to transform genetic sex into a fluid or "living" category.

The relation between genetic sex and gender is frequently conveyed by the mantra "X-X is a girl, X-Y is a boy," which is chanted in popular magazines, birth clinics, and until recently at the Olympic Games. This separation of the human population into the biological entities of female and male plays an important part in current society, marking the institutional structures of their birth, marriage, and passport. As Dean (2004) notes, exploring the techne of government poses the question, "by what means, mechanisms, procedures, instruments, tactics, techniques, technologies and vocabularies is authority constituted and rule accomplished?"(p. 31). Thus drawing on Foucault's discussion of government in terms of "the regulation of conduct by the more or less rational application of the appropriate technical means" (Hindess, 1996,

p. 106), This chapter explores three institutional structures that allow medical and juridical bodies to constitute authority with regard to the sexing of the human body.

The first of the institutions is that of birth registration. From the moment a person is born he or she encounters the governance of sex-gender through the registration of his or her sex. While the infant's self-awareness of their sex is debatable, the subsequent actions of parents, from naming the child to choosing clothes and toys become institutionally sexed and gendered. As Dreger (1998) has detailed, the registration of sex at birth indicates the medical community's establishing authority in "finding" and "revealing" the person's true sex. Throughout its history, the Western medical institution has been compelled to establish reliable indicators of sex, which has led to various approaches and debates. During what Dreger terms the "Age of the Gonads," a person's true sex was determined by the gonads, and this lead to the difference between female and male becoming located within reproductive differences (Hird, 2002). Currently an infant's sex is assigned based on the visual appearance of the genitals. However, in cases of "ambiguous genitalia" a number of "signs," such as genital, chromosomes, reproductive capacity, and sexual function are taken into consideration. In these cases establishing the genetic sex through the technology of karyotyping is also routinely done.[1] However, assigning sex to an infant with ambiguous genital is not clear-cut, and Dreger has observed that the need to label "hermaphrodites" as either female or male stems from the medical and social requirement for one body to have a single sex. The idea of a person's body having only one fixed and static sex has become institutionalized within the birth certificate, which can be altered only if the doctor, that is the medical institution, has made a "mistake." Intersex activists are challenging this structure, which has the potential to label them transsexual if they do not agree with the sex assigned to them as babies. Clearly, the idea of sex as a biologically fixed category is critical to the stability of the current institutional procedure that governs the first stages of a person's life and marks them as belonging to the biological realm of either female or male, and the social realm of women or men.

The second institutional structure, which acts in the governance of sex-gender, is the marriage tradition and the integration of heterosexuality as a norm of "real" women and men within the legal system. Dreger (1998) has noted that, historically, the main motivation of doctors in hermaphrodite cases was a fear of homosexual practices. This fear of homosexuality is apparent in the case of marriage, which is regulated by law so that marriage is restricted to the union of a female woman and a male man. The United Kingdom's legal view of sex is based on the divorce case of *Corbett v. Corbett* (1970) where Lord Justice Ormrod set the legal definition of *sex* as comprising chromosomal factors, gonadal factors, genital factors, psychological factors, and in some cases, hormonal factors. The idea of scientific knowledge as truth, and the idea of sex as a biological category discoverable through scientific evidence intertwine in these juridical deliberations and the resulting "sex test" (MacNamee, 2004). The increasing importance attributed to sex chromosomes since the *Corbett* judgment can be seen in a ruling by the Texas appeals panel in 1999, which determined that Christie Lee Littleton as a postoperation transsexual was still a male. In the legal judgment the Chief Justice stated, "the male chromosomes do not change with either hormonal treatment or sex reassignment surgery. Biologically a postoperative female transsexual is still a male" (*Littleton v. Prange*, 1999). Thus, biology is rooted in the chromosomes, regardless of the body's sex development or sex performance. This illustrates a marked geneticization of the body and society, which has resulted in the "sex" chromosomes being given a controlling and deterministic role over the other factors that the legal "sex test" set. At the heart of this is the idea that the sex chromosomes are the biological "reality" of the person's sex. Central to the Chief Justice's argument is the idea of a biological sex, defined by static binary sex chromosomes. The two "sex" chromosomes seem to have surpassed their status of biological markers and become the female and male chromosomes.

The third example of institutional governance of sex-gender is an interesting contrast to birth registration and marriage that both seek to denote a person's sex as either female or male. The U.K. passport application asks for the person's sex but incorporates the realization that in the human adult, gender is adaptable. The question that asks for the person's sex (female or male) carries the clarification, "If you permanently live in a different gender to that which you were born, it may be possible for this acquired gender to be shown in your passport; indicate your new gender here" (U.K. Passport Service, 2004). This wording seems to indicate that a person is born "in a gender" rather than a sex. However, the U.K. Passport Service exhibits an apparent institutional willingness to allow transsexuals to assume a new gender, but not register a change in sex. This raises significant questions regarding the split between gender and sex within institutional governance structures, and how they lead to the governmentality of sex and consequently gender.

Feminists argued in the 1970s that a distinction should be created between sex and gender in an effort to counter the idea that "sex was destiny" and to separate the culturally constructed gender from the biologically constructed sex. Sex has since become seen as the "raw" natural biology, which contrasted with the culturally "cooked" gender (Butler, 1990). The naturalness of binary sex is supported by the "fact" that the human species seem comprised of two genetically distinct kinds.[2] The examples of birth registration, marriage, and passport seem to indicate that the dialectic between gender and sex has enabled the state to retain the static institutionalization of female and males. However, the current heterosexual system of biopolitics, which holds sex as biological, natural, binary, and fixed, is being challenged by a variety of unconventionally sexed actors, including those people with intersex conditions, homosexual couples who wish to marry, and transsexuals who aim to assume a new sex as well as gender.

As noted, the belief that humans exist in two distinct forms, female and male, is critical to the idea of a fixed sex. Yet, feminists have deconstructed this seemingly "biological fact" and shown that the human body and its phenotype of sex are not static or fixed into two distinct classes of humans (i.e., Dreger, 1998; Fausto-Sterling, 2000). Both Dreger, who has focused on the historical account of hermaphrodites, and Fausto-Sterling, who has detailed the recent methods of constructing sex, have challenged the authority of the medical community to determine a person's sex. Both have shown that in many cases the gonads and sex chromosomes were generally disregarded in favor of surgically constructing a body that could "function" in the heterosexual sex act. Thus, the medical gaze reads the body within cultural and social situations, and observes and measures the gonads, genitals, and chromosomes in relation to the social expectations of reproduction and sexual life. This has led some feminists to question the very existence of a binary sex model as representing a scientific reality because what counts within the laboratory as female or male is tightly connected with what society holds as woman and man, with the result that sex itself is always a gendered category (Butler, 1990). As a result, many feminists argue that the sex binary, which science seems to reveal, is the consequence of scientists presupposing gender binary upon their research (Butler 1990, 1993; Fausto-Sterling, 2000) and that the sex/gender division is not a feasible theoretical framework (Hood-Williams, 1996).

This chapter explores and questions what is often considered the ultimate guarantee or blueprint for the biological origin of maleness and femaleness: genetic sex. Through analysis of newly emerging research on X chromosome inactivation and imprinting, I examine how the historically cemented framework of the sex-binary has guided genetic science and how new scientific advances challenge this framework. A clearer understanding of how the concept of "genetic sex" is constrained by binary sex in science, and how the current scientific evidence complicates this, will both illuminate and propose a new mindset for feminist study. To do so, this chapter follows Fausto-Sterling's lead in recognizing that live organisms are active processes. In her book, *Sexing the Body* (2000), Fausto-Sterling remarks that organisms are moving targets, from fertilization until death, thereby stressing the idea of an organism's life cycle. She (2005) strengthened this "call to arms" in a recently published paper noting:

> The sex-gender or nature-nurture accounts of difference fail to appreciate the degree to which culture is a partner in producing body systems commonly referred to which culture is a partner in producing body systems commonly referred to as biology—something apart form the social. (p. 1516)

The view of the body as an active process is widespread in the discussions of the paradigm shift from studying single genes in genetics to studying genetic networks in genomics (Moss, 2002). Some see the paradigm of classical genetics, which explains a trait as the result of a single gene as being overtaken by genomics, which places greater emphasis on the newfound complexity at work in genetic pathways. This paradigm shift seeks to challenge the determinism and reductionism that has plagued genetics; however, its eventual success is, as yet, unknown. This chapter follows Fausto-Sterling's lead and offers a "life-course systems approach" to the analysis of sex/gender, with particular reference to genetic sex.

The secondary aim of this chapter is to illuminate the idea of a static, fixed "genetic sex" is a governing technology of the state. Feminist arguments surrounding the gender binary have influenced institutional structures. For instance, in the United Kingdom, Parliament has passed the Gender Recognition Bill, which enables a person to be issued a completely new birth certificate that registers the congruent sex for the person's "new gender."[3] Thus, as presented here, an exploration of the possibility of understanding "genetic sex" as a fluid object propose interesting new questions and challenges for institutions based on governing sex/gender.

Finally, the discussion of "genetic sex" will also touch on the relation between genetic sex and gender, and thus will push further Judith Butler's (1990) idea of "gender performance." Butler has noted "gender ought not to be conceived merely as the cultural inscription of meaning on a pre-given sex (a juridical conception); gender must also designate the very apparatus of production whereby the sexes themselves are established" (p. 7). In Butler's view, sex/gender should be conceptualized in terms of "doing" gender. Her concept of the performative gender draws on Foucault's discussion of prisoners, in which he maintains that the law is not internalized, but incorporated. As Butler notes, the body does not express an inner sex/gender; rather it performs, both intentional and performative. So, drawing on the earlier example of sex registration at birth, one can see that the sexed body of a newborn infant incorporates the imposed sex, to develop their gender identity. To explore the idea of performativity of gender and sex, I draw on the field of endocrinology where sex is viewed as relatively fluid and capable of being perceived in terms of a body's biological performance of sex. I then contrast this with the current view of "genetic sex" as fixed, which is based on the idea that "sex" is an adult phenotype determined by an underlying genotype. Drawing on Butler's notion of performativity, I suggest placing the concept of "genetic sex" within the performance of "doing sex," to show how genetic processes facilitate and enable the body in its "doing" of gender.

Endocrinology and Genetic Sex: Fixed or Fluid?

Genetic sex—the apparent fundamental biological cause of the two female and male human varieties—is a twentieth-century construct. Looking down the microscope, the stained chromosomes are concrete countable entities that lend themselves easily to genetic determinism. Because the chromosomal composition of a person is generally fixed at the time of conception, when a Y- or X-bearing sperm is united with the X-bearing egg, a person's genetic sex is taken as permanent and unchanging throughout their life.

Genetic sex, as a fixed and static characteristic, contrasts with the image of sex taken by endocrinology, where it seems more dynamic and fluid. In endocrinology, sex and sex hormones account for the wide variation in gender and gender roles that humans exhibit. As mentioned in the introduction, the distinction between the fixed natural sex and fluid social gender is often associated with feminism. However, in her study of sex hormones, Oudshoorn (1994) traces the origin of this distinction back to the research dispute between genetics and endocrinology over sexual development. She notes that during the 1910s physiologists suggested that the determination of sexual characteristics was affected by environmental and physiological conditions during the embryo's development. Geneticists suggested, however, that sex was irrevocably fixed at the conception by nuclear elements: the sex chromosomes (p. 21). The two research fields resolved the dispute by endocrinology limiting its study to sex differentiation (the biological process the organism underwent to become a certain sex) and genetics limiting its focus to sex determination (the cause of the biological process). Prior to this split, various experiments had indicated that in higher vertebrates the early embryo was morphologically female, until the testis were formed and secreted hormones to masculinize the embryo. Endocrinology viewed the "becoming" of female as passive and the result of "lacking" the active ingredients testosterone. Alfred Jost, a French developmental endocrinologist, was one of the first to describe the male's struggle against the internal "default female" stating "becoming a male is a prolonged, uneasy and risky adventure: it is a kind of struggle against inherent trends towards femaleness" (quoted in Fausto-Sterling, 2000, p. 119). The scientific study of sex differentiation became defined in terms of the active physical processes leading to the formation of the testis. Because the female was seen as "default," these masculine processes were defined as a movement away from the female basic body plan, and "becoming a male" was dependent on a "chemical messenger" produced by the testis, testosterone.

Within endocrinology, sex differentiation is an ongoing active process—because "sex hormones" are important through out an organism's life—with two significant stages of development: in the early embryo and at sexual maturity. This has allowed endocrinologists to conceptualize sex morphologies as linear, with the ideal female and male bodies on opposite poles, and a range of morphologies in-between. Animal experiments involving castration that illustrate this linear binary model are well documented (e.g., Fausto-Sterling, 2000), but human examples also support the idea of the linear endocrine sex model. During the cold war, East German sporting officials gave 142 female athletes steroids to improve their performance in sporting competitions, which resulted in many of them developing "male characteristics." One of the athletes who had been given steroids at age 16 later underwent a sex change operation as a result and blamed the East German sport doctors for "killing" her female self (Longman, 2004). Immediately apparent from this example is that in every day circumstances sex is important, not as a scientific entity, but as a lived experience where passing for the female or male norm can be an objective. As I mentioned, endocrinology considers that two major stages of sex development exists, the period in the womb, which leads to an infant labeled phenotypically male or female, and sex maturation during teenage years. During this latter stage, separating the influences of sex differentiation into nature and nurture, instead a person's biology, is continually and dynamically interacting with the environment, which includes social and political factors, is impossible (Birke, 1986). As indicated by the example of the

East German athletes, sex development can be viewed as a developmental process that is bound to, and part of, the process of "doing gender." What remains stubbornly fixed is the concept of genetic sex determination, the chromosomes.

X-X and X-Y: Fixing Genetic Sex

Regardless of the disputes between genetics and endocrinology, neither could answer what "makes" the human body follow the path of active male development or remain in the "default" female morphology. When the chromosomal difference between female and male mammals became known in the 1920s, two candidates were possible; the dosage of the X chromosome (as in flies where the number of X chromosomes determined sex) and the presence of the Y chromosome. Through studying Klinefelter's syndrome, a condition in which a person has additional X chromosome(s), researchers found that the number of X chromosomes did not seem to affect the phenotype of sex; rather it was the presence of the Y chromosome that determined the body's morphology (Fausto-Sterling, 2000). The idea of sex chromosomes as an easily discoverable "genetic sex" fitted neatly into the established endocrinological binary sex model where two opposite poles of morphologies (female and male) exist. Those individuals viewed by the medical establishment as inhabiting the middle ground between the female and male poles as could then be understood as the result of genetic mutations or a developmental abnormality (Fausto-Sterling, 2000)

The biological cause of sex became viewed as "genetic sex," and fixed as the X-X karyotype for female, and the X-Y karyotype for male. This structure of genetic sex has proved a successful construct for governing gendered action, particularly visible in the cases of certain sports governed along gender/sex lines. During the 1950s the public, and competing female athletes, grew suspicious of the lean, athletic bodies of female athletes in the Olympic Games. In an apparent effort to safeguard the female nature of women's sports, the Olympic Committee initiated nude parades in front of doctors, requiring participants to show their genitals and breasts (Fausto-Sterling, 2000). Understandably, a more scientific test was soon called for, and the officials implemented the "Barr-body test."

The Barr-body test resulted from the discovery in 1949 that female cat cells had dark blobs that were a type of "sexual chromatin" not found in male cat cells, which was later identified as the remains of one of the X chromosome (Lyon, 1963). The observation that in female cells the second X chromosome did not look like the other chromosomes indicated that they were unused by the cell, and hence were inactive. Researchers had been concerned with the double dosage of the X chromosome in females' cells because use having an additional chromosome had been recognized to cause Down's syndrome. The observation that the extra X chromosome was inactive explained why it did not cause a major defect. Gradually the physical entity of the "second" X chromosome became termed the *Barr body*." This apparently static and inactive construct became the identifying determination of a genetic female, which lent "sex" new scientific credibility and social legitimacy.

The Barr-body test, which was used to detect the presence of the second, inactive X chromosome in the Olympic Games, is an example of what Dean (2004) terms technologies of governmentality. Dean differentiates between the technologies of agency, in this case the structure that lent support to the separation of the Olympic Games into female and male sports. This type of technology "enhances and improves our capacities for participation, agreement and action . . . and allows the formation of more or less durable identities, agencies and will" (p. 173). The creation of the female athlete as an identity rested on the generally held assumptions that women were slower, weaker, and could not compete on an equal basis with male athletes. The Barr-body test acts as a technology of performance, "which made possible the indirect regulation and surveillance of these entities" (p. 173), and it did so by shaping the notion women could be separated from men on the basis of their inactive biologically.

Governing female athletes based on their cells was rooted in the principle that mammalian females only required one functioning X chromosome. This defined human females in terms of their inactive and nonfunctioning genetic unit. However, this assessment strategy proved difficult because several women had undiagnosed intersex conditions, and they became publicly stigmatized by the tests as not "real" women. Under pressure, the testing changed to define as female those who did not possess a gene called Sex Region on the Y chromosome (SRY), which, as will be detailed later, leads to the formation of the testis. This, too, defined female as a lack of a gene. Recently this has been abandoned due to the high rates of "false positives" and the argument that sport clothing and officially monitored drug tests decrease the likelihood of "illegally passing" as a female (Simpson, Ljungqvist, Chapelle, et al., 1993). Rather than having sex governed by a routine sex test and awarding of a "certificate of sex," the culturally imposed elements of the everyday activity of female athletes, their clothing, and drug testing, are seen as sufficient to regulate their participation.

Genetic sex determination in sports builds on the view of sex taken in endocrinology, where the female body is the default and inactive morphology, and the male body is actively responding to the action of the SRY gene. The concept of the male being the result of an active development away from the default female has a long history that has been explored within a historical context by Schiebinger (1987) and Laqueur (1990) and within a social context by Fausto-Sterling (2000). The idea that all vertebrates are inherently female can be seen popular science. One of the most interesting being the first *Jurassic Park* film, in which Ian Malcolm asks, "But again, how do you know they're all female? Does someone go into the park and, uh . . . lift up the dinosaurs' skirts?" Dr. Henry Wu gives the answer, "We control their chromosomes. It's not that difficult. All vertebrate embryos are inherently female anyway. It takes an extra hormone at the right developmental stage to create a male, and we simply deny them that" (Kennedy, Molen, Spielberg, & Crichton, 1993). Through studying Intersex conditions researchers found that only a single gene from the Y chromosome was required to produce a male morphology in an individual with X-X karyotype. The DNA sequence of this gene has since identified and labeled as the SRY (Sinclair et al., 1990). Thus, a conflict exists between the view held in endocrinology and in genetics. In endocrinology sex is seen as a process that requires testosterone and other hormones to continually act as chemical messengers to maintain the active process of sex difference, while, the view within genetics that the SRY acts as a "master switch," set to an on or off position by its presence or absence.

The binary sex model is integral to the identity of the SRY gene. Its existence was first suggested in 1927 by Danish geneticist Øjvind Winge (1927). He hypothesized that those genes that were beneficial to the male sex and disadvantageous to the female sex tended to accumulate near a testis-determining factor (TDF) on the Y chromosome. Winge proposed the existence of TDF as a hypothetical Mendelian gene with a set of expected characteristics based on the view of female and male as two distinct genetic entities. Through Y chromosome mapping studies the sequence was narrowed, and in the early 1990s a DNA sequence was identified that fit the characteristics of the hypothesized TDF. The history of the TDF/SRY gene shows how established paradigms not only pose a certain set of questions but also frame new scientific knowledge in line with the existing model. Thus, one of the main feminist critiques of research into sex determination problematizes the focused on the male as the active, and thus more interesting (Butler, 1990).

Detailing the extent to which research questions and findings have been hampered by the view of sex taken with genetics is outside the scope of this chapter. However, I briefly discuss two main examples. The first is the case of viewing the early embryo and its gonad as morphologically female. Researchers now understood that the early embryonic gonad is bipotent with regard to becoming an ovary or testis. Indeed, there is not one "genetic switch" but a group of genes required to function within a cascade network to turn the bipotential gonad into an ovary or testis. As with the skeletal diagrams Schiebinger (1987) discussed, the existing paradigm may have "blinded" observers to the "reality" of the organs that they viewed. However, the second example supports the view that the "default" nature of the female directed genetic research away from certain questions. As mentioned, the TDF/SRY gene was tracked down over a 70-year period, yet the first gene required for female development was only discovered, quite accidentally, in 1998. *New Scientist* (1999) reported the discovery with the news article, "There's More to Being a Woman Than Not Being a Man," which detailed how a well-characterized gene, Wnt-4, was found to play a previously unappreciated role in the development of the female morphology. The experiment, reported first in *Nature* (Vainio, Heikkilä, Kispert, et al., 1999), consisted of breeding mice with a defect in Wnt-4, which was known to produce a protein important in the development of the fetal kidney. As expected the mutant mice of both sexes did not develop kidneys and died soon after birth from toxins from their blood. However, the female mutant mice also had differences in their reproductive system; the Müllerian duct (precursor to uterus and vagina) lay dormant, and the sperm carrying Wolffian duct matured instead. This discovery emphasized that the early embryo has prestructures of both female and male humans (the early Müllerian and Wolffian reproductive ducts) and that development of male or female morphology requires, in both sexes, active degeneration of these structures (Knower, Kelley, & Harley, 2003). Thus unlike the traditional view of the male as the active development, sex development for all humans is an active process.

One of the most important effects of the discovery of a gene required for female development was as Eric Vilain stated in the *New Scientist*, "(a) shift from being obsessed with the testis to becoming more interested in the ovary" (quoted in Knight, 1999). As the research focus changed, it revealed a greater complexity in sex genetics, emphasizing that sex genes were not bound to the sex chromosomes. As one *Scientific Review* article states, "(the) testis development process involves several steps controlled by other non-OY-linked genes, such as Wilms tumor gene 1 (WT1), EMX2, LIM1, steroidogenic factor 1 (SF-1), SRY box-related gene 9 (SOX9)." The abstract goes on to state, "since other genes, such as Wnt-4 and DAX-1, are necessary for the initiation of female pathway in sex determination, female development cannot be considered a default process (Sinisi, Pasquali, Notaro, & Bellastella, 2003). Thus, not one just one causal factor exists for female or male, but rather a wide number of genes are required to form the morphologies.

Genetic research on the development of the ovary has raised questions regarding how female humans differ through their genetic processes from male humans. The realization that the embryo does not have a default setting to become female, but rather that it is bipotent and that active biological processes are ongoing in both the female and male form, means that sex cannot be located in a single gene. Thus, slowly the genetic view on sex has given way to the genomic understanding of sex as a morphology that relies on a network of genes, which are located across the genome.

From Genetics to Genomics

This section explores how new genetic and genomic knowledge, which is currently understood within the traditional genetics, has the potential to transform the current static and fixed idea of genetic sex used to govern within institutional structures. A good starting point to explore the possibility of sex being more fluid and dynamic is the idea that the female and male human as being genetically different. The basic difference in DNA sequences between the genomes of human females and human males is relatively easy to establish. Dr. David Page, a leading figure in sex research has been famously quoted in the *New York Times*, stating that "men and women differ by 1 to 2 percent of their genomes, which is the same as the difference between a man and a male chimpanzee or between a woman and a female chimpanzee" (p. 1). He went on to note that "we all recite the mantra that we are 99 percent identical and take political comfort in it. But the reality is that the genetic difference between males and females absolutely dwarfs all other differences in the human genome" (quoted in Wade, 2003, p. 1). What Dr. Page is referring to is not genetic processes in female and male cells but the genetic "script" of DNA bases in the genomic sequence. However, this is rather like comparing the words "cat" and "rat" and concluding that they are 66.7 percent similar with no knowledge of how the letters *c* and *r* function within that word or that word within the sentence. Indeed, in the case of comparing a human to a chimpanzee, there has been renewed concern over what such percentages can reveal. Recent research on the chimpanzee 22 chromosome and the human counterpart 21 chromosome compared the expression patterns of genes and found that 20% of genes had different activity patterns (Watanabe et al., 2004). Thus, even if the DNA sequences in human and chimpanzees may be similar, they may work in strikingly different ways. Therefore, genetic difference cannot be reduced to the mere presence or absence of a gene; rather how the cells use the genes has a larger significance. To view genetic sex as only being related to the X- and Y-chromosomes is thus misleading, and genetic difference must take into account the whole genome. What is especially important to this view of difference is how and where the cells use the genes (i.e., how they are regulated).

One of the most important impacts of the change from genetics to genomics has been the growing recognition that genetic processes can be modified through other processes not dependent on base changes of the DNA (i.e., mutations). One such process is epigenetic regulation and inheritance, defined as the transmission of information from one generation to the next or during the organism's development through fertilization and cell division and not contained or "encoded" within the holy grail of nucleotide bases of an organism's DNA or RNA. Most of the research has concentrated on a system called methylation marking, where the presence of methyl (CH_3) groups on some cytosines or other nucleotides are transmitted through one cell generation to the next. This is a type of chemical tip-ex or white out, where the cell modifies the backbone of the DNA so the cellular systems do not "read" the gene, rendering those genes in the cell inactive. The methylation marking system is relevant for sex development in two important ways. First, methylation is the cellular process that female cells use to inactivate their second X chromosome. Second, the methylation process is connected with the "imprinting" of certain genes, which refers to a kind of parent-specific methylation, where the cell selectively, and not randomly, uses genes that are inherited either from the mother or the father. The rest of this chapter details how research on methylation is harnessed to support the binary sex model and the view of genetic sex as fixed and static, suggesting that methylation challenges the binary sex model and supports the idea of genetic sex as a dynamic process.

X-Inactivation: From Genetic Sex to Genomic Processes

X chromosome inactivation has become the cornerstone that supports a dichotomous, genetic notion of sex, even if inactivation could be understood in genomic terms to challenge the binary sex model. As discussed earlier, the idea of the inactive female used in the Barr-body test played an important role the technology of performance for Olympic female athletes. Yet, to what extent science supports the view that the X chromosome is something that is nonfunctioning and nonrequired is debatable. Prestigious science journals, such as *Nature*, portray X-inactivation using metaphors, such as shutting up the X or A gene that gags the X chromosome keeps females alive that lend support to the binary sex model (Clarke, 2001). The popular and scientific media coverage of X chromosome inactivation has a penchant to use verbs and nouns associated with sound, such as "shutting up," "a molecular gagging order," "muffles," and "silence," to describe the research, expanding the metaphor of DNA as information to the area of oral communication. Verbs, such as *silencing* and *gagging* indicate a situation where genes are either "silenced" or "vocal" and either "passive" or "active."

However, these metaphors do not do proper justice to the active processes involved in the inactivation of the second X chromosome. Researchers now recognize the second X chromosome is inactivated into a Barr body at the 64-cell stage of the human female fetus. Evidence from studies of mice has shown that the first step of X chromosome inactivation is the methylation (i.e., tip-ex) of most of its genes, through the production of RNA from the Xist gene. The second step is the modification of the histones, which causes the X chromosome to condense. Within one to two cell cycles most of the genes on the X chromosome seem silenced. The newfound importance given to chromosomal RNA in this mechanism is typical of the change from genetics to genomics. Genes can no longer be viewed as complete and self-standing DNA sequences or the first step of the linear dogma that understands DNA to code for RNA, which codes for proteins. Instead, DNA is increasingly analyzed within an interactive structural cellular network, in which factors such as chromosomal RNAs play an important part. Metaphors with connotations of abrupt events such as "gagging" do not do justice to this interactive and processional nature of inactivation.

Furthermore, current research has revealed that the X chromosome is not simply "gagged" but that 19% or one-fifth of the second X chromosome is active (Graves, 2000). Those remaining active genes could result in double dosage of gene products, thus, the genetic difference created by the inactivation of the X chromosome should not only be seen as one of different gene products, but as one of different levels of gene product. Currently these genes are called "escapees," which brings into mind improper and unnecessary entities. However, the importance of these active genes is illustrated by Turner's syndrome. This is a condition where a person has only one X chromosome—no second X chromosome or Y chromosome (X-O). These people are generally women of short stature, who lack some factors connected with reproduction and who may have poor spatial ability attributed to the nondominant (usually the right) hemisphere (e.g., Netley & Rovet, 1982). Turner's syndrome indicates that the genes on the second X chromosome that remain active are not irrelevant leftovers, but play an important role in the development and functioning of the organism.

The current conception of genetic sex emphasizes the differences between the X and Y chromosomes. However, they do share homologue genes, which in some cases undergo inactivation. Researchers generally believe that 19 of the genes that "escape" inactivation on the second X chromosome have a related DNA sequence on the Y chromosome. While the male Y chromosome has been historically characterized as active, parts of the Y chromosome are now known to be inactivated. One example of this is the gene synaptobrevin-like 1 gene, which is found on the X and Y chromosomes. It is inactivated both on the second X chromosome in female X-X cells, and on the Y chromosome in male X-Y cells (Matarazzo, De Bonis, Gregory, et al., 2002). Therefore, the same process of silencing or inactivation happens in the Y chromosome, drawing attention to the way in which the X and Y chromosomes may be different at the karyotype level, yet share similar processes and genes.

In conclusion in the current science, X chromosome inactivation seems to conform neatly to the old idea of female as the default developmental pathway, and metaphors, such as "muffling," reinforce the old idea of femininity as something passive and voiceless, and masculinity as active and vocal. Similarly, the notion of "silencing" or "gagging" gives the impression of an "event," consolidating the idea of sex determination as a decisive happening. However, what is radical about the research on methylation and X chromosome inactivation is that it draws attention to its processional nature, making sex determination not an event but a process of sexing the early embryo. Additionally, both the X chromosome and the Y go through the process of methylation; this process is never complete but results in some of the genes on the chromosome remaining active while others are inactivated. However, the idea of inactivation or sexing as a precarious and always incomplete process that affects both the X and the Y is overlooked when it is explained in the historically and culturally loaded terms of silencing the X or the woman.

Battle of the Sexes

This section explores the use of genetic sex as a technology of action, that is, as a technology that forms identities, agencies, and wills. As mentioned earlier, technology of action holds human females and males as distinct biological beings, and indeed in the example of the Barr body this is used to govern the segregation of their sport performance. The difference between women and men has been the basis of many popular books, one of the best known was perhaps John Gray's (1993) self-help relationship bestseller *Men Are From Mars, Women Are From Venus*. This portrays women and men as being from different planets and speaking different languages, inferring that this stemmed from a biological difference between the two sexes. I argue that genetic sex as a technology of action frames the identities of genetic females and males in terms of conflict and the "genetic battle." This battle rests on a process called *cellular imprinting*, a process which involves parent-specific methylation. When an embryo forms, it receives half of its chromosomes from the female and half from the male, and is thus diploid. The embryo has two copies of every gene on the nonsex chromosomes. Which copy is used by the cell appears random; however, this is not the case with imprinted genes. When the chromosomes are being packaged into sperm or egg cells, the cellular machinery "covers over" certain genes with a chemical modification of the DNA backbone, which "hides" or whitens out that gene from the cellular mechanism. This process, called *imprinting*, accounts for the fact that in some cases the cell uses specific genes because they are inherited either paternally or maternally.

The main framework for understanding the evolution of this cellular mechanism is "genetic conflict theory," which relies heavily on the binary sex model where the female and male are two distinct kinds with opposing genetic interests. Dr. Shirley Tilghman, the researcher who first discovered an imprinted mammalian gene in 1999, explains the general idea of the theory thusly, "This is an arms race where the weapons in the race are genes, where the protagonists are the parents, and where the battlefield is the placenta and the uterus" (quoted in Potier, 2002). The imprinted mammalian gene Tilghman discovered is supportive of this gendered assumption because it produces the protein insulin-like growth factor II, a growth-stimulating hormone that plays an important role in embryonic growth. Researchers first discovered imprinting in insect genetics, but in mammalian genetics it was quickly translated into supporting the culturally laden assumption that a mother wishes for the offspring to be small to minimize her burden, while the father wants a large offspring to maximize the potential of his genes to survive. The spread of this theory into the mass media can be seen in the BBC's article, "Gene Battle 'May Cause Small Babies'" (BBC, 2002). This article first discussed the health application of screening mothers, and then developed the gene conflict view, stating:

> the more babies a woman has, the more chance there is that her genes will pass on to a further generation. However, having a[n] infant places immense stresses on the body, and in times of poorer

nutrition and health, having a bigger infant might reduce a woman's chance of surviving to give birth to many more. So, in theory, it would be advantageous to have higher numbers of slightly smaller babies. Equally, if a man was having babies with a number of different partners, it would be better for him to have as large a[n] infant as possible with each. This means that the man and woman are in unknowing competition for the survival of their genetic code.

The article goes on to describe the IGF gene that comes from the father, terming it his "weapon" in boosting the size of his infant. The heavily gendered presumptions underpinning the language of such reports are quite clear and gloss over the location of this gene on chromosome 11. This means that both sexes carry the gene, and if both copies were active it may result in an overexpression and potentially offspring too large to give birth to, while if both of the copies were inactive the underexpression would affect the formation of a healthy infant.

An apparent example of the genetic battle comes from behavioral genetics and research on "nurturing genes." Nurturing genes entered the mass media in 1998, when scientists at Cambridge published a report in *Science* on the action of Mest. The BBC reported the findings under the headline, "Genes for Better Mothers," which stated, "Researchers from Cambridge University say they have found a mothering gene in mice. . . . Writing in the *Nature Genetics* journal, the Cambridge researchers say this might be nature's way of ensuring females put full effort into caring for their young" (BBC, 1998). In 1999 a similar report of another gene, PEG 3, appeared under the title, "Second 'Good Mother' Gene Found." This article noted "that males appear to have the upper hand when sexes battle over how much time to spend with the babies" (Fox, 1999). Genetically modified mother mice without PEG 3 do not exhibit nurturing behavior, and their pups normally die. In 2001, Susan Murphy and Randy Jirtle (2003), researchers at the Duke University Cancer Center, reported in an issue of *Genomics*, that the related gene in humans is paternally imprinted as seen in mice. Initially, this seems to reveal that imprinting has an important role in the behavioral expression, and thus have important implications for the biology of gender roles; however, the gene may also be a possible mechanism for autistic behavior, which would account for the observed lack of nurturing behavior. The idea that nurturing genes are imprinted as a result of the "conflict theory" has also come under criticism. A recent article (Hurst, Pomiankowski, McVean, et al., 2000) points out the "nurturing gene" affects not the offspring but the grand-offspring and "grand-offspring are equally related to their maternal grandmother and to their maternal grandfather. So there is no evolutionary reason to expect differential expression of paternally and maternally inherited genes that affect the fitness of grand-offspring through maternal care behavior." The article concludes by pointing out that other issues must be drawn on to explain imprinting of genes that influence maternal care (p. 1167a).

The findings of both these imprinting examples related to the size of the offspring and the idea of nurturing having a genetic "cause," and are clearly politically and emotionally powerful. The genetic conflict theory views the "genetic battle" in terms of having evolved to control sex-specific gene expression in early embryos, and some researchers have expanded its impact to later developmental stages where the offspring is still reliant on parental protection.

What the story about imprinting tells us is how new biological knowledge easily gets interpreted in terms of old social tropes, such as the "battle between the sexes." The idea that paternal imprinting aims to render the fetus large or female fetuses nurturing is culturally appealing because it conforms to a cultural idea of "what men want" as well as the populist idea of genetics and evolution in terms of "selfish" genes propagated by Richard Dawkins (2006). However, imprinting can also be seen as a molecular process that enables diploid cells to express only one copy of a gene, where the expression of both copies would have resulted in overabundance of the gene product. This indicates a mutually beneficial outcome for both paternal and maternal points of view. Furthermore, what is interesting about imprinting is that it, again, highlights that DNA sequences tell us only part of the story because cells do not use all their genes all the time and that the way they use their genes varies among tissues and during the organism's life cycle. Thus, the truly novel idea of viewing the meaning and role of genes not as part of a stand-alone blueprint, but as pieces of the genetic and cellular processes, becomes lost in the rather stale stories about sex wars and weaponry.

From Genetic Sex to Living Sex

In the end, new genomic knowledge that might challenge old notions of sex determination is seemingly interpreted within old social discourses underpinned by the binary sex model. Perhaps new metaphors are required to replace the existing ones, such as "switching on and off" and "silencing" or "battle between the sexes." Porta (2003) has suggested that rather than describe DNA in terms of blueprint we should think of it as a "jazz score," which rather than determine performance leaves ample room for playing or jamming the score differently in different contexts.

The fact that a cell does not use all the genes in its genomes at once problematizes the concept of genetic sex as a static and fixed object. An example of this is those X-X individuals who have the SRY (which is typically found on the Y chromosome) on one of their X chromosomes. Because the genes required for the typical male phenotype are not on the Y chromosome, this gene is able to activate typical male genetic processes in X-X cells and leads to a male phenotype. A notion of genetic sex related to the genetic process would appreciate the situation in terms of the person being a genetic male because their genetic processes are that of a typical male although his karyotype is nontypical male. Clearly, the concept of genetic sex is tightly linked within both society and science to the karyotype, and is thus extremely resistant to change. However, devising a concept of a living genomic sex, where the stress is placed on the genetic processes of the body, might be useful.

Moving toward a concept of living genetic sex follows Fausto-Sterling's (2000) call to recognize that nature and nurture cannot be separated. Within genomics, genetic processes cannot be separated from the cellular environment in which they occur, nor can they be separated from the local (tissue) and global (body) biological environment that they occur. One example that brings to light the typically hidden genetic processes that take place during puberty is 5 alpha-reductase deficiency. This syndrome is caused by the body being unable to produce the enzyme 5 alpha-reductase, which is needed to process testosterone into its stronger from, dihydrotestosterone. Numerous genes lead to the person being born with an X-Y karyotype and ambiguous female genitalia. Two genes have been shown to be implemented in the deficiency, with more than 20 mutations having been characterized, again stressing the inadequacy of focusing on the DNA sequence. Once the person reaches sexual maturity she is likely to begin developing male characteristics as their testis descend and their voice drops. Historically, scientists viewed these individuals as genetically male, even in childhood. Because this condition may only be recognized when the child fails to menstruate, this can cause a conflict between her self-identity and what science seems to say has been their "true" genetic sex. I argue that a view of genetic sex should be rooted in the body's genetic processes, as opposed to being a characteristic dictated by the X and Y chromosomes. This would allow us to understand how the body responds and develops as novel genetic processes are set in motion, as well as the influence of hormones on existing genetic processes. This last influence is especially relevant in the case of transsexuals who transform their biology by choosing to remove their body's hormones and take hormone substitutes.

The genetic mechanisms and knowledge explored here suggests that the concept of genetic sex should be seen in terms of a lived process and life cycle, where different genes are expressed in various levels interacting with the cellular and outer environment. This would recognize that a person's sex is not an inert mark on his or her birth certificate, but a composite of self-identity and changing biology which is in fact constantly used when applying for jobs, using public toilets, and taking medicine. Instead of forcing congruency between the four properties of sex (gonads, genitals, chromosomes, and brain), a deeper understanding should be developed of how they relate and mutually influence each other (e.g., the influence of hormones on the brain).

Such an idea would also incorporate the biological changes that take place during sexual maturation, pregnancy, transgender surgery, menopause, and so forth. This holds the potential to recast our study of sex and the body from objects into actors, and to transform the sex chromosomes from static sex markers into parts of the genome, which as dynamic genetic entities interact with the physical body through biological processes.

Throughout, this chapter has questioned how to incorporate the idea of genetic sex as fluid and dynamic into current social and cultural concepts. In 2002, Alex MacFarlane won the battle to gain an Australian passport, which did not register sex as male or female, instead recognizing Alex's karyotype as X-X-Y and sex state as being undetermined, not being male or female (Butler, 2003). Alex argued that choosing to be male or female was impossible and doing so would be committing fraud. Although Alex's claim was most likely supported by karyotype validation, this is a drastic challenge to an institutional structure that rests on the idea of a binary "true sex."

The concept of a living genetic sex, based on genetic processes occurring in the human body throughout its life cycle would diminish the idea that a child is "sexed" in the same way as an adult, as well as restoring the link between genetic processes and the environment in which they occur. With the recent events in the Olympics, the era of genetic testing to prove femaleness is clearly at an end. In a proposal approved in 2004 by the International Olympic Committee, the executive board now recognizes the legitimacy of transgender athletes to compete in their "new" gender once they have undergone a sex change and undergone two years postoperative hormone therapy. Being born female or male no longer governs one's identity, and equally as biological cyborgs we do mutate our sexual biology from the seemingly slight changes through contraception pills to severe surgical operations, and these in turn influence our genetic processes.

Butler's (1990) theory of gender performance holds that gender is fluid and variable over time and place. People's everyday surroundings and activities shape their expression of sexuality and gender, and biology cannot be divorced from this play. Genetic processes are important actors within gender performance, which decry the passivity of the body and its biology. In Butler's later book, *Bodies That Matter* (1993), she argues that sex is a social and cultural norm, which is expressed on the surface of the body. This chapter has shown that the apparently fixed nature of sex biology is part of a scientific cultural norm, forming genetic sex as an "inner core" identity of fixed sex chromosomes and genetic sex. As such, the new genomic approach to genetic sex holds potential to recast sex in terms of genetic processes, which is deeper than the skin of gender performance, reaching, connecting, and molding both body and culture.

Notes

1. Karyotyping involves visualizing and counting the chromosomes to determine the chromosomal composition of an individual's cells.
2. Humans generally exhibit two sex karyotypes, X-X and X-Y, which typically correspond to female and male morphologies respectively, although this does not necessarily result into two distinct genetic kinds.
3. The original birth certificate is modified to show that a new certificate has been issued in line with the Gender Recognition Register.

References

Birke, L. (1986). *Women, feminism and biology.* Brighton, England: Wheatsheaf.

British Broadcasting Corporation. (1998, September 29). Genes for better mothers. *BBC News Health.* Retrieved September 21, 2003, from http://news.bbc.co.uk/1/hi/health/182310.stm

British Broadcasting Corporation. (2002, June 2) Gene battle "may cause small babies." *BBC Online Health.* Retrieved September 21, 2003, from http://news.bbc.co.uk/1/hi/health/2072597.stm

Butler, J. (1990). Gender trouble feminism and the subversion of identity. London: Routledge.

Butler, J. (1993). Bodies that matter: On the discursive limites of "sex." London: Routledge.

Butler, J. (2003, January 11). X marks the spot for intersex Alex. *The Western Australian.*

Carrel, L., Cottle, A. A., Goglin, KC & Willard, HF. (1999). A first-generation X-inactivation profile of the human X chromosome. *Proceedings of the National Academy of Sciences, 96*(25), 14440–14444.

Clarke, T. (2001, 23 July). Shutting up the X. *Nature Science Update Online.* Retrieved from http://cmbi.bjmu.edu.cn/news/0107/195.htm

Corbett v. Corbett, Probate, Divorce and Admiralty Division (United Kingdom 1970).

Dawkins, R. (2006). *The selfish gene*. Oxford: Oxford University Press.

Dean, M. (2004). *Governmentality, power and rule in modern society*. London: Sage.

Dreger, A. D. (1998). *Hermaphrodites and the medical invention of sex*. Cambridge, MA: Harvard University Press.

Fausto-Sterling, A. (2000). *Sexing the body: Gender politics and the construction of sexuality*. New York: Basic.

Fausto-Sterling, A. (2005). The bare bones of sex. *Sings: Journal of Women in Culture and Society, 30*(2), 1491–1527

Fox, M. (1999, April 9). Second "good mother" gene found. Retrieved August 17, 2009 from: http://www.fact.on.ca/newpaper/yn990409.htm

Graves, J. A. M. (2000). Human Y chromosome, sex determination, and spermatogenesis—A feminist view. *Biology of Reproduction, 63,* 667B–676.

Gray, J. (1993). *Men are from Mars, women are from Venus*. New York: HarperCollins.

Grosz, E. (1994). Volatile bodies: Toward a corporeal feminism (Theories of representation & difference). Bloomington: Indiana University Press.

Hindess, B. (1996). Discourses of power. From Hobbes to Foucault. Oxford: Blackwell.

Hird, M. (2002). Unidentified pleasures: Gender identity and its failure. *Body & Society, 8*(2), 39–54.

Hood-Williams, J. (1996). Goodbye to sex and gender. *Sociological Review, 44*(1), 1–16.

Hurst, L. D., Pomiankowski, A. & McKean, G. T. (2000). Peg 3 and the conflict hypothesis. *Science, 287*(5456), 1167a.

Kennedy, K., & Molen, G. R. (Producer), Spielberg, S. (Director), & Crichton, M. (Writer). (1993). *Jurassic Park*. [Motion picture]. United States: Universal Studios.

Knight, J. (1999). The female gene. *New Scientist, 161,* 9.

Knower, K., Kelly, S., & Harley, V. R. (2003). Turning on the male--SRY, SOX9 and sex determination in mammals. *Cytogenetic and Genome Research, 101*(3–4), 185–198.

Laqueur, T. (1990). *Making sex body and gender from Greeks to Freud*. Cambridge, MA: Harvard University Press.

Littleton v. Prange, 288th Judicial District Court, Bexar County (Texas, United States, October 27, 1999).

Longman, J. (2004, January 26). Drug testing; East German steroids toll: They killed Heidi. *New York Times*, sect. D. p. 1.

Lyon, M. (1963). Lyonisation of the X-chromosome. *Lancet, II,* 1120–1121.

MacNamee, E. (2004). Girls and boys. *Law and Critique, 15,* 25–43.

Matarazzo, M. R., De Bonis, M. L., Gregory, R. I. , Vacca, M., Hansen, R. S., Mercandante G, et al. (2002). Allelic inactivation of the pseudoautosomal gene SYBL1 is controlled by epigenetic mechanisms common to the X and Y chromosomes. *Human Molecular Genetics, 11*(25), 3191–3198.

Moss, L. (2002). *What genes can't do*. Cambridge, MA: MIT Press.

Murphy, S. K., & Jirtle, R. L. (2003). Imprinting evolution and the price of silence. *BioChapters, 25,* 557–588.

Netley, C. & Rovet, J. (1982). Atypical hemispheric lateralization in Turner's syndrome subjects. *Cortex, 18*(3), 377–84.

New Scientist (1999, February 06). *There's more to being a woman than not being a man,* p. 9

Oudshoorn, N. (1994). *Beyond the natural body: An archaeology of sex hormones*. London: Routledge.

Porta, M. (2003). The genome sequence is a jazz score. *International Journal of Epidemiology, 32,* 29–31

Potier, B. (2002, March 21). "Genetic arms race" described. *Harvard Gazette Archives.* Retrieved September 15, 2003, from http://www.news.harvard.edu/gazette/2002/03.21/12-tilghman.html

Schiebinger, L. (Ed.). (1987). *Skeletons in the closet; The first illustrations of the female skeleton in eighteenth-century anatomy. The making of the modern body, sexuality and society in the nineteenth century.* Berkeley: University of California Press.

Simpson, J. L., Ljungqvist, A, de la Chapelle, A., Ferguson-Smith, M. A., Genel, M., Carlson, A. S., et al. (1993). Gender verification in competitive sports. *Sports Medicine, 16,* 305–315.

Sinclair, A., Palmer, S., Hawkins, R., Griffiths, B. L., Smith, M. J., Foster, J. W., Frischauf, A. M, et al. (1990). A gene from the human sex-determining region encodes a protein with homology to a conserved DNA-binding motif. *Nature, 346,* 240–245.

Sinisi, A., Pasquali, D., Notaro, A., & Bellastella, A. (2003). Sexual differentiation. *Journal of Endocrinological Investigation, 26*(3), Suppl. 23–8.

United Kingdom Passport Service. (2004). *United Kingdom Passport Application.*

Vainio, S., Heikkilä, M., Kispert, A., Chin, N., McMahon, A. P. (1999). Female development in mammals is regulated by Wnt-4 signalling. *Nature, 397,* 405–409.

Wade, N. (2003, June 19). Y chromosome depends on itself to survive. *New York Times,* p. 1.

Watanabe, H., Fujiyama, A., Hattori, M., Taylor, T. D., Toyoda, A., Kuroki, Y., et al. (2004). DNA sequence and comparative analysis of chimpanzee chromosome 22. *Nature, 429,* 382–388.

Winge, Ø. (1927). The location of eighteen genes in Lebistes reticulatus. *I Genet, 18,* 1–43.

CONTRIBUTORS

Lisa Blackman is a Senior Lecturer in the Department of Media and Communications, Goldsmiths College, U.K., and works at the intersection of media studies and critical psychology. Her recent books include *Mass Hysteria: Critical Psychology and Media Studies* with Valerie Walkerdine (Palgrave, 2001) and *Hearing Voices: Embodiment and Experience* (Free Association Books, 2001). She is currently working on a genealogy of self-help.

David Breshears is a doctoral candidate, an Assistant Instructor in the Department of Communication Studies, and Assistant Director of Debate at the University of Texas-Austin. During the summer he is a Senior Instructor at the University of Texas National Institute in Forensics. His specializations include rhetorical and cultural studies. He is recipient of the Jesse H. Jones Fellowship in Communication and has published in the *Journal of Law in Society*. He is currently writing a dissertation about the alterations in the mentalities of racial governance in the United States during the twentieth century.

Laura Briggs is Associate Professor of Women's Studies at the University of Arizona. She holds a joint appointment in the Department of Anthropology and courtesy appointments in Department of History and Comparative Cultural and Literary Studies Program. Her primary areas of interest are in the cultural contexts of science, history of gender and science, postcolonial studies, and critical race theory. She has published articles on the history of birth control in Puerto Rico and the question forced sterilization in journals such as *differences* and *Signs*. She is the author of *Reproducing Empire: Race, Sex, and Science in the U.S.*

Imperial Project in Puerto Rico (University of California Press, 2002), which grapples with the specifically sexual and gendered content of struggles for political legitimacy in Puerto Rico. Her other research interests are eugenics and reproductive technology.

Ronald Walter Greene is an Associate Professor in the Department of Communication Studies at the University of Minnesota, Twin Cities. His areas of specialization include rhetorical/argumentation studies, cultural studies, and critical/interpretive theory. He is the author of *Malthusian Worlds: U.S. Leadership and the Governing of the Population Crisis* (Westview, 1999) and has published in journals such as *Quarterly Journal of Speech, Critical Studies in Media Communication, Communication and Critical/Cultural Studies,* and *Argumentation and Advocacy.* He is currently writing a book on the role of communication education in forging neoliberal citizens.

Joshua Gunn is an Assistant Professor in the Communication Department at Louisiana State University. He has published essays in the *Journal of Communication Inquiry* and *Southern Communication Journal.* He is currently completing a book on the rhetoric of the occult.

Ingrid Holme is a Research Assistant at the Institute for Social Marketing, University of Stirling, U.K. She has a degree in biology, but has followed her interests into science and technology studies and gender studies. She is completing a dissertation exploring how genetics and genomics have influenced concepts of "sex determination," both for those who study the biological phenomena and those separated as variant by the scientific research (i.e., intersex conditions, transgender, etc.).

Samantha King is Associate Professor at the School of Kinesiology and Health Studies, Queens University, Canada. She teaches and researches on the cultural politics of sport, leisure, and health. Her publications include, "An All Consuming Cause: Breast Cancer, Corporate Philanthropy, and the Market for Generosity," *Social Text* (2001); "Consuming Compassion: AIDS, Figure Skating, and Canadian Identity" in the *Journal of Sport and Social Issues* (May 2000); and "Documenting America: Racism, Realism and Hoop Dreams" in *Multiculturalism in the United States* (Kivisto & Rundblad, Eds., Sage, 2000). She is the author of *Pink Ribbons Inc: Breast Cancer and the Politics of Philanthropy* (University of Minnesota Press, 2008).

Barbara Mennel is Associate Professor at the Department of English, University of Florida. She has published several essays addressing film, culture, and the body in books and journals such as the *Quarterly Review* *of Film and Video, Camera Obscura,* and *Triangulated Vision(s): Women in Recent German Cinema* (SUNY, 2000). She is the author of *The Representation of Masochism and Queer Desire in Film and Literature* (Palgrave, 2007) and *Cities and Cinema* (Routledge, 2008).

Isabel Molina is Associate Professor of Latina/o Studies at the University of Illinois, Urbana-Champaign. Her primary areas of interest are in transnational cultural studies, particularly in the intersections between the production of global diasporas as they relate to the formation of cultural identities.

Lori Reed is an independent scholar, and she has taught at the University of Illinois, University of Rhode Island, and Southern Illinois University. Her primary interests are in new media studies, and in social and cultural studies of science and technology. She has published essays in journals such as *The European Journal of Cultural Studies* and *Critical Studies in Media Communication.* She is currently completing a book on the history, culture, and politics surrounding definitions of pathological computer use, titled *High on Technology: Computer Addiction and Cultural Regulation* (Routledge, forthcoming).

Paula Saukko is a Senior Lecturer in Sociology at the Department of Social Sciences, Loughborough University, U.K. Her research is informed by science and technology studies and medical sociology and has explored the use of genetic information to prevent common diseases and the lived and political dimensions of diagnostic discourses on eating disorders. She is the author of *Doing Research in Cultural Studies: An Introduction to Classical and New Methodological Approaches* (Sage, 2003) and *The Anorexic Self: A Personal, Political Analysis of a Diagnostic Discourse* (SUNY Press, 2008). Her essays have been published in, for example, *Qualitative Inquiry, Social Science & Medicine,* and *Critical Studies in Media Communication.*

Kristin Swenson is Assistant Professor at the Department of Communication Studies, Butler University, Indianapolis, IN.

Karen Throsby is an Associate Professor at the Department of Sociology, University of Warwick, U.K. Her research interests focus on issues of gender, and on technology and the body, with particular interest in reproductive technologies. She is the author of *When IVF Fails: Feminism, Infertility and the Negotiation of Normality* (Palgrave, 2004) and has published in journals, such as *Narrative Inquiry* and *Men and Masculinities.*

Angharad N. Valdivia is Research Associate Professor in the Institute of Communications Research at the University of Illinois at Urbana–Champaign. She holds joint appointments in Women's Studies and Latina/o Studies. She is the author of many scholarly essays as well as *A Latina in the Land of Hollywood: And Other Essays on Media Culture* (University of Arizona Press, 2000), and the editor of *The Blackwell Companion to Media Studies* (Blackwell, 2003), *Geographies of Latinidad* (with Marie Leger, Sage, forthcoming), and *Feminism, Multiculturalism, and the Media: Global Diversities* (Sage, 1995).

Mary Douglas Vavrus is an Associate Professor in the Department of Communication Studies at the University of Minnesota. She is the author of *Postfeminist News: Political Women in Media Culture* (SUNY Press, 2002), which received the 2003 Diamond Anniversary Book Award from the National Communication Association. She has published articles on media political economy and feminism, which have appeared in journals such as *Critical Studies in Mass Communication, Political Communication,* and *Women's Studies in Communication.*

INDEX